Aging and Neuropsychological Assessment

Asenath La Rue
University of California, Los Angeles
Los Angeles, California

PLENUM PRESS • NEW YORK AND LONDON

Library of Congress Cataloging-in-Publication Data

La Rue, Asenath, 1948-
Aging and neuropsychological assessment / Asenath La Rue.
p. cm. -- (Critical issues in neuropsychology)
Includes bibliographical references and index.
ISBN 0-306-44062-8
1. Geriatric neuropsychiatry. 2. Neuropsychological tests.
I. Title. II. Series.
[DNLM: 1. Aging. 2. Basal Ganglia Diseases--in old age.
3. Brain--anatomy & histology. 4. Brain--physiology. 5. Cognition--in old age. 6. Depressive Disorder--in old age.
7. Neuropsychological Tests--in old age. 8. Organic Mental
Disorders, Psychotic--in old age. WT 150 L336a]
RC451.4.A5L25 1992
618.97'68--dc20
DNLM/DLC
for Library of Congress 92-21649
CIP

ISBN 0-306-44062-8

A Division of Plenum Publishing Corporation
233 Spring Street, New York, N.Y. 10013

Printed in the United States of America

Foreword

It is a privilege to be asked to write the foreword for so excellent a book, so timely and so much needed by the field. Not only is it most unusual these days to have a single-authored volume on so broad a topic, but Dr. La Rue has done a superb job of providing both a scholarly treatise and a practical handbook.

With a burgeoning elderly population and the corresponding increase in geriatric psychopathology, the needs of mental health services are exceeding by far the supply of appropriate providers. In an effort to meet this need, psychiatry, medicine, neurology, pharmacology, psychology, nursing, and social work have all made the provision of training in geriatrics and gerontology a high priority—but I fear we are losing the race. For example, multidisciplinary teams that assess, diagnose, and treat mental health disorders in elderly patients are incomplete without clinical psychologists and neuropsychologists, and yet there is barely a handful of clinical psychologists trained in dealing with geriatric patients. We can count on our fingers the additional ones graduated each year. In hospitals, clinics, and private practices across the country, otherwise skilled psychologists are unprepared to respond to the special mental health needs of the elderly. A few CME programs are helping to address this need, but they are clearly not enough.

Books are even rarer. To illustrate, we need only look at two major books in the field. The first, Muriel Lezak's *Neuropsychological Assessment* (1983) is an outstanding clinical handbook but oriented primarily to a younger patient population; in the third edition (now in press), there may well be more emphasis on assessing the elderly. The second book, *Geriatric Neuropsychology*, edited by Marilyn Albert and Mark Moss (1988), has excellent chapters, literature reviews, and discussions of the predominant issues in the field, but does not focus on assessment or the evaluation of findings. Dr. La Rue has combined these approaches, providing a solid clinical handbook about testing and evaluating the performance of elderly patients, as well as thoroughly researched background chapters.

Aging and Neuropsychological Assessment will benefit a broad audience. It is a "must" for psychologists without special training in neuropsychology or aging. They will find in it information to assist them in assessing their elderly patients—and so will neuropsychologists and clinical psychologists being trained in gerontology. Geriatric psychiatrists, geriatricians, and neurologists, too, will profit from the extensive and knowledgeable review of the changes occurring with normal aging. The complex subjects of cognition in normal aging, its changes with psychopathology, and the attempts to define both with the aid of neuropsychological assessment are dealt with most lucidly. The case examples illustrate some of the difficulties we face when assessing the elderly patient, as well as the caution and wisdom we need to exercise when making a diagnosis.

Dr. La Rue and I have worked together for more than a decade; when we first met, she was in child development, and I worked very hard to convince her to change her focus to the other end of the age spectrum. It is, therefore, especially gratifying for me to see this book, which I believe will be recognized as a major contribution to her "new" area of interest. She has done an outstanding job, and we will all benefit from it.

Lissy F. Jarvik

University of California, Los Angeles, and
West Los Angeles VA Medical Center
Brentwood Division

Preface

This book provides an introduction to the neuropsychological aspects of aging and to some of the prominent neuropsychiatric disorders of later life. It is a clinically oriented text, written for psychologists, psychiatrists, and other mental health professionals who have interests in working with older clients but who lack expertise in gerontology and geriatrics.

The first aim of the book is to increase the reader's knowledge about changes in brain and behavior that occur in later life. The second is to provide a guide to the psychological assessment of older patients. Specific tests and techniques are described, recommendations are made for interpretation, and case examples are provided to demonstrate the application of different techniques. The two aims are interrelated, since the technical process of assessment must be directed by an understanding of older people and the problems they are likely to encounter.

Neuropsychological evaluation is emphasized because brain changes play a prominent role in the psychological disabilities of later life. The great benefit—and challenge—of a neuropsychological approach, however, is that it encourages an integrated explanation of behavior, combining hypotheses about altered brain function with an understanding of an individual's personality, current stressors, and social relationships.

The first part of the book, Chapters 1 through 5, examines normal aging. The great majority of older adults do not have neurological or psychiatric disorders, but many have milder cognitive or behavioral problems that may be related to altered brain function. Learning about these normal changes is interesting in its own right and also provides a background for understanding pathological change. Chapter 1 provides an overview of aging processes and characteristics of contemporary old people. Chapters 2 and 3 explore normal brain changes and cognitive developments, and Chapter 4 describes clinical neuropsychological measures for older adults. Chapter 5 gives guidelines for interpreting neuropsychological results and presents examples of assessment findings in normal older individuals.

The second part, Chapters 6 through 12, discusses common neuropsychiatric conditions of later life. No attempt has been made to cover the full range of illnesses that can lead to cognitive or emotional problems. Rather, the focus is on a few of the most prevalent conditions in which neuropsychological assessment can make a valuable contribution to diagnosis or patient management. Chapter 6 reviews the clinical syndromes of delirium and dementia. Chapters 7 through 9 examine Alzheimer's disease, Parkinson's disease, and vascular dementia, respectively, and Chapter 10 presents case examples of individuals with dementing disorders. Chapter 11 is devoted to depression in old age. Here, too, accurate detection is important, since depressive symptoms are often overlooked, or taken for granted, in older patients. Cognitive sequelae of depression are identified, and recommendations are made for distinguishing dementia and depression. Chapter 12 presents case examples that illustrate the range of neuropsychological findings that can be seen in depressive conditions.

Although a text such as this cannot do justice to the treatment of mental disorders in old age, overviews of relevant therapies have been included, and references are provided for more detailed readings on specific interventions. Also, in the discussion of case examples, an attempt has been made to illustrate how test findings can be applied in selecting treatments and evaluating their usefulness.

ACKNOWLEDGMENTS

Many people have given me encouragement and assistance in preparing this book. Lissy Jarvik provided support when I first became interested in aging and has continued to do so for years; her knowledge of and dedication to the field have been an unparalleled source of inspiration for me and many others. Anna Waldbaum made countless trips to the library on my behalf and has been a constant reminder of the positive side of aging. Art Montana's enthusiasm for the project and his technical knowledge have been greatly appreciated. Sandy Westerman's careful editing made the text more readable and organized than it would otherwise have been, and Lynne Newton helped with the typing and editing of the long list of references. Thanks to the many excellent students with whom I have had the pleasure of working over the years; their questions provided the impetus for this book and helped to shape its content. Thanks to Eliot Werner, Executive Editor, whose long association on many projects at Plenum Publishing provided me with continued support and sound advice. Thanks also to Judith DeCamp, Senior Production Editor at Plenum, for her diligence and great care throughout the book's production cycle. Final thanks go to Nolina, whose companionship made the long hours pass more quickly.

Asenath La Rue

Los Angeles

Contents

Part II. COMMON NEUROLOGICAL AND PSYCHIATRIC DISORDERS

I

Normal Aging

1

Introduction to Aging and Older Adults

In countries such as the United States, growing old has become a common experience. Average life expectancy at birth is now about 78 years for women and 71 years for men. Even those who are currently old can expect to live many more years; for example, at age 65, mean life expectancy is nearly 19 years for women and 15 years for men.

As aging has become more predictable, the process of growing old has attracted great attention; also, attitudes toward the elderly have become more diverse and, at times, more positive. Accomplishments of exceptional old people are widely publicized, and many middle-aged people are adjusting their lifestyles to increase the odds of aging successfully. The drawbacks of aging have also assumed a new importance, as many families confront the burdens imposed by chronic medical illnesses and neuropsychiatric conditions such as Alzheimer's disease.

The field of mental health has been slowly accommodating to the trend toward an aging society. Training programs in psychology, social work, medicine, and nursing have increased their coverage of gerontology and geriatrics. However, most practicing clinicians lack this training, and as a result, many do not feel equipped to evaluate or treat older patients.

This book provides a basic background in neuropsychological aspects of aging. The first part aims to increase appreciation of the variability and limits of normal aging change. A foundation in normal development can suggest ways of dealing with everyday problems of older clients (e.g., forgetfulness or aches and pains) and can enhance detection of treatable psychiatric and neurological conditions. It can also help to counteract the common tendency to overdiagnose organic mental disorders in older people.

This chapter establishes a framework for discussing aging and older adults. The first section examines conceptual and methodological issues in gerontology and clarifies how terms such as *old* and *normal* will be used. The second section provides an overview of biological, social, and psychological aspects of aging. The final section summarizes demographic characteristics and health care needs of older people in the United States.

BASIC ISSUES IN GERONTOLOGY

Ambiguity of Terms: Who Is Old?

Americans often change their opinion about who is old depending on their own current age. Gerontologists, too, have been inconsistent in defining what they mean by *old age*.

The common practice of designating 65 years as the lower limit of old age began in Germany in the 1880s, when Otto von Bismarck started a program of social benefits for the aged (Butler & Lewis, 1973). A century later, 65 is still the qualifying age for full Social Security benefits in the United States. As legislators are well aware, a much greater percentage of people are now living to age 65 and beyond than was the case in the 1880s, and beginning in the year 2000, the qualifying age for Social Security will gradually be raised to 67 years. Many other conventional delimiters of old age (e.g., mandatory retirement) have been legally challenged and are gradually being eliminated.

Most biological and psychological age changes develop gradually and continuously. The rate of change often accelerates at some time late in life, but the point of inflection varies for different biological and behavioral systems. Chronological age provides a rough marker for these developmental events, even though specific chronological boundaries for old age are arbitrary. Investigations that sample people in their 60s or 70s (sometimes referred to as the *young old*) usually show minimal age effects compared to those that focus on 80- or 90-year-olds (the *old old*, *very old*, or *oldest old*). Abrupt decompensations in physical or mental ability ("threshold effects") are usually seen only in advanced old age.

In this book, the term *old* generally refers to ages 60 years and above. Adjectives such as *older*, *elderly*, and *aged* are used interchangeably, and terms such as *young old* and *old old* may be used to highlight contrasting subgroups. When particular investigations are discussed, an effort has been made to note specific ages and to identify points on the chronological scale where significant age effects are observed.

Variability in Aging Trends

Development across the life span has been compared to an opening fan, implying that the uniqueness of the individual increases with the passage of time. There are many studies of aging that seem to support this idea, reporting larger variances for older adult samples than for younger groups.

Recently, considerable attention has been paid to the possibility that variance may be inflated in aged samples because of the inclusion of medically ill subjects. Some geriatric specialists argue that only completely healthy subjects (i.e., those with no identified illnesses, no suggestion of subclinical pathology, and no medications) should be included in research on normal aging. Others point out that such research will not generalize to the average old person; if results are used as normative reference points, a majority of old people may be classified as ill or impaired. In effect, two literatures on normal aging are emerging, one for the very fortunate aged who have no physical problems ("optimal" or "healthy" aging) and another for those who have acquired some of the chronic medical conditions prevalent in later life ("typical" aging).

In this book, *normal* connotes the absence of neurological or psychiatric disease, but not necessarily medical disease. Medical illness is treated as one of the many factors that can affect psychological and neurobiological findings, and care is taken to identify the medical status of normative samples. This is sometimes impossible to do, however, since a surprising number of gerontological studies do not provide adequate descriptions of subject characteristics or sampling criteria (Camp, West, & Poon, 1989; Poon, Krauss, & Bowles, 1984).

Limitations in Research Design

Most studies of aging use cross-sectional research designs, comparing separate groups of younger and older adults at a particular point in time. The limitations of this approach have been discussed in detail by Baltes, Reese, and Nesselroade (1977), Schaie and Hertzog (1985), Nesselroade and Labouvie (1985), and others.

The primary problem is that groups differing in age also differ in other ways. Of particular concern is the confounding of age and generation (birth cohort) effects. Each generation is exposed to unique combinations of experience, ranging from major events (e.g., wars, financial depressions) to changing technology (e.g., television, computers) to shifting dietary and exercise patterns. The cumulative effects of these experiences—shared by all members of a generation—may be as important in determining characteristics in old age as intrinsic biological or behavioral age changes. Because all of these effects are combined in cross-sectional comparisons, the resulting age differences tend to overestimate the degree of change that individuals will experience with advancing age.

Longitudinal investigations, which track the same individuals over years or even decades, also have limitations. Subjects who remain in studies through many successive testings are likely to be exceptional people, having fewer physical health problems and scoring higher initially on many cognitive measures. As a result, longitudinal investigations often underestimate the typical effects of age. Also, age trajectories based on a single longitudinal study may not generalize to other samples.

It would be helpful to have studies of both types available to allow a consensus view of normal aging. As Chapters 2 through 4 demonstrate, however, most of what we know about aging is based on cross-sectional research.

Implications of Basic Issues

The chronological span of latter life is decades long, and there is no clear point of entry into old age. Depending on the range and upper limit of ages sampled, advanced chronological age can have either a prominent or a negligible impact on variables of interest. Generally, it is the very old who are most likely to experience significant reductions in physical and psychological capability, with relatively minor changes observed in midlife to early old age. However, what *very old* means may change in the coming decades.

The rapidity of social and medical changes affecting later life makes it particularly important to consider possible cohort effects as a confounding factor in the literature on aging. Results of studies conducted decades ago may not be appropriate for contemporary old people, who tend to be healthier and more physically and mentally active than previous generations.

Some people age at a much slower rate than others. The reasons for this variability are just beginning to be understood. Currently, great attention is being paid to the influence of medical illness on aging trends, but many other factors also contribute to heterogeneity in older age groups.

Each of these issues makes arriving at an estimate of normal aging a complex and creative endeavor. A skeptical stance is needed in reviewing gerontological research, and a "benefit of the doubt" approach may be best in certain clinical situations (see Chapter 5).

DIMENSIONS OF THE AGING PROCESS

Biological Aging

Biological aging has been defined as "the process of change in the organism, which over time lowers the probability of survival and reduces the physiological capacity for self-regulation, repair and adaptation to environmental demands" (Birren & Zarit, 1985, p. 9). Numerous theories have been proposed to explain biological aging, and great effort and energy have been expended in attempts to reduce its unwanted effects (for historical accounts, see Comfort, 1979; Walford, 1983).

Biological aging is partly primary or intrinsic (i.e., built into the organism, most likely on a cellular level) and partly secondary (reflecting accumulated environmental insults, such as inadequate nutrition or injuries). The following paragraphs note some contemporary models of primary aging (see Warner, Butler, Sprott, & Schneider, 1987, for details).

Models of Primary Aging

Genetic Theories. Genetic factors appear to play a central role in primary biological aging. Maximum life span differs reliably across species, suggesting general genetic programs that set the upper limits of life span. As many as 100 or more genes are believed to be involved in the control of longevity (Schneider, 1987). Differences in life span also tend to cluster within families, suggesting variations within the species in genotypes for aging.

The mechanisms whereby genes enforce longevity limits are not known (Johnson, 1988). There may be genes that directly control longevity or special "life elongation genes" that increase fitness in childbearing years and have residual benefits in the postreproductive phase (e.g., Cutler, 1982). Alternatively, aging changes may be the result of accumulated errors involving mutations of genes or defects in their transcription. For example, errors may occur as information in DNA is transcribed by RNA and carried to ribosomes, causing the synthesis of defective cellular proteins that cannot carry out their functions properly. With increasing age, defects may accumulate, eventually resulting in cellular death (e.g., Orgel, 1963).

Molecular Theories. Many nongenetic theories of aging have also been proposed. Several emphasize accumulated changes in molecules and structural constituents of cells (Shock, 1977). Age-related cell death may stem from the damaging effects of free radicals (chemical compounds containing oxygen in a highly activated state) that may combine with cellular proteins and alter their structure or function (Harman, 1968). Alternatively, aging may result from cross-linkages within or between molecules that alter their physical and chemical properties (Bjorksten, 1968). A third hypothesis concerns possible disruptive effects on cellular metabolism of age-related increases in lipofuscin, a fatty pigment that accumulates with advancing age in the cells of many body tissues, such as neurons and muscle fibers of the heart (Dowson, 1982; Strehler, 1964).

Physiological Theories. Physiological theories view aging as a product of changes in organ systems or physiological control mechanisms. Early versions of these theories focused on single organ systems, such as the cardiovascular system or pituitary gland. As Shock (1977) pointed out, these theories cannot explain why aging and death occur in phylogenetically simple species that lack these organs. Models that emphasize immune system function or hormonal or nervous system regulatory mechanisms are considered more tenable. For example, because of age-related declines in antibodies, the immune system may lose the ability to recognize and destroy mutated cells (e.g., Makinodan, 1974). Alternatively, special antibodies may develop with age that attack and destroy normal cells (e.g., Walford, 1969).

Impact of Aging on Structure and Function

Although the causes of biological aging are unclear, there is agreement that its effects are widespread. As the summary in Table 1.1 indicates, all major organ systems are affected to a degree. A useful overview of these changes was provided by Foster (1988); more detailed discussions can be found in Reichel (1989), in Timiras (1988), and in selected chapters from Birren and Schaie (1985, 1990) and Finch and Schneider (1985).

TABLE 1.1. Age Changes in Structure and Function of Organ Systems[a]

System	Structure	Function
Cardiovascular		
Heart	Decreased size. Lipofuscin and fat deposition in myocardium. Calcification of aortic and mitral valves.	Resting data conflict. Under stress, reduced maximal heart rate, stroke volume, cardiac output and oxygen consumption.
Arteries	Changes in elastin in arterial walls; calcification.	Loss of elasticity; increased systolic blood pressure.
Respiratory		
Lungs	Enlargement of alveolar ducts and alveoli; loss of elasticity.	Reduced ventilatory capacity, especially during exercise.
Musculoskeletal	Increased chest wall and joint rigidity; cartilage calcification.	Reduced ventilatory capacity, especially during exercise.
Gastrointestinal	Loss of smooth muscle cells of intestine; atrophy of gastric mucosa and increased gastric pH. Reduced hepatic blood flow.	Reduced eliminatory efficiency; constipation. Reduced metabolism of drugs (see Chapter 6).
Genitourinary	Loss of renal mass, including loss of glomeruli. Reduced intrarenal arterial tree. Reduced bladder elasticity. Menopause. Prostate enlargement.	Reduced glomerular filtration rate and renal plasma flow. Loss of bladder-emptying capacity.
Endocrinological	Atrophy and fibrosis; loss of vascularity. Changes may be minimal.	General decline in secretory rate, but resting hormone blood levels may remain constant since clearance also declines.
Immunological	T suppressor cells increase; helper T cells decrease. Increased IgA and G; decreased IgM. Increased autoantibodies. Changes in thymus gland.	Susceptibility to infection, and cancer increased.
Musculoskeletal	Reduced muscle and bone mass. More fat in muscles, calcium in cartilage. Loss of elasticity in joints.	Loss of muscular strength and stamina.
Neurological	Reduced brain weight and volume. Loss of neurons and changes in dendritic arbors, varying by region. Neurofibrillary tangles, neuritic plaques, and other microscopic changes (see Chapter 2).	Inconsistent findings regarding reduced cerebral blood flow and metabolism of glucose and oxygen. Possible intellectual changes (see Chapters 2 and 3).
Sensory	Gradual changes in the cochlea, inner ear, and auditory pathway. Lens and retinal changes.	Reduced sound clarity and comprehension. Reduced visual acuity, dark adaptation.

[a]From Spar and La Rue (1990, pp. 29–30). Copyright 1990 by American Psychiatric Press, Inc. Adapted by permission.

Many of the age changes noted in the table double as symptoms of disease. Old people suffer from chronic medical disease much more often than younger adults (see "Health Problems and Medical Care," below). Many others have preclinical changes that are not severe enough to warrant diagnosis but are clearly on a continuum with disease. This overlap between aging and illness complicates research on normal aging, as discussed above. It is also at the heart of many personal fears about growing old.

Promoting Healthy Lifestyles

There is great variability between individuals in the rate of physiological aging, due in part to genetic factors but also to differences in lifestyle. Great effort is being directed at control of risk factors for disease through lifestyle changes, both within the medical profession and in the culture as a whole. Many popular health-enhancement books are aimed specifically at older adults, encouraging changes in diet, exercise, or stress management.

Research on effects of healthier lifestyles is too limited to permit firm conclusions, but some preliminary trends are apparent (see Fries, Green, & Levine, 1989, for an interesting discussion). Lifestyle changes of recent decades have not raised the upper limit of the life span, but they may have contributed to the fact that more and more people are surviving into old age (see "Demographic Trends," below). Health promotion also appears to be extending *active* life expectancy (i.e., the time during which a person is free of disabling medical conditions).

Clinical Implications of Biological Aging

The causes of biological aging are poorly understood (Schneider, 1987). However, consideration of different theories serves to underscore the fact that biological aging is a predictable process shared by nearly all living things.

The net effect of biological aging is reduced physiological capacity and increased risk of chronic disease. However, the rate at which these changes occur can be influenced by lifestyle factors which the individual can partly control.

Physical aging changes complicate neuropsychological assessments in several ways (see Chapters 4 and 5). Because of slowing and loss of stamina, formal testing must often be kept to a minimum; sensory impairments can further restrict the quality of information obtained. When cognitive and emotional problems are observed, effects of medical illness and medications must be carefully weighed in diagnostic interpretation.

In psychotherapy with older adults, it is important to be alert to the meaning of biological changes for the individual. Nearly everyone is sensitive to the "body messages" of aging, such as wrinkling of skin, loss of stamina, or stiffness of joints and muscles (Karp, 1988). Most people adjust their self-image to incorporate these changes, but for a few, the loss of youthful appearance or physical prowess can contribute to serious depression. For others, physical complaints may substitute for direct admissions of depression or loneliness (see Chapter 10).

The fields of health psychology and behavioral medicine are very relevant to gerontology and geriatrics. Texts in these areas (e.g., Friedman & DiMatteo, 1989; Sweet, Rozensky, & Tovian, 1991) are an excellent source of techniques for maintaining effective health habits and for treating common physical problems such as pain and insomnia.

Social Aspects of Aging

Old age is accompanied by role change and, often, role loss. Most people can expect transformations in occupational, family, and community responsibilities, and for many, the number of different roles declines in later life.

Work and Financial Status

A majority of elderly adults are retired from full-time work. In 1986, only 25% of men in the age range of 65 to 69 years were working for pay, and among those aged 70 years and above, only 10% were employed (U.S. Senate Special Committee on Aging, 1987–1988). Participation of older people in the labor force has declined sharply over recent decades, primarily because of improvements in private pension plans (Ruhm, 1989). However, about 15% to 25% of retired men and women have part-time paid employment (Ruhm, 1989), and about one in five is active in volunteer work (U.S. Senate Special Committee on Aging, 1987–1988).

Retired people report that they miss the money, the sense of accomplishment, and the opportunities for social contact that everyday work provides. However, most take retirement in stride, adopting new routines and activities to take the place of work (Atchley, 1975). This is particularly likely when retirement is predictable or self-imposed, and when postretirement income is adequate. Physical and mental health problems usually do not increase in the weeks or months following retirement; however, retirement that occurs much earlier or later than the norm (which is at or slightly before age 65) may be associated with greater symptoms of mental distress (Bosse, Aldwin, Levenson, & Ekerdt, 1987).

Because of Social Security and other pension programs, a majority of older people are financially independent of younger relatives. Social Security provides about 38% of total income for Americans 65 and older (U.S. Senate Special Committee on Aging, 1987–1988). An additional 16% comes from other pension funds, 26% from investment income, and 17% from current earnings. About 3% comes from other sources, including contributions from children.

Marriage and Widowhood

Satisfaction with marital relationships may be greater in old age than at earlier times of life (Weishaus & Field, 1988). However, most women, and many men, must face the death of a spouse in old age. About one-half of women 65 years and older are widows, and another 11% are single, divorced, or living apart from their spouses. For those aged 75 years and above, two out of three are widowed and less than one-quarter are married and living with their husbands. By contrast, 75% of men aged 65 years and older, and 68% of those 75 years or older, are living with their wives (U.S. Senate Special Committee on Aging, 1987–1988).

Bereavement often results in increased depressive symptoms and a decline in positive affect, although normal bereavement generally does not produce a loss of self-esteem or exaggerated guilt (Gallagher, Thompson, & Peterson, 1981–1982). Normal grieving tends to resolve within a year or two of a spouse's death (e.g., Clayton, 1973; Murrell & Himmelfarb, 1989; Reich, Zautra, & Guarnaccia, 1989). However, men, and women with few friends, may have a harder time adjusting to widowhood (Anderson, 1984; Goldberg, Comstock, & Harlow, 1988).

Children, Siblings, and Friends

Compared to younger people, the elderly tend to have smaller social networks and less frequent interpersonal contacts (Morgan, 1988). Older people also rely more heavily on family members and long-term friendships for input on important matters.

About 80% of older adults have at least one living child, and at least two-thirds report that they have seen their children within the past week; others maintain frequent contact by telephone (Harris, 1975; Kovar, 1986). For most older people, contact with children is a highly valued source of emotional gratification (Field & Minkler, 1988).

The elderly are also actively involved with their siblings. As a person's subjective sense of aging increases, sibling relationships appear to increase in importance, with sisters playing a particularly active role in maintaining kinship networks (Cicirelli, 1989; Field & Minkler, 1988).

Intimate, confiding relationships may be most valuable to well-being and mental health in old age (Lowenthal & Haven, 1968). About four out of five old people report having confidants, and many have several (Babchuk, 1978; Kendig, Coles, Pittelkow, & Wilson, 1988). When available, spouses are most likely to be listed as confidants, followed by friends, children, and siblings (Kendig *et al.*, 1988; Simons, 1983–1984). Emotional support from significant others helps to bolster self-esteem and serves as a buffer against physical and personal losses of later years (Krause, 1987).

Assistance across Generations

One of the most prominent fears of old people is the specter of becoming a burden on their children (U.S. Senate Special Committee on Aging, 1987–1988). Research substantiates that the elderly receive much assistance from their children, but the reverse is also true (Ingersoll-Dayton & Antonucci, 1988). In one national survey (Harris, 1975), more than one-half of the respondents aged 65 years and older reported helping younger family members when ill and taking care of grandchildren, 45% provided loans or gifts of money, and 16% had taken in a grandchild, niece, or nephew to live with them.

Assistance from children is more readily accepted by those who are satisfied with the contributions that they have made to their children's welfare in the past (Beckman, 1981). In general, however, children are more willing to give assistance than older people are to receive it. Some older people may need to be encouraged to look at help from younger relatives as withdrawal from a "support bank" (Antonucci, 1985) to which they have contributed throughout their lives.

Clinical Implications of Social Change

Mental health professionals need be prepared to identify sources of social support for isolated older people and to promote reciprocity within existing social networks. Programs that maximize social opportunities and help to build interpersonal skills are particularly helpful, and marital and family therapy can be useful in certain situations. For older people with very restricted social resources, therapists must sometimes be willing to provide support on a long-term basis.

Because older women are frequently widowed and may outlive other kin, they are especially likely to find themselves alone in advanced old age. Women are often more adept than men at forming new friendships in later life, but this strength can be offset by physical disability or practical obstacles such as a lack of transportation. Women also bear most of the burden of caring for other aging family members, and many need encouragement to continue their lives outside of the caregiving role (see Chapter 6).

Psychological Aging

Psychological aging pertains to changes in self-regulatory processes, including cognition and personality (Birren & Zarit, 1985). Cognitive changes in later life have been extensively studied and are reviewed in detail in Chapter 3. Personality has not been as thoroughly researched, but the available data suggest that some normative age trends may be present.

Stability and Change in Personality

Many basic personality dispositions develop early in life and persist throughout adult years (e.g., McCrae & Costa, 1984; Neugarten, 1977); however, there is also evidence for change in adult personality. One study (Haan & Day, 1974) traced the relative prominence of different personal qualities (e.g., assertiveness, cheerfulness, hostility) from early adolescence to midlife and early old age. Most qualities retained their original degree of importance within the personality, including basic tempo or activity level, styles of cognitive engagement, modes of self-presentation, and pathological tendencies. Other characteristics underwent "ordered transition," shifting upward or downward in a consistent way with increasing age. These orderly changes were more common among women than men and included such shifts as increasing aspiration levels and declining reliance on conventionality. In addition, there were some aspects of personality that changed erratically over the years, increasing at one point, then fading in prominence at others. Another study (Ryff, 1989) found that older people were subjectively aware of stability in personality but at the same time perceived themselves as becoming more tolerant, confident, relaxed, and self-accepting.

Precise patterns of ebb and flow in personality probably vary with generations, since each cohort encounters a unique set of pressures and opportunities in successive life phases. However, certain causal processes appear to be consistently important.

One influential developmental force is the "social clock" (Neugarten, 1970). Most societies have rather firm beliefs about the age-appropriateness of various actions. Some of these beliefs are formalized through minimum age laws or standards (e.g., for marriage, voting, or retirement), but most are informally imposed. The social clock sets the pace for psychosocial development within a given generation and provides a standard that individuals may internalize as a "normal, expectable life cycle" (Neugarten, 1970). Norms about age-appropriate behaviors have loosened considerably in this society; however, even the most recent studies find a continuing sensitivity to contextual reminders of age (Karp, 1988).

A second important force is the individual's desire for continuity in personal past and present. Continuity has been described as "a grand adaptive strategy" promoted by individual preference and reinforced by social approval (Atchley, 1989). The search for continuity may be at the heart of reminiscence, which occurs at all ages, and of the process of life review that is so common among elderly adults (Butler, 1974).

Individual and social influences may combine to produce ordered transitions or stages in adult personality. Erikson's widely cited theory (1959) depicts development as progressing through eight age-correlated phases. Each stage is associated with a primary developmental task, and accomplishment of each task has a bearing on subsequent stages. In late adulthood, the primary task concerns integrity versus despair; that is, each person is faced with making sense of his or her actions over a lifetime, and with judging the purpose and impact of these behaviors. Morale in old age may depend upon success in accomplishing this task, in addition to those of earlier life phases (Erikson, 1959; Erikson, Erikson, & Kivnick, 1986). Many other stage theories of adult personality have also been proposed, including those of Buhler (1968); Gould (1978); Levinson, Darrow, Klein, Levinson, and McKee (1978; see also Levinson, 1986); and Valliant (1977).

Stress and Coping

Specific losses that accompany old age (e.g., bereavement, disability, retirement) can also affect morale and subjective well-being (Bengtson, Reedy, & Gordon, 1985; Kuypers & Bengtson, 1973). The aged may be particularly vulnerable to such losses because of negative age stereotypes, which may be internalized at times of high stress; negative messages about aging may lead, in turn, to erosion of self-esteem and atrophy of basic competence. In this view, emotional problems in old age result from a cyclic process set in motion by societal biases and the loss of social roles, rather than from disruptions of intrapsychic development. However, this model may exaggerate the strains that are normally experienced with aging, since most older people do not appear dissatisfied with themselves or their lives (see below).

Older adults tend to cope with stressful events in different ways from younger adults, relying more often on emotion-focused forms of coping, as opposed to active, problem-solving approaches (Folkman, Lazarus, Pimley, & Novacek, 1987; Lazarus & DeLongis, 1983). Emotion-focused coping is more passive than confrontive, more individual than interpersonal, and oriented more toward control of distressing feelings than altering of stressful situations. Examples of emotion-focused coping include distancing from the problem, accepting responsibility, or positive reappraisal. The elderly also tend to see their situations as less changeable than those of younger adults, and to the extent that this is true, their preferred forms of coping may be highly adaptive. However, both old and young adults often use several different approaches to cope with specific problems.

Locus of control is another dimension that affects response to stressful situations. For example, older people who believe that their health is controlled by powerful others adjust better to acute-care hospitals and high-constraint long-term care than those who see their physical well-being as under their own control (Cicirelli, 1987). In the community, belief in external locus of control is associated with increased visits to physicians during times of very high stress (Krause, 1988). Regardless of preexisting control orientation, however, studies of long-term care show that sense of well-being tends to increase when residents are given greater opportunities to regulate their own environment (Langer & Rodin, 1976).

Although old age presents many personal and social obstacles, poor morale has been found to be the exception rather than the rule among older adults. In one recent poll of relatively healthy people, 60% of respondents aged 50 years and older said they were "very satisfied" with their lives, compared to 53% of those between the ages of 18 and 49 (Roark, 1989). Most respondents over 50 said that theirs was the "ideal age," compared to people between 18 and 49, who generally thought the best age to be 29 years or younger. Another study (Ryff, 1989) asked people to indicate what they would change about themselves or their lives if they could. Middle-aged people (30 to 64 years old) listed a variety of desired improvements (e.g., exercising more, accomplishing more, having more friends). By contrast, the most frequently occurring answer among people over the age of 65 was "nothing"! Whether this reflects acceptance, satisfaction, or resignation is unclear.

Clinical Implications of Psychological Aging

Continuity in psychological capacities, and especially in personality, makes it possible for people to adjust to the many physical and social changes of later life. The fact that most of these changes are gradual, and predictable to a degree, also promotes adjustment.

Because core features of personality remain stable in adulthood, any marked change in mood or interpersonal behavior should raise a question of pathology. However,

Aging and Neuropsychological Assessment

CRITICAL ISSUES IN NEUROPSYCHOLOGY

Series Editors

Antonio E. Puente
University of North Carolina, Wilmington

Cecil R. Reynolds
Texas A&M University

Current Volumes in this Series

AGING AND NEUROPSYCHOLOGICAL ASSESSMENT
Asenath La Rue

BRAIN MECHANISMS IN PROBLEM SOLVING AND INTELLIGENCE:
A Lesion Survey of the Rat Brain
Robert Thompson, Francis M. Crinella, and Jen Yu

BRAIN ORGANIZATION OF LANGUAGE AND COGNITIVE PROCESSES
Edited by Alfredo Ardila and Feggy Ostrosky-Solis

HANDBOOK OF CLINICAL CHILD NEUROPSYCHOLOGY
Edited by Cecil R. Reynolds and Elaine Fletcher-Janzen

HANDBOOK OF HEAD TRAUMA: Acute Care to Recovery
Edited by Charles J. Long and Leslie K. Ross

HANDBOOK OF NEUROPSYCHOLOGICAL ASSESSMENT:
A Biopsychosocial Perspective
Edited by Antonio E. Puente and Robert J. McCaffrey

NEUROPSYCHOLOGICAL EVALUATION OF THE SPANISH SPEAKER
Alfredo Ardila, Monica Rosselli, and Antonio E. Puente

NEUROPSYCHOLOGICAL FUNCTION AND BRAIN IMAGING
Edited by Erin D. Bigler, Ronald A. Yeo, and Eric Turkheimer

NEUROPSYCHOLOGY, NEUROPSYCHIATRY, AND BEHAVIORAL NEUROLOGY
Rhawn Joseph

THE NEUROPSYCHOLOGY OF ATTENTION
Ronald A. Cohen

THE NEUROPSYCHOLOGY OF EPILEPSY
Edited by Thomas L. Bennett

RELIABILITY AND VALIDITY IN NEUROPSYCHOLOGICAL ASSESSMENT
Michael D. Franzen

A Continuation Order Plan is available for this series. A continuation order will bring delivery of each new volume immediately upon publication. Volumes are billed only upon actual shipment. For further information please contact the publisher.

more subtle reordering of personal priorities, and shifts in coping styles, is not inconsistent with normal aging. It is particularly important not to measure older people's coping by youthful standards. Emotion-focused coping may be a sign of wisdom rather than regression, particularly if the problem being faced is hard to resolve through action or information.

Older people can benefit from the full range of psychotherapies used with younger adults (see Chapter 11). Some highly educated and thoughtful old people are candidates for long-term, insight-oriented therapy. For many others, cognitive behavioral approaches or situational interventions, aimed at modifying real-life problems, may be more helpful (Knight, 1986). Cognitive changes, such as a reduced rate of learning or concreteness in reasoning, may result in a slower clinical improvement for certain older patients. Often, this can be dealt with effectively by increasing the length or number of therapy sessions (Knight, 1988).

CONTEMPORARY OLDER ADULTS

Demographic Trends

According to recent population estimates, one in five Americans is 55 years or older, and one in eight is at least 65 years old (U.S. Bureau of the Census, 1987). Within the total U.S. population of approximately 242 million, there are 51 million people (21%) who are at least 55 years old and 29 million (12%) who are age 65 or older.

Projections for the coming decades suggest that older people will compose an even larger portion of the population. By 2030, one in three Americans is expected to be 55 years or older, and one in five will be at least 65 years old (see Figure 1.1). If fertility and immigration patterns remain as they are today, people aged 55 and older are the *only*

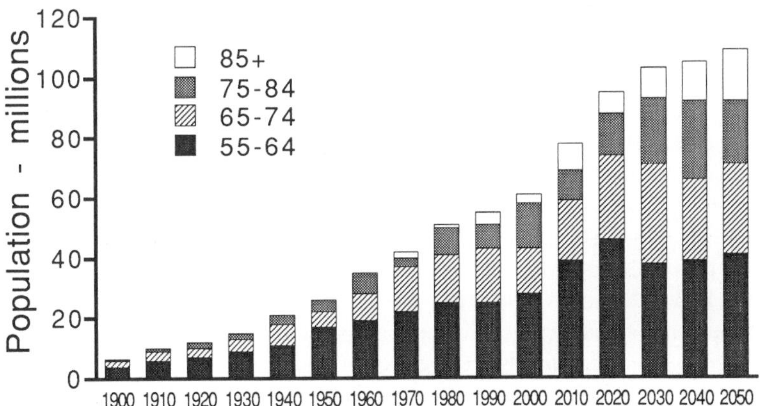

FIGURE 1.1. Population 55 years and older by age: 1900 to 2050. From U.S. Senate Special Committee on Aging (1987–1988, p. 11).

segment of the population that is expected to grow significantly in the near future (U.S. Senate Special Committee on Aging, 1987–1988).

Very old people (85 + years) constitute one of the fastest growing groups in this country (see Figure 1.1). In 1900, there were only about 123,000 people 85 years and older, compared to an estimated 2.2 million in 1980. By the year 2050, there will be 16 million people in this very-old group, or 5% of the total population. Life expectancy at age 85 is growing, too, having increased by 24% since 1960. Even living to be 100 years or older will not be such a rare event early in the 21st century!

Women outnumber men in the upper age ranges, in ratios of 3:2 at the age of 65 years and 5:2 at age 85. The average life expectancy for a woman born today is 78.2 years, compared to 71.2 years for men (National Center for Health Statistics, 1986). At age 65, a woman can expect to live an average of 18.6 years longer, compared to 14.6 years for men.

Nonwhite adults are underrepresented in the older U.S. population. They compose about 15% of the total population, but only about 10% of the people aged 65 years and older (U.S. Special Senate Committee on Aging, 1987–1988). However, because of recent immigration and increased life expectancy, a rapid increase in minority elderly is predicted, with nonwhites expected to constitute about 30% of the older population in the 21st century.

Health Problems and Medical Care

The likelihood of suffering from a chronic or disabling medical condition increases rapidly with age. More than four out of five people over the age of 65 years have at least one chronic medical illness, and many have multiple conditions. Heart disease, cancer, and stroke are the primary causes of mortality and morbidity in the elderly (see Figure 1.2). In addition, approximately 48% of people aged 65 years and older suffer from arthritis, 17% from orthopedic conditions, 30% from hearing loss, and 10% from visual impairment.

Older people are hospitalized twice as often as younger adults, make more outpatient visits to physicians (in a ratio of 3:2), and use twice as many prescription drugs (National Center for Health Statistics, 1987a). In 1985, persons over the age of 65 years accounted for 30% of all hospital discharges and 41% of all short-stay hospital days. People aged 75 years and above, who constitute only 5% of the current population, accounted for 16% of hospital discharges and 22% of short-stay hospital days (National Center for Health Statistics, 1987c). An average of 4.0 discharge diagnoses are assigned to elderly patients as opposed to only 2.4 diagnoses for younger patients (National Center for Health Statistics, 1987b).

Although older people make frequent use of medical facilities and personnel, many of their day-to-day needs for assistance are met by relatives and friends. Many older people are limited in their ability to perform basic activities of daily living as a result of chronic medical conditions. Among the very old (85 + years), more than 25% need help in walking or going outside the home, 17% require assistance in bathing, and 10% in

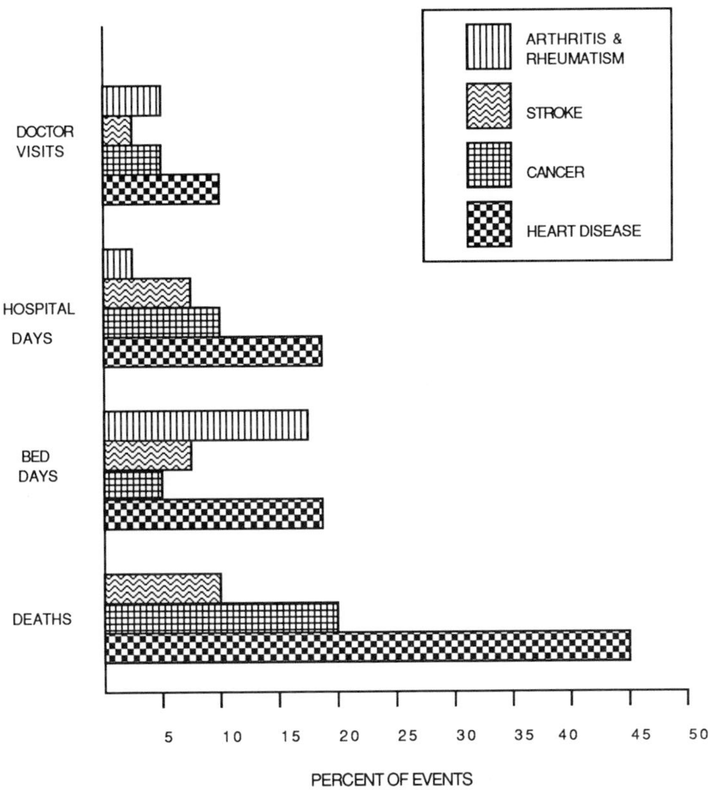

FIGURE 1.2. Proportion of medical events caused by selected conditions for persons age 65 years and older: 1980. (From U.S. Senate Special Committee on Aging, 1987–1988, p. 11.)

toileting. For old people living in the community, relatives provide 84% of routine care. About 80% of family caregivers provide assistance on a daily basis, and 64% do so for at least a year (U.S. Senate Special Committee on Aging, 1987–1988). Wives, daughters, and other female relatives are the predominant providers of informal care (U.S. Senate Special Committee on Aging, 1987– 1988).

Elderly people with chronic needs that cannot be met at home generally receive care in nursing homes. At any given time, only about 5% of the elderly population are residing in nursing homes, but the lifetime risk for this type of institutionalization is much higher, estimated at 52% for women and 30% for men who have reached the age of 65 (U.S. Senate Special Committee on Aging, 1987–1988).

People over the age of 65 years account for one-third of the country's total personal health-care expenditures. Per capita spending in 1984 was $4,200 per old adult, of which 45% was spent for hospitalization, nearly 21% for physician services, and an additional

21% for nursing-home care (U.S. Senate Special Committee on Aging, 1987–1988). Medicare provides the largest single source of funding for health care costs of older people, and the greatest proportion (69%) of the Medicare funds are spent on short-stay hospital care. For older people in nursing homes, one of the primary funding sources is Medicaid, which covered 42% of the costs of long-term care in 1985. It is also important to note that the elderly paid one-third of their own medical costs in 1984 through direct payments or through insurance premiums, and that more than half (52%) of nursing-home costs in 1985 had to be covered by direct patient payments (U.S. Senate Special Committee on Aging, 1987–1988).

Mental Health Needs and Services

Prevalence and Distribution of Mental Disorders

Mentally ill older people constitute a significant subgroup of the aged population. However, specific prevalence estimates vary widely depending upon the samples studied and the methods used for evaluating mental problems (Gurland & Cross, 1982; La Rue, Dessonville, & Jarvik, 1985).

The Epidemiologic Catchment Area Survey by the National Institute of Mental Health (see Regier, Myers, Kramer, Robins, Blazer, Hough, Eaton, and Locke, 1984, for a description), which focused on community residents, suggested that older adults may have a slightly lower rate of mental illness than younger people. For example, the one-month prevalence rate for all forms of mental disorder was reported to be 12.3% for people aged 65 years and older compared to 17.3% for the age range of 25 to 44 years (Regier, Boyd, Burke, Rae, Myers, Kramer, Robins, George, Karno, & Locke, 1988). This is one of the few studies of mental disorder that examined a large, multiethnic sample of older people (n = 5,702 aged 65 years and older) from several geographic localities in the United States. Also, both community-residing and institutionalized persons were included. However, most of the findings published to date (e.g., Regier *et al.*, 1988) have included only community residents, and as a result, the available figures cannot be generalized to high-risk populations of older people (e.g., those with acute medical problems). Also, diagnostic interviews were conducted by lay examiners (using the structured Diagnostic Interview Schedule; see Robins, Helzer, Croughan, & Ratcliff, 1981) as opposed to trained professionals, and only a brief screening test (the Mini-Mental State; Folstein, Folstein, & McHugh, 1975) was given to evaluate cognitive problems.

Mental illness appears to be very common among elderly people hospitalized for medical conditions and among residents of nursing homes. Estimates suggest that at least 40% to 50% of older patients in acute-care hospitals have significant psychiatric problems (Small & Fawzy, 1988), and in nursing homes, 70% or more of patients reportedly suffer from mental impairment (U.S. Senate Special Committee on Aging, 1987–1988). However, some of these estimates may be biased by poor methodology (e.g., relying on chart review for diagnoses or focusing only on patients referred for psychiatric consultation).

Rapp, Parisi, and Walsh (1988a) provided a relatively careful look at mental disorder in medically ill older adults. More than 300 elderly inpatients (age $\geqslant$ 65 years) on medical/surgical services of a Veterans Administration hospital were screened for participation. Nearly a third of these patients had possible cognitive impairment, as estimated by Mini-Mental State scores and were excluded from further assessment. With the use of Research Diagnostic Criteria (Spitzer, Endicott, & Robbins, 1978), more than a quarter of those who remained were found to have other psychiatric disorders. Limitations in this study included the brief procedure for assessing cognitive problems (conducted for screening purposes only) and the fact that the sample was restricted to men and veterans.

Rovner, Kafonek, Filipp, Lucas, and Folstein (1986) used similar methods to study mental disorders in a nursing home. Subjects (n = 50) were randomly selected from residents of an intermediate-care nursing home and nearly all were over the age of 65 (mean = 83 years). Based on a semistructured psychiatric examination (the Geriatric Mental State Schedule; Copeland, Kelleher, Kellett, Gourlay, Gurland, Fleiss, & Sharpe, 1976) and the Mini-Mental State, nearly all participants (94%) were found to have mental problems. The advanced age of the subjects and the brief screening procedures may have contributed to the high estimates of impairment.

Table 1.2 summarizes the distribution of mental disorders found in the studies described above. The values in this table portray a broad spectrum of psychiatric problems in older patients, but they also demonstrate that cognitive and depressive disorders are especially common.

The high frequency of cognitive impairment is in agreement with the larger literature on mental disorders of aging (see Chapters 6 through 12). Cognitive loss

TABLE 1.2. Mental Disorders of Older Adults in Three Settings

	Relative frequency (%) of illness		
Category of illness[a]	Community residents[b]	Medical inpatients[c]	Nursing-home residents[d]
Cognitive impairment	4.9	30.2	84.0
Depressive disorders	2.5/8.0[e]	18.5	8.0
Anxiety disorders	5.5	5.2	0
Alcoholism	0.9	2.6	0
Schizophrenia	0.1	0	0
Somatization	0.1	0	0
Personality disorders	0	8.3	0
Other disorders	0	7.9	2.0

[a]General categories of illness are reported because specific diagnostic breakdowns varied from study to study. Zero scores may reflect limitations in measurement instruments.

[b]Regier *et al.* (1988).

[c]Rapp *et al.* (1988a).

[d]Rovner *et al.* (1986).

[e]Higher estimate of depressive disorder is from Blazer *et al.* (1987).

underlies many of the day-to-day problems of older people and is the principal reason why elderly individuals (or concerned family members) seek help from mental health professionals.

A relatively low prevalence of depression (2.5%) was reported for older people in the Epidemiologic Catchment Area Survey (see entry for "Community Residents," Table 1.2). However, further analysis of data from this study suggested that at least 8% of the elderly respondents had significant depressive symptoms and nearly 19% had less severe dysphoric symptomatology (Blazer, Hughes, & George, 1987). The revised estimates are in line with those of previous research, suggesting that depression is also a widespread problem in older age groups (see Chapter 11).

Barriers to Mental Health Services

There is general consensus that older people are poorly served by the mental health system. Elderly people account for only 2% of the patients seen by private therapists and only about 6% of those served by community mental health centers (Roybal, 1988). Among clinical psychologists, fewer than 1% report a primary focus on aging, and less than 5% of all psychological services are delivered to clients over the age of 65 years (VandenBos & Stapp, 1983).

The gap between mental health needs and services has been attributed to several factors. The most tangible, and probably the most important (Gatz & Pearson, 1988; Knight, 1986), are limited reimbursement, limited access, and staffing patterns. Medicare reimburses for mental health services at a lower level than for many medical interventions, and payments for psychologists and other nonphysician specialists are currently extremely limited. Problems with transportation and medical illness (in the patient or an aging spouse) place significant practical constraints on care delivery. And in a majority of hospitals and clinics, very few staff members have been trained in gerontology or geriatrics.

Attitudes may also play a role in quality and availability of service. There is little evidence that mental health practitioners, or Americans in general, are strongly or pervasively ageist (see reviews by Gatz & Pearson, 1988; Kite & Johnson, 1988). However, age bias seems to influence specific aspects of care. For example, American psychiatrists and other professionals tend to overdiagnose organic mental disorders in the aged (Gurland & Cross, 1982) and are likely to refer older patients less often for psychotherapy than younger clients (Ford & Spordone, 1980; Gatz & Pearson, 1988).

There is also growing concern that ageism may be assuming new forms. Braithwaite (1986) described an "antidiscrimination response," where, in an attempt to avoid discrimination against the aged, health care professionals may exaggerate the competencies and excuse or overlook the deficits of their elderly patients. A trend toward "compassionate stereotyping" has also been observed, where older people in general are perceived to need support because of helplessness and infirmities (Binstock, 1983; Revenson, 1989). An additional area of concern is that both the general public and health care professionals may be forging too strong an association between old age and possible

Alzheimer's disease. Gatz and Pearson (1988) cited evidence that older adults, college students, and caregivers of patients with dementia all greatly overestimated the prevalence of Alzheimer's in the aged. Finally, recent emphasis in the media on the affluence of older Americans may be diverting attention from the continuing need for improved services for the disadvantaged aged, including those with mental illness (Minkler, 1989).

Elderly patients themselves contribute to underutilization of mental health services. Contemporary old people are more likely to consult medical specialists, such as their family doctor, a general practitioner, or an internist, than they are to seek out the services of a mental health professional (Gatz, Popkin, Pino, & VandenBos, 1985). Many elderly patients focus heavily on the reporting of physical phenomena, as opposed to psychological events, and if psychological complaints are raised, these, too, are most often communicated to a primary-care physician (e.g., Shapiro, Skinner, Kessler, Von Korff, German, Tischler, Leaf, Benham, Cottler, & Regier, 1984).

Unfortunately, in medical settings, mental disorders are generally overlooked when input from mental health professionals is not available. This problem is particularly common for elderly patients for a number of reasons (German, Shapiro, Skinner, Von Korff, Klein, Turner, Teitelbaum, Burke, & Burns, 1987): the elderly rely more heavily than younger patients on primary-care physicians; their multiple medical illnesses may divert physicians' attention from psychiatric signs and symptoms; depression and anxiety may be viewed as normal in older people with serious medical illness; and physicians with neither psychiatric nor geriatric training may find it hard to distinguish normal aging changes from signs of mental disorder. In one study (Rapp & Davis, 1989), medical residents were found to be aware of the possibility of depression in elderly medical/surgical patients and strongly motivated to treat depressive symptoms; however, their knowledge of the basic diagnostic criteria was so limited that they identified fewer than 10% of patients with clinically significant depression.

The Challenge of Mental Health Care in an Aging Society

As the number of older people grows, an increasing percentage of clinicians' clientele will consist of elderly persons. Therefore, the importance of understanding aging and common disorders of later life can hardly be overstated.

Mental health professionals can contribute to the care of old people in two complementary ways. The first is to provide education, support, and preventive interventions to strengthen older people and their families in managing common stresses of aging, including chronic medical illness and bereavement. The second is to effectively identify and treat specific cognitive and emotional disorders.

Working effectively with older adults requires specialized knowledge and a flexible clinical approach (see Table 1.3). An understanding of normal aging can suggest ways to promote well-being and can help to minimize diagnostic errors. Knowledge of mental disorders that preferentially affect the aged is required, as is awareness of the ways in which aging can influence other psychiatric conditions. Learning to adjust specific treatments for age effects is another important skill.

TABLE 1.3. Working Effectively with Older Patients[a]

Important areas of knowledge
1. Normal aging: biological, psychological, and social changes
2. Mental disorders of old age (e.g., Alzheimer's disease)
3. Effects of aging on other psychiatric disorders (e.g., depression and anxiety)
4. Adjusting treatments for aging changes (e.g., altering the format and pace of psychotherapy)
5. Managing social and physical problems of later life (e.g., bereavement, role loss, pain, sleep disturbance)
6. Information and referral: familiarity with community agencies, geriatric medicine specialists, Medicare regulations

Personal qualities and professional approaches
1. Willingness to provide broadly based, flexible management
2. Patience and skill in providing medical information and assisting in decision making
3. Willingness to explore one's own feelings about aging
4. Openness to discussing patients' concerns about younger professionals
5. Comfort in working closely with other health professionals
6. Ability to maintain therapeutic optimism when the long-term prognosis is poor

[a]From Spar and La Rue (1990, pp. 8–9). Copyright 1990 by American Psychiatric Press, Inc. Adapted by permission.

Certain personal qualities and professional approaches are equally important. Although some older people can manage the complexities of modern medical and social services, many more lack the energy and information needed to negotiate the system. Mental health professionals must often be willing to play a case-management role, helping with a variety of medical, social, and situational problems. Patience and skill in explaining diagnoses and treatments are other valuable assets, since many older people tend to defer to professionals without a thorough understanding of benefits and risks (Haug, 1979; Woodward & Wallston, 1987). It is helpful to have a willingness to explore one's own feelings about aging and to be open to discussing older patients' reservations about the wisdom of youth. Elderly patients may be inclined to view younger therapists or physicians as similar to their children, and in response, clinicians may need to deal with reverse transference (Berezin, 1972; Robiner, 1987). A final, and important, quality is the ability to take pleasure from gradual improvements and small gains in quality of life, since some common conditions of old age cannot be reversed with the available treatments.

SUMMARY AND CONCLUSIONS

Aging is a lifelong process reflecting the combined effects of normal biological development, the impact of illness and injury, cultural standards and expectation, changes in social networks, and continuous psychological growth and accommodation. There is no single point when old age begins, but by tradition, gerontologists have focused on people in their 60s and older.

Most of what we know about aging comes from cross-sectional research, with important contributions from a few longitudinal studies. Cross-sectional data may overestimate age-related changes because they confound age and generational differences, while longitudinal studies may be biased by selective attrition.

Another complication in research on aging is marked interindividual variability in older age groups. Medical illness contributes to this variation, and in general, physically healthy and active old people have fewer of the negative sequelae typically associated with aging. Many of the generalizations about declines in abilities with age in this and subsequent chapters do not apply for optimally healthy individuals in their 60s. In effect, these individuals are not yet "old." By contrast, persons in their 80s who have experienced some of the illnesses and losses common to that phase of life may show sizeable changes in neuropsychological performance and other functions. Even in advanced old age, however, some individuals retain an impressive array of mental and physical abilities, and, as the health-conscious middle-aged persons of today grow old, these exceptions will become more numerous.

The number of people living to old age has increased dramatically in this country in the past few decades, and this trend is projected to continue into the 21st century. Currently, about 12% of the U.S. population is 65 years or older.

Contemporary old people have a higher rate of chronic medical illness and utilization of medical services than younger adults. By contrast, rates of mental illness do not differ greatly for the young and the old. At least one out of every eight older people in the community has a diagnosable mental disorder, with much higher rates observed in hospitals and long-term care settings. The two most prevalent categories of mental illness in later life are organic mental disorders (e.g., delirium and dementia) and depression.

Older people have had limited access to mental health care, and historically, many have been reluctant to consult mental health professionals. However, with the increasing attention paid to aging and health promotion, and with recent changes in Medicare reimbursement policies, a working knowledge of gerontology and geriatrics may well become a necessity for mental health professionals.

Stability in basic personality characteristics provides a buffer against the effects of illnesses and social losses that are common in later life. However, losses can sometimes contribute to depression or other mental health problems. Older people benefit from the same psychotherapeutic approaches used with younger adults, although certain adjustments in technique and approach (e.g., increasing the number of sessions and being willing to fill a case-managerial role) may be needed for some elderly clients.

2

The Aging Brain

This chapter provides an overview of some of the changes in brain structure and function that have been observed with normal human aging. Information about neuroanatomical changes is presented first, followed by discussion of selected neurotransmitter changes and neurophysiological investigations. Each section is organized in two parts, with descriptions of biological measures and their age-related changes preceding reviews of studies that attempt to relate biological and behavioral measures.

Because only a brief discussion is provided for each topic, readers are encouraged to consult other sources for additional information. A good overview of human neuroanatomy can be found in Barr and Kiernan (1988). Wiederhold (1988) and Weiner and Goetz (1989) have covered the basics of human neurology for nonspecialists, and more detailed information is provided in Adams and Victor (1989). Reviews by Berg (1988a) and Scheibel (1992) are helpful sources with respect to aging changes, as are several of the chapters in Albert's *Clinical Neurology of Aging* (1984), Albert and Moss's *Geriatric Neuropsychology* (1988), and Katzman and Rowe's *Principles of Geriatric Neurology* (1992). For more detailed information, the multivolume Aging Series published by Raven Press and the *Handbook of the Biology of Aging* (Finch & Schneider, 1985; Schneider & Rowe, 1989) are recommended.

NEUROANATOMICAL CHANGES

Gross Neuroanatomy

One of the best documented brain changes with age is an overall decrease in brain weight and volume (see Table 2.1; Berg, 1988a; Dekaban & Sadowsky, 1978; Kemper, 1984). In a study correcting for cohort trends in brain and body size, Miller, Alston, and

TABLE 2.1. Neuroanatomical Age Differences[a]

Measure	Direction of change	Comments
Gross neuroanatomy		
Brain weight/volume	Decrease	Cohort differences.
Ratio of gray to white matter	Increase	Reflects myelin loss.
Width of gyri	Increase	Noted on autopsy and CT.
Width of ventricles	Increase	Noted on autopsy and CT.
Periventricular lucencies	Increase	May reflect cerebrovascular illness.
Microscopic findings		
Neuron number	Decrease	Varies by region; large neurons most affected.
Dendritic arbors	Inconsistent	Some increasing arbors.
Neuritic plaques	Increase	
Neurofibrillary tangles	Increase	Few in cortex.
Granulovacuolar degeneration	Increase	Rare in cortex.
Lewy and Hirano bodies	Increase	Infrequent.
Lipofuscin and melanin	Increase	

[a]From *Handbook of Neuropsychological Assessment: A Biopsychosocial Perspective* (pp. 86, 93) by A. Puente and R. McCaffrey, 1992, New York: Plenum Press. Copyright 1992 by Plenum Press, Inc. Adapted by permission.

Corsellis (1980) reported no change in the volume of cerebral hemispheres between the ages of 20 and 50 years, followed by a 2% decrease per decade through age 98 for both sexes.

The ratio of gray to white matter increases in the cerebral hemispheres with age, an effect suggesting an age-related loss of myelin (Miller *et al.*, 1980). Myelin loss in old age is greatest in regions where myelinization is completed relatively late in the developmental cycle (e.g., association and limbic cortices, as opposed to motor, someshetic, visual, and auditory regions; Kemper, 1984).

The walls of major cerebral blood vessels thicken and become less flexible in old age, but the extent of these changes varies considerably among individuals; in addition, vascular pathology tends to occur later in the brain than in systemic vessels such as the coronary arteries (Scheibel, 1992).

Other gross changes in brain morphology that have been observed in autopsy studies are gyral atrophy and ventricular dilation (Berg, 1988a). *Gyral atrophy* refers to the declining mass of brain tissue in prominent cortical regions, with corresponding widening of sulci between these regions. Atrophic changes have been reported most often in the convexities of the frontal lobes, parasagittal region, and temporal and parietal lobes; the base of the brain and the occipital pole exhibit less decline (Kemper, 1984). Ventricle dilation increases with age but is not closely correlated with gyral atrophy.

Atrophic changes in aging brains can be visualized noninvasively by means of computerized tomographic (CT) procedures, which provide X-ray images of cross-sectional "slices" of the brain and other organs. Nearly all CT studies have documented increased ventricular size with advancing age, but there are discrepancies across studies in the age at which significant enlargement is observed. Studies of optimally healthy older adults and those using automated or highly standardized measurement procedures show that ventricular size does not increase substantially until about the seventh decade (Albert & Stafford, 1988).

Magnetic resonance imaging (MRI), which provides structural brain images of higher resolution than CT, is also useful for visualizing atrophy and for detecting cerebral white matter changes. MRI scans of older brains often report small areas of hyperintensity around the ventricles which may reflect a loss of white matter tissue. Whether these findings should be considered part of normal aging or a sign of ischemic disease is unresolved (see Chapter 8 for a discussion). However, it is not unusual to observe periventricular hyperintensities on MRI in fairly healthy, mentally normal old people (Berg, 1988a).

Microscopic Changes

Neuronal Loss

Age-related neuronal loss has been documented in many areas of the human neocortex, although some regions show much larger age differences than others (Berg, 1988a; Bondareff, 1985; Brody, 1955; Kemper, 1984; Timiras, 1988).

In the neocortex, as shown in Figure 2.1, the most pronounced losses are in the frontal polar cortex (area 10), the premotor cortex (area 6), and an association region in the temporal lobe (area 21). The temporal limbic region (area 38) and association areas of the somesthetic and visual cortex (areas 40 and 18, respectively) also show losses in cell count with age, but to a lesser degree (Kemper, 1984).

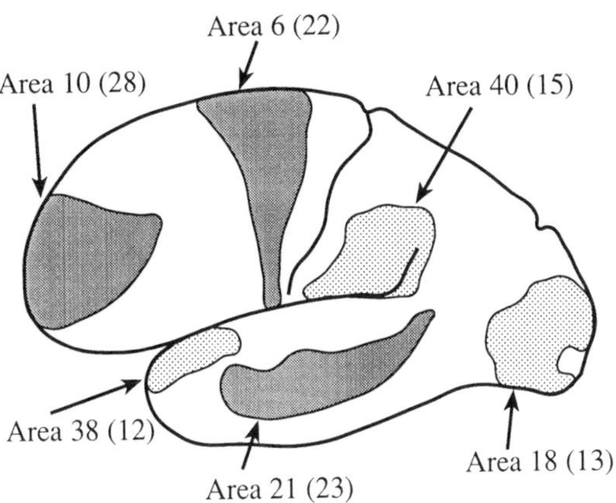

FIGURE 2.1. Regional distribution of neuronal cell loss in the human neocortex. Numbers in parentheses indicate the percentage of cell loss in a given region. (From Kemper, 1984, p. 14. Copyright 1984 by Oxford University Press. Adapted by permission.)

Many areas of the hippocampal formation show age-related neuronal loss, but in the amygdala, subcortical forebrain, brain stem, and cerebellar formations, changes are more selective (Kemper, 1984). The locus ceruleus and substantia nigra exhibit the most reliable declines in neuronal counts with age (Berg, 1988a; Bondareff, 1985), whereas in nucleus basalis of Meynert, an important site of cholinergic neurons, cell loss is still unclear (Berg, 1988a; Cummings & Benson, 1987; Scheibel, 1992).

Terry and Hansen (1988) noted the usual decrease with age in the number of large neurons in selected cerebral areas. However, small neurons in the same brain regions actually increased in number with age. This finding suggests that the total population of neurons may remain stable later in life, but that large neurons may shrink into smaller neuron classes. The significance of this finding is unclear; however, failure to take neuron size into account may have contributed to inconsistencies in past studies of brain cell populations (see Flood & Coleman, 1988, for a review).

Scheibel (1992) pointed out a number of other methodological limitations in studies of neuron loss with age and emphasized that it is unclear how many surviving neurons are required to permit adequate performance of behavior.

Dendritic Changes

Scheibel and colleagues (e.g., Scheibel, Lindsay, Tomiyasu, & Scheibel, 1975, 1976; cf. Scheibel, 1992) described a characteristic pattern of degenerative changes in dendritic processes with age, with swelling of the cell body and apical shaft preceding loss of dendritic branches. These changes were most clearly noted in the large Betz cells of the motor cortex but were also observed in the hippocampal region and in neocortical pyramidal cells. Loss of dendritic branches reduces the number of interconnections between brain cells; however, as in neuronal loss, it is not clear how important dendritic debranching is in age-related cognitive change or how extensive these changes would have to be in order for behavioral effects to be observed.

Other evidence suggests that dendritic branching increases with normal aging in certain cell populations (Buell & Coleman, 1979; Coleman & Flood, 1988), and in rats, dendritic branching has been related to the degree of stimulation available in everyday environments (Carughi, Carpenter, & Diamond, 1989; Volkmar & Greenough, 1972). Continued dendritic arborization may help to compensate for decremental brain changes (Bondareff, 1985), although how this occurs remains to be determined (Coleman & Flood, 1988).

Amyloid Accumulation

Amyloid is a complex, glycoprotein-rich material that is rarely observed in tissues of healthy young adults. Infiltration of amyloid into the lining of cerebral blood vessels and free deposits of amyloid within brain tissue are observed with increasing frequency in advanced old age. In one autopsy series of more than 100 geriatric patients, the percentage of subjects with vascular amyloid increased from 8% in the seventh decade to 58% after the ninth decade (Tomonaga, 1981).

Excess brain amyloid occurs in nearly all patients with Alzheimer's disease, in other neurodegenerative disorders (e.g., kuru, scrapie, and Creutzfeldt-Jakob disease), and Down's syndrome. Causal associations have been hypothesized between amyloid deposition and the formation of neuritic plaques and tangles, but a direct role has yet to be established (see Chapter 7 for further discussion).

Neuritic Plaques

Neuritic plaques are distinctive intercellular structures visible on microscopic examination. A typical mature plaque consists of a central core of amyloid surrounded by glial cells, macrophages, degenerating axons, and occasional dendrites (Kemper, 1984).

Neuritic plaques increase with age from about the fifth decade onward, with two-thirds or more of brains in the ninth decade having occasional neuritic plaques (Jordan, 1971). Plaques are generally more numerous in brains of patients with Alzheimer's disease than in those of normal older adults and have been observed in other neurodegenerative diseases such as Pick's disease and Creutzfeldt-Jakob disease (Kemper, 1984).

Neurofibrillary Tangles

A neurofibrillary tangle is an intraneuronal structure composed of twisted bands or filaments that often displace the cell nucleus (Kemper, 1984). It is not clear why neurofibrillary tangles form, or what their effects are upon cell processes. Neurofibrillary tangles occur as early as the third decade and are noted at least occasionally in nearly all brains in the ninth decade and above (Jordan, 1971; Matsuyama & Nakamura, 1978).

In normal aging, tangles are rarely observed in the neocortex (Matsuyama & Nakamura, 1978). The highest concentrations in normal old brains are in certain regions of the hippocampus, parahippocampal gyrus, and brain stem (Kemper, 1984). In the locus ceruleus, neurofibrillary tangles were reported in 10% to 20% of patients dying between the ages of 60 and 90 and in all patients over 100 years of age in one investigation (Tomonago, 1979).

Neurofibrillary tangles are noted in much greater concentration and with wider distribution in Alzheimer's disease than in normal aging and have been observed in other neurological disorders including dementia pugilistica and Down's syndrome.

Granulovacuolar Degeneration

Granulovacuolar degeneration refers to the accumulation of distinctive vesicles with a central dark core within the cytoplasm of neurons. This degenerative change is uncommon before age 60 but has been reported to be present in 75% of brains after age 80 (Tomlinson & Kitchener, 1972). Granulovacuolar degeneration is generally restricted to certain regions of the hippocampus, and in normal older people, the proportion of affected cells is quite low ($\leqslant 10\%$), even in areas of greatest concentration (Tomlinson & Kitchener, 1972).

Hirano and Lewy Bodies

Hirano bodies are minute, crystalline-appearing inclusions found within the neuronal cytoplasm. Like granulovacuolar degeneration, they are observed primarily in portions of the hippocampus. Hirano bodies increase in frequency with age but are observed in higher mean concentrations in Alzheimer's disease, Pick's disease, and the Parkinson dementia complex of Guam (Kemper, 1984).

Lewy bodies are intracellular structures composed of packed filaments with a granular core which occur most often in the substantia nigra and locus ceruleus. They increase slightly with age but are much more common in Parkinson's disease (see Chapter 8) and cortical Lewy body disease (Gibb, 1989).

Lipofuscin and Melanin Deposits

Lipofuscin, a fatty pigment, reliably accumulates in brain cells with increasing age (Berg, 1988a). Melanin pigment also increases with age in certain brain areas, particularly the locus ceruleus and substantia nigra. Rates of accumulation do not appear to be affected by dementia or by conditions of accelerated aging such as Down's syndrome or progeria (Kemper, 1984).

Microvascular Changes

In some very old individuals, and more noticeably in patients with Alzheimer's disease, there is a loss of innervation to cerebral capillaries and the development of small openings in portions of the capillary wall (Scheibel, 1992). Structures similar to senile plaques are often clustered around these denervated capillaries, a finding leading to the hypothesis that microvascular changes may play a role in the development of Alzheimer-type pathology (Scheibel, 1992). In older individuals with risk factors for stroke (e.g., hypertension or diabetes), narrowing or blockage of capillaries may produce a localized hypoxic state that could result in small areas of tissue loss (see Chapter 9 for further discussion).

Neuroanatomical Changes and Cognitive Performance

Lesion Studies

There is an extensive neuropsychological literature on cognitive functions of patients with focal brain lesions (for reviews, see Kolb & Wishaw, 1984; Lezak, 1983;

Strub & Black, 1988). The value of this literature for the understanding of normal brain–behavior relations is a matter of considerable debate. Even when a brain injury is limited to a single structure, the function of distal brain regions may be affected because of the connectivity and interaction of neural systems (Luria, 1974; Riege, Harker, & Metter, 1986). In aging, many brain changes are generalized or involve several regions rather than being localized to a given area; thus, it may be especially difficult to apply lesion studies to the understanding of neuropsychological processes in the elderly.

Neurodegenerative Markers

There have been several cross-validation studies relating measures of cognitive performance to neurodegenerative markers (see Fuld, 1986, for a review). The best known of these investigations is that of Tomlinson, Blessed, and Roth (1968), who administered a quantitative mental status questionnaire to dementia patients and normal controls and subsequently examined postmortem the number of neuritic plaques. A significant correlation was obtained ($r = .63$), suggesting that problems with concentration, orientation, and memory may reflect degree of neurodegenerative change. This result has since been replicated in other research (e.g., Katzman, Brown, Fuld, Peck, Schechter, & Schimmel, 1983). However, as a more recent study (Katzman, Terry, DeTeresa, Brown, Davies, Fuld, Renbing, & Peck, 1988) illustrates, some individuals have normal cognitive function despite increased plaque counts.

Katzman *et al.* (1988) studied 137 very-old (mean age = 85 years) residents of a nursing home who were given brief cognitive testing on a yearly basis; after death, autopsies were performed examining cell counts, numbers of neuritic plaques and neurofibrillary tangles, and selected neurotransmitters. The cognitive tests consisted of a mental status examination (Katzman *et al.*, 1983) and a multitrial object recall test (Fuld, 1981). Neuroanatomical data were obtained from eight brain regions, including the midfrontal, superior temporal, and inferior parietal cortex, hippocampus, substantia nigra, and locus ceruleus.

Subjects were separated into groups based on their cognitive test scores. Of 29 cognitively normal individuals, more than one-third ($n = 10$) had brain findings consistent with Alzheimer's disease, including moderate levels of neuritic plaques and decreased choline acetyltransferase (see "The Cholinergic System," below). Brains in this group were heavier on the average than those of other subjects, and they also contained more large neurons in several brain regions. The investigators speculated that these subjects may have had "incipient Alzheimer's disease" but did not show it behaviorally because of "greater brain reserve." A second important finding was that, in general, brains of demented and nondemented patients in this very-old sample did not differ by as great a margin as has been noted in younger groups. A final, humbling, result was that for 11% of the clinically demented subjects, there was no evidence on autopsy of Alzheimer-type pathology or other cerebral pathology that might have been the cause of poor performance.

This study illustrates that a broad range of neuropathological findings can be observed in older people with normal cognitive performance. How some function well despite having Alzheimer-type brain changes is a question that needs to be explored.

Studies of plaque counts may yield variable outcomes because of the use of different histological stains. The amount of elapsed time between cognitive testing and postmortem examination can also affect results. Similar problems apply to research relating other microscopic brain changes to behavioral variables. In general, therefore, it is premature to draw conclusions about the strength of associations between antemortem cognitive performance and specific age-linked neuropathological changes.

CT Investigations

Studies using CT procedures provide an opportunity to correlate signs of atrophy with cognitive function in living subjects. Many studies have compared dementia patients to age-matched controls on CT measures, but relatively few have focused on normal aged samples.

In an early investigation, Earnest, Heaton, Wilkinson, and Manke (1979) examined 59 elderly residents of retirement communities who were free of obvious neurological disease. Several measures were computed from the CT scans, including widths of the four largest sulci and ventricle-to-skull diameter ratios. Neuropsychological tests evaluating speeded perceptual-motor functions and nonverbal memory were administered approximately one year after the CT scans. Age differences were observed between younger and older subgroups (60 to 79 vs. 80 to 99 years, respectively), with poorer cognitive performance, wider sulci, and higher ventricle-to-skull ratios in the older groups. However, correlations between CT measures and cognitive test performance were not significant when age differences were partialed out, a finding suggesting that cerebral atrophy and cognitive decline may be independent correlates of advancing age.

More refined analyses of CT scans have produced somewhat stronger evidence for brain–behavior relations. Stafford, Albert, Naeser, Sandor, and Garvey (1988) obtained quantitative CT measures for 69 optimally healthy men (aged 31 to 87 years) who also completed a lengthy neuropsychological battery. A highly significant relationship was observed between fluid volume measures of the ventricles and sulci and performance on tests of naming and abstraction. Weaker associations were noted between CT number (a measure related to attenuation of brain material at a particular scanning location) and tests of memory and attention.

These findings suggest that quantitative CT measures may be related to cognitive performance in normal aging, but that the strength and pattern of relationships vary considerably for different CT measures. The measurement difficulties and inherent limitations of CT have led a number of reviewers to be cautious in judging the value of CT as a differential diagnostic measure and as a tool for understanding the effect of atrophic brain changes on behavior (e.g., de Leon, George, & Ferris, 1986; Riege *et al.*, 1986). Under some circumstances, ventricle enlargement appears to be reversible, so that brain shrinkage as visualized in CT may not be directly proportional to neuronal death or deactivation (Jernigan, Zatz, Feinberg, & Fein, 1980).

Summary of Neuroanatomical Findings

According to Kemper (1984), age-related neuroanatomical changes can be organized into contrasting groups. Changes in the first group—including decreased brain weight, loss of neurons, loss of myelin, gyral atrophy, ventricular dilation, and amyloid accumulation—all show relatively strong correlations with age; each of these changes is further accentuated in Alzheimer's disease, but there is considerable overlap in distributions for normal aging and dementia. Changes in the second group—including granulovacuolar degeneration and neurofibrillary tangles—also increase with age but appear only in small numbers and restricted distribution in the healthy older brains; in Alzheimer's disease, these changes are more widespread throughout the brain and much more numerous. Neuritic plaques fall between these two groups, bearing a modest relationship to both age and Alzheimer's disease.

Although neuronal atrophy is clearly a part of normal aging (Bondareff, 1985), recent neuroanatomical studies have placed increasing emphasis on growth and development in the aging brain. The mechanisms underlying brain plasticity in old age are just beginning to be explored (Berg, 1988a; Coleman, Higgins, & Phelps, 1990; Russell, 1988; Scheibel, 1992); however, continued study of natural compensatory mechanisms may help to identify ways to forestall or counteract atrophic change.

Cross-validation studies show a rough correlation between selected neuroanatomical findings (e.g., cortical plaque counts) and cognitive performance, especially when normal individuals are compared to severely demented patients. However, a significant proportion of mentally healthy old people also have cortical plaques and other pathological microscopic brain changes.

Because neuroanatomical findings of Alzheimer's disease are present in the brains of clinically normal old people, the neuropathological distinction between these conditions must be made on quantitative grounds (see Chapter 7). Certain changes (e.g., neurofibrillary tangles) are markedly more common in dementia than in normal aging, so it can be argued that the Alzheimer's process is a disease rather than an accentuation of normal aging (Berg, 1985; Kemper, 1984). Similar arguments have been made for other disorders that cause dementia, including cerebrovascular conditions and Parkinson's disease (see Chapters 8 and 9). However, similarities between normal aging and these conditions probably contribute to the difficulties that neuropsychologists have in distinguishing cognitive aging from dementia in its various forms (see Chapters 7 through 9).

NEUROTRANSMITTER CHANGES

Communication between neurons results from the transfer of neurotransmitters from one cell to another. A few neurotransmitters have been recognized for many years, but recently, many more substances have been added to the list of possible neurotransmitters. Also, research suggests that different neurotransmitters may act in tandem, either across neural networks or within the same neuron, greatly increasing the possibilities for chemical communication.

Knowledge of age differences in neurotransmission is very incomplete, particularly in the human brain (Rogers & Bloom, 1985; Timiras, 1988; Whitehouse & Au, 1986). The present discussion focuses only on relatively well-studied changes in the cholinergic and catecholaminergic systems that may have implications for cognitive performance. Rogers and Bloom (1985) provided a comprehensive overview of neurotransmission in aging, and Whitehouse and Au (1986) examined receptor changes with age. Excellent discussions of interrelations between behavior and neurotransmitter changes in old age include those of Bartus, Dean, Beer, and Lippa (1982) and Kubanis and Zornetzer (1981).

The Cholinergic System

Figure 2.2A, from Timiras (1988), provides a simplified model of a junction (synapse) between two cells and identifies components of the cholinergic neurotransmitter system. Acetylcholine (ACh), the neurotransmitter, is created in the presynaptic neuron from choline and acetyl coenzyme A; the synthetic enzyme choline acetyltransferase (CAT) acts as a catalyst for ACh formation. ACh is taken up by receptors located on the membrane of the postsynaptic neuron and is later decomposed into choline and acetate by acetylcholinesterase (AChE). The highest concentrations of cholinergic neurons are found in the nuclei of the basal forebrain; from there, ACh is distributed to many brain regions, including the neocortex.

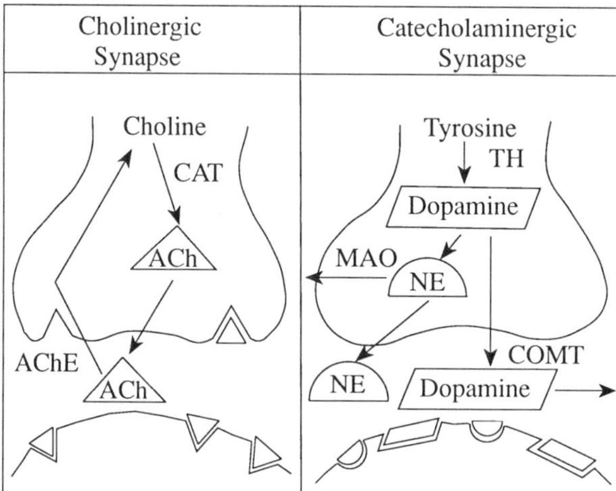

FIGURE 2.2. Simplified diagram of chemical events in neurotransmission at the cholinergic and catecholaminergic synapses. (From Timiras, 1988, p. 135. Copyright 1988 by Macmillan Publishing Company. Adapted by permission.)

Age Changes in the Cholinergic System

Most investigations have monitored levels of CAT as a marker for cholinergic metabolism. Some studies of normal elderly adults have reported decreases in CAT compared to that in younger subjects, particularly in the neocortex, striatum, and hippocampus; however, others studying the same brain regions have found no change with age (Rogers & Bloom, 1985). Bartus and colleagues (1982) suggested that age-related changes in CAT may be small and, therefore, hard to measure; further, investigators examining large brain sites (e.g., neocortical regions or the hippocampus) may inadvertently sample different cell populations. Other investigations indicate that there may be a reduction in the density of cholinergic receptors in normal aging, especially muscarinic receptors (Whitehouse & Au, 1986).

In contrast with the literature on normal aging, virtually all studies examining CAT in patients with Alzheimer's disease have reported reliable declines compared to control samples (see Chapter 7). However, definitive data are still lacking on cholinergic receptor changes (Whitehouse, 1987).

Cholinergic Changes and Cognitive Performance

The cholinergic neurotransmitter system is important for learning new information, and deficiencies in this system have been hypothesized to underlie both age-related memory changes and the more dramatic memory deficits observed in dementia (Bartus *et al.*, 1982; Giacobini, 1990).

Perry, Tomlinson, Blessed, Bergmann, Gibson, and Perry (1978) found a significant correlation between cortical CAT levels and mental status scores prior to death, but the analysis did not include data for normal subjects. Fuld (1986) reported a correlation between cortical CAT and learning and memory scores, but again, data for normal old people were not provided. Katzman *et al.* (1988), discussed above, found that in cognitively normal old people, more than a third had moderate reductions in CAT, a finding suggesting that associations between CAT and cognitive status may be weak within the normal range.

Indirect evidence of the importance of the cholinergic system in cognitive function in aging is provided by studies of normal young adults in which temporary problems with learning, memory, and performance IQ have been induced by administering drugs (e.g., scopolamine) that block ACh uptake at the receptor. These deficits are similar in some respects to those observed in normal aging, a finding suggesting, perhaps, a common cholinergic basis (for discussions, see Drachman & Leavitt, 1974; Howard & Howard, 1989).

Treatment strategies designed to enhance ACh by increasing the amount of available choline (e.g., by taking choline tablets or lecithin) have generally not been successful, either for normal older people or for those with Alzheimer-type dementia (Bartus *et al.*, 1982). Arecoline (a drug the enhances the function of cholinergic receptors) and physostigmine (a drug that slows the breakdown of ACh) have sometimes resulted in memory improvement, but the data base in normal aging is very limited (see Chapter 7 for studies with dementia patients).

Multiple points in the cholinergic pathway may need to be altered before reliable cognitive increases are observed; or it may be necessary to change the balance between cholinergic system function and other neurotransmitters in order to produce improved behavior (Bartus *et al.*, 1982; Giacobini, 1990; Timiras, 1988; Whitehouse, 1987).

The Catecholaminergic System

Dopamine (DA) and norepinephrine (NE) are the principal neurotransmitters in the catecholaminergic system (see Figure 2.2B). Brain DA is created from dietary tyrosine through the action of several enzymes, including tyrosine hydroxylase (TH) and aromatic amino acid decarboxylase (DOPA decarboxylase). NE is created from DA by means of dopamine beta-hydroxylase (DBH). Both DA and NE are broken down by catabolic enzymes, the most important of which is monoamine oxidase (MAO).

Age Changes in Catecholamines

Like ACh, DA is widely distributed throughout the brain. Fairly consistent decreases in DA in old age have been observed in the striatum (including the caudate nucleus and putamen), but evidence for age changes in other brain areas is more variable (Rogers & Bloom, 1985). For NE, consistent old-age declines have been reported in the locus ceruleus (Kubanis & Zornetzer, 1981; Rogers & Bloom, 1985), septum, and substantia nigra, but findings are less clear in other regions (Rogers & Bloom, 1985). Pronounced declines in TH, the enzyme that stimulates synthesis of catecholamines, have been observed in the human brain, particularly in the striatum (McGeer & McGeer, 1975, 1976). By contrast, MAO-B, important in the breakdown of catecholamines, may increase with age by as much as 50% (Robinson, Nies, Davies, Bunney, Davis, Colburn, Bourne, Shaw, & Coppen, 1972). The number of catecholaminergic receptors and the response of these receptors to stress appear to decrease with age in several brain regions (Kubanis & Zornetzer, 1981). However, even in old age, catecholaminergic neurons seem to possess considerable reserve capacity (Carlsson, 1986). If neural numbers decrease, the remaining neurons may increase their firing rates and utilize more of their enzymatic synthesizing capacity. Therefore, there may be little functional consequence of mild neuronal loss.

Catecholaminergic Changes and Cognitive Performance

Behavioral effects of altered catecholamine activity have been studied much more extensively in animals than in humans. In rodent species, changes in NE have been implicated in decreased neural plasticity, inability to curb arousal, altered feedback control of the hypothalamic-pituitary-adrenal system, and problems with selective attention (see Kubanis & Zornetzer, 1981, for a review). Orienting behavior, exploratory activity, and strategic behavior may be diminished by disruptions in normal catecholamine activity (Clark, Geffen, & Geffen, 1987a). Alterations in these functions could, in turn, result in changes in learning and memory or other complex cognitive processes (Kubanis & Zornetzer, 1981; Zornetzer, 1985; see Wenk, 1988, for a contrasting opinion).

When healthy young adults are given drugs that block catecholamine activity, they experience negative changes in mood and motivation and problems with learning and memory; by contrast, drugs that enhance catecholamine activity (e.g., amphetamines) may elevate mood and improve memory scores (Weingartner, 1984). Effects on attention have also been observed; for example, in difficult divided-attention tasks, amphetamines such as methylphenidate tend to increase available attentional capacity and may facilitate allocation of attention to specific events (Clark, Geffen, & Geffen, 1987b).

DA deficiency may play a role in the cognitive deficits observed in Parkinson's disease (see Chapter 8) and other neurodegenerative conditions (e.g., progressive supranuclear palsy) that selectively impair dopaminergic neurons. Also, altered catecholamines may contribute to depression and its accompanying cognitive changes (see Chapter 11).

Cognitive performance of normal old people is similar in some respects to that of patients with depression or Parkinson's disease (see Chapters 3, 8, and 11). In all of these conditions, learning and memory deficits are greatest on "effortful" processing tasks, and there are declines on tests of psychomotor speed. Whether these similarities reflect a common neurochemical substrate (e.g., dopamine depletion) is a matter of speculation at this point. There are a few studies with healthy elderly adults (e.g., Newman, Weingartner & Smallberg, 1984) showing facilitation of memory with dopamine enhancement drugs, but more research is needed to determine the strength and pattern of beneficial effects.

Summary of Neurotransmitter Findings

Reductions in levels of neurotransmitter substances and changes in associated enzymes and receptors have been demonstrated in the aging human brain. Dopamine neurons appear to be more age-sensitive than many other neurons, but important changes also occur in the cholinergic system and in numerous other neurotransmitters not included in this discussion.

Associations between cognition and neurotransmitter variables have not been extensively studied in normal older people. At present, there is clearer evidence for correlations in pathological conditions such as Alzheimer's disease or Parkinson's disease, where the neurotransmitter changes are more pronounced and behavioral impairment is more severe.

Researchers have only begun to examine imbalance among neurotransmitters as a possible cause of aging change, although many believe that interactions between systems will prove to be more important than alterations in single neurotransmitters (Timiras, 1988; Whitehouse, 1987). Also, the ways in which neurons may compensate for declining availability of neurotransmitters are being increasingly studied (Russell, 1988). Other current research is exploring the role of calcium and nerve growth factor (NGF) in maintenance of neuronal function (Berg, 1988a).

At present, one of the most important clinical implications of neurotransmitter changes in aging concerns the increased risk of adverse side effects of psychoactive medications. Older patients often experience anticholinergic side effects from tricyclic antidepressants and may have adverse responses to many pain medications, sleeping pills, and antihistamines (see Chapter 6 for additional information on cognitive side effects of medications).

NEUROPHYSIOLOGICAL CHANGES

A number of procedures have been developed in recent decades that permit *in vivo* examination of metabolic processes in the human brain. These offer the opportunity of observing brain regions that are activated by performance of specific cognitive acts and of studying the functional interplay between different areas of the brain. Cerebral blood flow and emission tomography studies provide relatively direct means of tracing cerebral metabolic processes. Electroencephalographic methods are less direct but can provide important information about the time course of different sensory and cognitive processes.

Brain Metabolism

Among the procedures currently used to measure human brain metabolism, two of the most prominent are regional cerebral blood flow (rCBF) and positron emission tomography (PET). Metter (1988) provided an excellent description of these methods as applied to the study of aging, and Phelps and Mazziotta (1985) gave an informative overview of emission-tomographic methods and their application to brain–behavior questions.

Most recent investigations of rCBF have used a procedure in which radioactive xenon gas is either injected or inhaled. The xenon is carried throughout the brain by blood flow, and its distribution in various areas is monitored through multiple detectors placed over the skull. Cerebral blood flow can also be measured by PET (Phelps & Mazziotta, 1985). One of the assumptions made in studying rCBF is that changes in neuronal metabolism are directly reflected in cerebral blood flow, lessened blood flow indicating lower metabolic rates (de Leon *et al.*, 1986).

PET also involves the injection or inhaling of small quantities of radioactive tracers. Many different tracers have been used (see Phelps & Mazziotta, 1985), but the most common in aging studies has been 2-deoxy-2-[^{18}F] fluoro-D-glucose (FDG), a glucose compound labeled with a radioactive form of fluorine [^{18}F]. Glucose provides the primary energy source for most brain metabolic processes, and brain tissues use FDG as if it were ordinary glucose. As a result, FDG accumulates most rapidly in tissues that have a high metabolic rate. As the radioactive substance decays in these tissues, it emits positrons that are recorded by detectors and analyzed by computer to provide quantitative estimates of metabolic rates for various brain regions.

Age Differences in rCBF and PET

Most studies of older persons report at least mild declines in global and regional blood flow relative to young adults (see Table 2.2; Metter, 1988; Meyer & Shaw, 1984). However, this age trend may be confounded by medical illness, since many studies have not excluded individuals with vascular conditions or heart disease. The effects of illness on rCBF are illustrated in Figure 2.3, which shows that optimally healthy older adults have higher cerebral blood flow than those with risk factors for cerebrovascular disease (e.g., hypertension, heart disease, or diabetes), who, in turn, have greater blood flow than those with a history of transient ischemic attacks (TIAs). Nonetheless, there is some decline in cerebral blood flow when subjects are followed longitudinally, even in the healthy group.

Studies using PET report conflicting evidence for age changes in cerebral glucose metabolism. Kuhl and colleagues (Kuhl, Metter, Riege, & Phelps, 1982; Kuhl, Metter, Riege, & Hawkins, 1984) reported about a 20% decrease in global glucose metabolic rates from age 24 to 74 years accompanied by a reduction in the normal trend toward high

TABLE 2.2. Neurophysiological Age Differences[a]

Measure	Direction of change	Comments
Brain metabolism		
Cerebral blood flow	Decrease	May vary by region; minimal age difference when risk factors for cerebrovascular illness are absent.
Metabolic rate for glucose	Inconsistent	May vary by region; age differences appear to be small.
Electrophysiology		
Dominant EEG frequency	Decrease	Minimal age difference in optimally healthy persons.
Alpha reactivity	Decrease	
Cortical coupling	Increase	May suggest decreased regional specialization.
Sensory evoked responses (latency)	Increase	
Sensory evoked responses (amplitude)	Increase	May suggest decreased cortical inhibition.
Event-related potentials (P300 latency)	Increase	Slowing of central decision processes; minimal age difference in optimally healthy persons.

[a]From *Handbook of Neuropsychological Assessment: A Biopsychosocial Perspective* (pp. 86, 93) by A. Puente and R. McCaffrey, 1992, New York: Plenum Press. Copyright 1992 by Plenum Press, Inc. Adapted by permission.

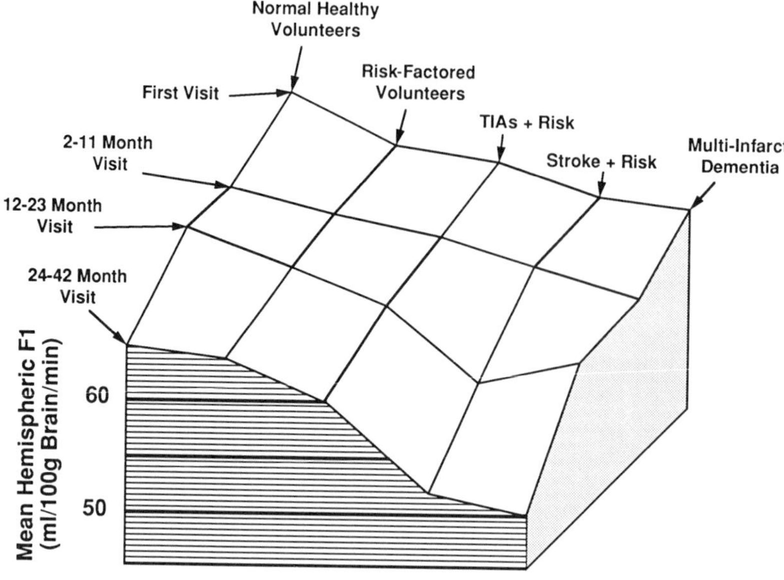

FIGURE 2.3. Cerebral blood flow measurements for optimally healthy volunteers and patients with varying degrees of cerebrovascular illness. F_1 is cerebral gray matter flow; risk factors included hypertension, diabetes, and other conditions related to cerebrovascular disease; the TIAs + risk group had a history of transient ischemic attacks in addition to risk factors. (From Meyer and Shaw, 1984, p. 188. Copyright 1984 by Oxford University Press. Reprinted by permission.)

metabolic rates in the frontal region. A number of other studies have found no significant age differences (e.g., de Leon, George, Ferris, Christman, Fowler, Gentes, Brodie, Reisberg, & Wolf, 1984; Duara, Margolin, Robertson-Tchabo, London, Schwartz, Renfrew, Koziarz, Sundaram, Grady, Moore, Ingvar, Sokoloff, Weingartner, Kessler, Manning, Channing, Cutler, & Rapoport, 1983). Metter (1988) attributed some of the inconsistency to sampling procedures. Kuhl and colleagues excluded subjects with neurological disorders, moderate hypertension, and severe heart disease but included individuals with milder levels of medical illness. Therefore, age-related declines may have reflected hypertensive and atherosclerotic change. By contrast, Duara and colleagues accepted only subjects who had no evidence of any disease, that is, optimally aging individuals.

The studies by Kuhl and Duara and their associates also used different resting states (e.g., vision and hearing not impeded vs. eyes and ears covered) that may have induced different types of internal mental activity. Cerebral blood flow and metabolism show habituation to testing environments, and regional patterns shift when subjects engage in different types of mental activity. Therefore, if older subjects habituate less quickly to the PET procedure than younger adults, or if they think different thoughts in the course of the assessment, age differences may reflect performance factors rather than tissue changes.

Brain Metabolism and Cognitive Performance

Riege *et al.* (1986) described a study of 23 adults (aged 27 to 78 years) free of cardio- or cerebrovascular disease who were examined with PET and tested on an extensive battery of memory measures. For most of the 18 brain regions studied, there were no significant age differences in glucose metabolic rates; however, the regional metabolic ratio in Broca's area decreased with age. This decrease was correlated with poorer performance on tasks that required retrieval of words, sentences, or designs from secondary memory. In addition, intercorrelations between metabolic indices for frontal and subcortical regions decreased in strength with age, a finding suggesting that older adults may have reduced interactions between these regions during memory activities. By contrast, Duara, Grady, Haxby, Ingvar, Sokoloff, Margolin, Manning, Cutler, and Rapoport (1984) found few relationships between regional brain metabolic measures and performance on intelligence and memory tests.

Both of these studies included only a small number of elderly subjects (e.g., $n = 8$ in Riege's old group), increasing the odds that sample variation might have affected the results. In addition, there were important procedural differences between the studies. For example, Duara *et al.* (1984) covered subjects' eyes and ears during PET, whereas Riege *et al.* (1986) left both unoccluded; and while Duara *et al.* (1984) used a small battery of standard psychometric measures, Riege and colleagues included many experimental learning and memory tests that may have been more sensitive to subtle cognitive differences than standard clinical measures.

Summary of rCBF and PET Findings

Metter (1988) emphasized that age differences in brain metabolism have been inconsistently observed with the use of rCBF and PET techniques. Regarding age effects, he concluded that "the overall patterns of the PET scans remain the same, and . . . if a decline occurs, it is of relatively small magnitude" (p. 241). Studies interrelating patterns of brain metabolism to neuropsychological performance have also produced inconsistent results, and it is not clear how age affects the functional interrelations between brain regions. Simultaneous study of behavioral and metabolic parameters offers great promise as a research technique but has not yet provided a definitive picture of brain–behavior relations. One obstacle to large-scale studies is the great expense of PET procedures; rCBF with xenon inhalation is less costly but also less versatile in terms of the metabolic processes that can be measured. Single-photon emission tomography (SPECT) is also less expensive and may have greater clinical potential than PET.

Cerebral Electrophysiology

Electroencephalography

Electroencephalograph (EEG) measures the ongoing electrical activity of the brain. Typically, EEG is recorded with multiple scalp electrodes to permit simultaneous evaluation of the activity of several brain regions. Various aspects of EEG output can be monitored, including frequency, consistency across time, and symmetry across brain regions. These parameters can be rated clinically (by visual inspection of the EEG tracings) or by computer-assisted methods (e.g., as in power spectral analysis and brain electrical activity mapping, or BEAM).

The most consistently reported late-life change in EEG (see Table 2.2) is a diffuse slowing of the dominant alpha rhythm from a mean frequency of 10 cps (cycles per second) to 8 or 9 cps (Obrist, 1963, 1975; Wang & Busse, 1969). The extent of slowing is related to general health, being greatest among persons with cardiac or cerebrovascular disease (Duffy & McAnulty, 1988). Other age-associated findings include increased occurrence of the slower delta (≤ 4 cps) and theta (5 to 7 cps) rhythms, a high incidence of focal findings (affecting approximately one-third of normal elderly persons), and decreased alpha reactivity or blocking (Duffy & McAnulty, 1988).

Although EEG slowing is a correlate of normal aging, age differences are small compared to those observed with dementia (see John, Prichep, Fridman, & Easton, 1988, for clinical applications of EEG). A majority of patients with primary degenerative dementia show slowing into the theta range, compared to only about 7% of normal aged persons (Wang & Busse, 1969). Delta activity is also much more common in dementia than in normal aging (Wang & Busse, 1969).

Recent studies with optimally healthy older adults suggest that only minimal age-related EEG change occurs in the absence of medical illness (Duffy & McAnulty, 1988). Mean alpha frequencies in the range of 9.5 to 9.8 cps (similar to values reported for young and middle-aged adults) have been reported for very healthy older people, with delta and theta activity either decreasing in old age (Katz & Horowitz, 1982) or showing no age-related change (Gianquinto & Nolfe, 1986). Even with optimally healthy older people, however, diminished alpha reactivity has been observed; that is, older subjects show less change in EEG between eyes-closed and eyes-open recording states (Duffy, Albert, McAnulty, & Garvey, 1984b; Katz & Horowitz, 1982).

Evoked and Event-Related Potentials

Other commonly used electrophysiological measures include evoked potentials (EPs) and event-related potentials (ERPs). Unlike clinical EEG, these measures are correlated in time with the processing of specific stimuli and are thought to represent a limited set of cognitive operations, most often sensory discrimination and decision making. Cortical electrical responses to external stimulation may last for 750 msec or longer, and early versus late components of the response are assumed to reflect different biological and psychological mechanisms.

Very early components of the EP (occurring at 20 msec or less after stimulation) represent the activity of brain-stem or thalamic structures. Age differences have been reported for both auditory brain-stem evoked responses and somatosensory evoked responses, with longer latencies observed at older ages. Much of this change has been attributed to decreased speed of nerve conduction.

EPs observed between 30 to 100 msec after stimulation are thought to reflect cortical activation arising from sensory-specific and more diffuse pathways. Advanced age also results in prolonged latencies of these EP components. Analysis of the pattern of EP changes in relation to increasing stimulus intensity suggests that elderly people may be stimulus "augmenters"; that is, they tend to show increased amplitudes of brain response to more intense stimulation. This effect contrasts with findings for young and middle-aged adults, most of whom tend to be stimulus "reducers." These differences could mean that with advancing age, there is reduced ability to inhibit responses to external stimulation (e.g., Dustman, Snyder, & Schlehuber, 1981).

Late components of the cortical response to stimulation are thought to reflect not only automatic effects of stimulus registration but internal reactions (e.g., recognition or surprise) as well. The term *event-related potential* has been adopted to refer to these components. The most widely studied ERP is the P300, a positive peak in the waveform that occurs in young adults at about 300 to 500 msec after stimulation, particularly when the person detects a rare stimulus within a series of more familiar stimuli (the so-called oddball paradigm). The P300 has been hypothesized to reflect activity in the temporal lobes, possibly in or near the hippocampus and amygdala (Duffy & McAnulty, 1988), but other brain regions may also be involved.

A number of studies using auditory oddball paradigms have observed an increase in mean latency and a decrease in mean amplitude of the P300 across the adult life span (e.g., Brown, Marsh, & La Rue, 1983; Goodin, Squires, Henderson, & Starr, 1978). Most investigations suggest that the latency increase accelerates in old age (e.g., Beck, Swanson, & Dustman, 1980; Brown *et al.*, 1983; Mullis, Holcomb, Diner, & Dykman, 1985). However, a study of optimally healthy older subjects failed to find a significant correlation between P300 latency and age (Duffy *et al.*, 1984b).

Electrophysiological Changes and Cognitive Performance

Significant correlations between EEG slowing and cognitive performance have been reported for patients with dementia (e.g., Kaszniak, Garron, Fox, Bergen, & Huckman, 1979). However, among healthy old persons, slight generalized slowing of the clinical EEG and certain focal changes (especially slow-wave activity in the anterior temporal region) are generally unrelated to performance on intelligence and memory tests (e.g., Birren, Butler, Greenhouse, Sokoloff, & Yarrow, 1963; Obrist, 1975).

Latency of the P300 also differs in dementia patients and normal elderly controls, with more exaggerated slowing observed in dementia (e.g., Duffy, Albert, & McAnulty, 1984a; Goodin *et al.*, 1978). This difference is most likely to be found when moderately demented patients are contrasted with normals; in mildly demented individuals, prolongation of the P300 is slight and may even be absent. Also, "forgetful" elderly subjects appear to have similar P300s to age-matched controls with normal memory (Loring, Levin, Papanicolaou, Larrabee, & Eisenberg, 1984). Therefore, like clinical EEG, P300 may be of limited use in studying normal cognitive aging.

By contrast, using computer-assisted BEAM methodology in optimally healthy subjects, Duffy *et al.* (1984b) found age shifts in several aspects of EEG topography (particularly in the temporal regions) and a number of significant intercorrelations between topographical patterns and performance on neuropsychological tests. The principal age trend was toward decreasing slow-wave activity (theta and delta) and increasing amounts of fast-wave activity (beta) in old age, a pattern that the investigators described as EEG desynchronization. This desynchronized pattern, in turn, was associated with poorer performance on cognitive tests. Most EEG features correlated with many different types of cognitive tests, and performance on particular tests was often associated with EEG features from several different cortical regions.

BEAM patterns induced by verbal versus spatial tasks appear to be similar for young and old adults, but there may be a reduction with age in the degree of asymmetry resulting from different tasks (Duffy & McAnulty, 1988). The latter finding could be explained by a breakdown in the functional autonomy of different cortical areas in old age. Dustman, LaMarche, Cohn, Shearer, and Talone (1985) found EEG power values to be less variable across electrode sites in older subjects (aged 55 to 70 years) than in young adults; in addition, cortical coupling, a measure designed to reflect functional communication between different brain areas, was higher among the older subjects. These results provide further evidence that the older brain may respond in a more homogeneous or global manner than the younger brain.

Summary of Electrophysiological Findings

Electrophysiological data suggest that at older ages, slowing occurs in the rate at which the brain registers sensory information and makes decisions about differences between stimuli. Mild slowing of the clinical EEG or of evoked-potential measures such as the P300 is not highly correlated with intelligence or memory scores in normal older adults; however, more sophisticated EEG measures (e.g., BEAM or spectral analysis) may show closer relationships with neuropsychological findings.

Age-related changes in electrophysiology provide intriguing clues to potential differences in modes of cognitive processing in young versus old adults. A loss of cortical inhibitory ability is suggested by the trend toward stimulus augmentation in older individuals. And higher cortical coupling in old age may suggest that tasks are processed in a less differentiated way than at earlier ages. These trends may result from neuroanatomical and neurochemical age changes such as increased cell loss in the anterior neocortex or declining levels of inhibitory neurotransmitters, including DA and NE (Dustman *et al.*, 1985); at present, however, these associations are speculative.

There are limitations in the use of electrophysiological measures that need to be recognized (Duffy & McAnulty, 1988). Electrical responses are diffused by the skull, so that it is difficult to localize the region generating a particular response; small individual differences in the location of particular brain regions can increase the variance of regional electrophysiological findings; and differences in the number and placement of electrodes can lead to contradictory results. However, procedures such as BEAM and spectral analysis have increased the clinical and research potential of EEG, and refinements in measurement and analysis are continuing.

SUMMARY AND CONCLUSIONS

Normal aging is accompanied by a wide range of changes in brain structure and function. Neuroanatomical differences include a decrease in brain weight and volume with advancing age, a loss of large neurons in selected brain regions, and an increase in certain microscopic findings associated with pathology (e.g., neuritic plaques and neurofibrillary tangles). Neurochemically, relatively large changes in brain catecholamines have been noted with normal aging, whereas cholinergic system changes are less clear. Findings from PET and rCBF studies are equivocal with respect to normal aging changes, but electrophysiological data indicate slowing in the rate at which the brain processes sensory information and arrives at decisions.

Research on human brain aging is exciting but very preliminary. According to Bondareff (1985), "The effects of age on human behavior are only beginning to be understood as they relate to chemical and structural changes in the brain" (p. 108). Berg (1988a) noted the rapid expansion in research on brain aging in recent years, but he also observed, "Literally all of the clues reported are accompanied by assertions that much more work is needed to obtain more convincing answers" (p. 12).

The fragmentary nature of current knowledge helps to explain why neuropsychological theories of aging are so limited (see Chapter 3). Attributing complex cognitive changes to isolated brain phenomena seems simplistic and potentially harmful. This is particularly true with normal aging, since most brain–behavior research has been directed at pathological conditions such as Alzheimer's or Parkinson's disease.

The neurobiological literature has not always distinguished aging changes from the effects of medical illness. On many metabolic and electrophysiological measures, age differences are small or absent when optimally healthy subjects are studied. This finding suggests that secondary aging processes (e.g., illness, trauma, and poor nutrition) play an important role in the degenerative changes we have come to associate with "normal" aging.

The next decade may dramatically alter our picture of human brain aging. Advances in neuroimaging and electrophysiology are making it possible to study dynamic brain–behavior relationships and to track individuals longitudinally. Also, in basic research, the emphasis is shifting away from some of the processes discussed in the present chapter (e.g., manipulation of precursors, enzymes, or receptors for neurotransmitters) toward investigations of membrane functions, cellular metabolism, and trophic factors, more emphasis being placed on plastic and regenerative aspects of central nervous system function (Coleman *et al.*, 1990).

At present, it is important to recognize that procedures such as brain scans do not provide a substitute for clinical assessment of cognitive and functional ability. Older neurodiagnostic techniques (routine CT and clinical EEG) are of limited utility in evaluating normal aging or in distinguishing age changes from those observed in mild dementia or depression. Newer techniques (e.g., MRI, PET, SPECT, and BEAM) are more sensitive, but there are technical problems with each of these measures and normative data are still quite limited. Even when positive findings are obtained on such tests, functional correlates need to be investigated, since behavior is often normal despite mild signs of brain change.

3

Cognition in Normal Aging

As interest in aging and the aged has increased, thoughts about the relationship between cognition and aging have undergone repeated revisions. At mid-century, the dominant perspective on this topic was expressed by David Wechsler (1958): "Nearly all studies . . . have shown that most human abilities . . . decline progressively after . . . ages 18 and 25" (p. 135). By the early to mid-1970s, the notion of inescapable age-related decline was being strongly challenged, with titles such as "Aging and IQ: The Myth of the Twilight Years" being used in reviews of the literature (Baltes & Schaie, 1974). Contemporary approaches emphasize the diversity of aging–cognition relations, plasticity in old-age abilities, and the marked individual differences that exist among older people.

This chapter presents a summary of psychometric and experimental research on aging and cognition. Changes in intelligence are discussed in the initial section, which is followed by reviews of specific cognitive domains (e.g., attention, language, and memory). Normative trends and individual differences are described, and situational influences on performance are examined. The final sections discuss neuropsychological hypotheses about normal aging and strategies for enhancing cognitive performance.

INTELLIGENCE

The Cattell/Horn Model

Perhaps the most influential model of the effects of normal aging on basic intellectual abilities is the fluid/crystallized conceptualization proposed by Cattell (1963) and subsequently expanded and revised by Horn (e.g., 1970, 1982). Part of the initial attraction of the model was its simplicity. Briefly stated, Cattell (1963) hypothesized that human intellectual abilities could be divided into two broad categories: (1) those dependent upon the accumulation of formal and informal educational experiences over the course of a lifetime ("crystallized" abilities) and (2) those reflecting maturational growth and decline of neural structures ("fluid" abilities). In normal aging, crystallized abilities were expected to improve or remain stable with the passage of time, but fluid abilities were predicted to decline because of decremental changes in the central and peripheral nervous system.

Figure 3.1 portrays one version of the fluid/crystallized model, illustrating hypothetical life-span trajectories of different components of intelligence and causal factors. The curve for crystallized abilities (Gc) parallels the function for educational exposure (E); both accelerate relatively sharply into early adulthood and then increase very gradually into old age. Fluid abilities (Gf) parallel the curve depicting maturational growth and decline of neural structures (M), rising steeply through childhood, but declining slowly from adolescence onward. Accumulated injury to neural structures is depicted as increasing linearly from infancy through old age. Thus, this model includes the notion that there are some normal declines in neural structures, as well as some decremental effects resulting from illness or injury that increase in likelihood with the passage of time.

Subsequent revisions of the fluid/crystallized model have treated these two classes of intellectual abilities as overarching constructs and have identified a number of more specific intellectual components that vary in relation to age, including short-term acquisition and retrieval (SAR) functions, tertiary storage and retrieval (TSR) functions, and clusters of abilities related to sensory function and cognitive speed.

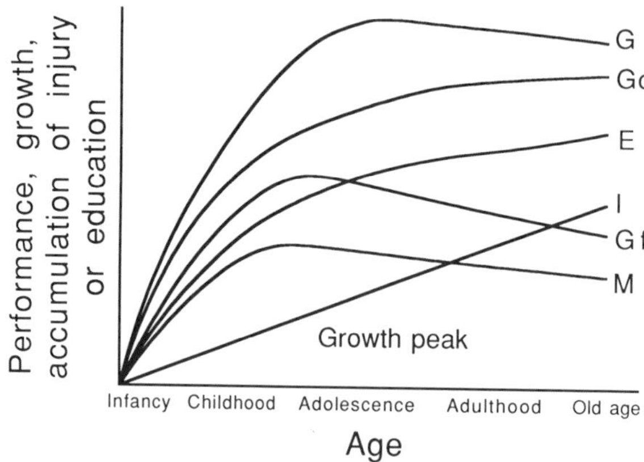

FIGURE 3.1. Development of fluid intelligence (Gf) and crystallized intelligence (Gc) in relation to maturational growth and decline in neural structures (M), accumulation of injury to neural structures (I), accumulation of educational exposures (E), and overall ability (G). (From Horn, 1970, p. 465. Copyright 1970 by Academic Press. Reprinted by permission.)

The primary data base for the fluid/crystallized model comes from cross-sectional studies of performance on standardized intelligence measures, subtests of which have been classified in terms of the intellectual components that they purportedly assess (Horn, 1985). For example, on the Wechsler Adult Intelligence Scales—Wechsler-Bellevue (Wechsler, 1944), WAIS (Wechsler, 1955), and WAIS-R (Wechsler, 1981)—Information, Comprehension, Similarities, and Vocabulary are considered measures of crystallized intelligence, all performance subtests are classified as fluid intellectual measures, and Digit Span and Arithmetic are assumed to measure the short-term acquisition and retrieval function. The increasing difficulty of performance subtests with advancing age and the comparative stability of verbal scores have been substantiated by many cross-sectional comparisons (see Botwinick, 1977, for a discussion) and by longitudinal studies (e.g., Jarvik & Bank, 1983; Sands, Terry, & Meredith, 1989).

Procedural Artifacts

Many researchers and clinicians have questioned whether observed declines on performance subtests may not be artifactual, that is, arising for reasons that have little to do with intelligence (e.g., reduced sensory acuity, differential familiarity with testing, or simple differences in motor speed). However, increasing the size of the stimuli for the Picture Arrangement and Picture Completion subtests does not substantially alter the performance of older subjects (Storandt & Futterman, 1982); also, correlations between measures of intelligence and visual or auditory acuity have been found to be relatively low in normal aging (e.g., Sands & Meredith, 1989). Similarly, providing training on the Digit Symbol subtest does not help older subjects more than younger ones (Erber, Botwinick, & Storandt, 1981). At least two studies (Doppelt & Wallace, 1955; Storandt, 1977) examined age differences on timed versus untimed administrations of the WAIS performance subtests. Removing time constraints did benefit old-age samples somewhat more than younger groups, but it did not raise the total scores of the old to the levels of the young; correlations between performance on the timed and on the untimed administrations were very high (*r*'s ranged from 0.88 to 1.00). Considered together, these studies suggest that performance subtests are genuinely difficult for older adults.

The apparent stability of scores on verbal subtests has also been questioned on procedural grounds. For example, Botwinick and Storandt (1974b) expanded the scoring categories for the Vocabulary subtest of the WAIS and found that old people were less likely than young adults to give perfect synonyms as responses and more likely to achieve their "full-credit" points by describing examples or uses of the words. Thus, if a more stringent approach were taken to scoring, even Vocabulary scores might be interpreted as showing some decremental age changes.

Generational Differences

Other lines of research have emphasized generational differences in intelligence test performance. A large-scale sequential investigation, the Seattle Longitudinal Aging Study (see Schaie, 1983, for a review), illustrated that rates of intellectual change across specific age intervals vary for different birth cohorts. For example, one analysis found that individuals born in 1917 tended to decline in intellectual performance between the ages of 39 and 46 years, whereas those born in 1924 improved in performance across the same age span (Schaie & Labouvie-Vief, 1974). Also, from age 67 to 74 years, decline in test scores was much greater for individuals born in 1889 than for those born in 1896.

Many factors probably contribute to these generational differences. Cohorts born earlier often received less education and less adequate nutrition and health care than more recently born groups. Types of work performed by people from different generations, or differences in leisure activities, may also contribute to the observed generational effects.

The most recent analyses of data from the Seattle Longitudinal Study (Hertzog & Schaie, 1986, 1988) continue to support cohort differences in intellectual performance. However, fairly consistent outcomes have accumulated which show that the basic trend in intellectual abilities over time is for slight improvement in early adulthood, stability in the middle years, and decline in later years. Decline begins at some point between ages 55 and 70, with individual differences in the age of onset. Because the tests used to measure intelligence in this study (Primary Mental Abilities; Thurstone & Thurstone, 1949) place a premium on perceptual and decision-making speed (i.e., Gf abilities), these recent outcomes support the hypothesis of normative age decline in such skills (cf. Salthouse, 1985); however, the decline appears to begin later in life than was initially postulated in the Horn/Cattell model.

Training Effects

Generalizations based on the fluid/crystallized model must also be evaluated in light of the results of training studies, where performance of older people on Gf tasks has been shown to improve considerably with practice or training.

In one of the earliest studies to demonstrate plasticity in Gf (Plemons, Willis, & Baltes, 1978), the focus of training was on nonverbal analytic skills, using tasks that required the person to identify relations between figures in a pattern and to produce a missing element. Subjects ranging in age from 59 to 85 years were randomly assigned to a training group or to a control condition that provided no practice or instruction in figural relations. The training group was presented with examples of figural problems and with specific solution rules; there were eight 1-hour instruction sessions given over a period of four weeks. Effects of training were measured on posttests conducted one week, one month, and six months after training. On tasks that were similar but not identical to those used in training, scores of the training group exceeded those of the control group at each of the posttest times. Training benefits generalized to other nonverbal tests, but not to very different types of tasks, such as verbal comprehension. Control subjects also tended to improve on the figural relations tasks across successive testings, a finding indicating some nonspecific benefits of practice. More recent studies have continued to show beneficial effects of training on Gf tasks (e.g., Willis & Schaie,

1986), and in some cases (e.g., Baltes, Sowarka, & Kliegl, 1989), self-guided practice has been found to produce as much gain as direct tutoring.

Everyday Context

There is a growing endorsement of a contextual perspective of aging–cognition relations (e.g., Labouvie-Vief, 1985). This approach assumes that cognitive performance reflects social-environmental demands, and that these demands may differ in important ways for older and younger adults. Elderly people may be called upon less often than younger ones to perform complex, speeded, psychomotor tasks; they may be expected to learn new procedures less frequently; and, particularly if they have been retired for a number of years, they may be able to function with less detailed and less efficient modes of information processing. When asked to perform on a battery of cognitive tests, therefore, they would be likely to do best on those measures that most closely approximate a natural task and worst on those that are artificial compared to the day-to-day context of older adult life.

From the contextual perspective, models of aging changes derived from standard laboratory or intelligence tests may be of limited value because they tend to exaggerate late-life decline. This perspective may also help to explain variations in performance on standard tests by different subgroups of older adults (e.g., Craik, Byrd, & Swanson, 1987; Heaton, Grant, & Matthews, 1986; Manton, Siegler, & Woodbury, 1986). For example, low scores obtained by poorly educated or inactive people may reflect reduced opportunity in everyday life to use the types of information processing required by novel and abstract tests.

Terminal Decline

Data from several longitudinal aging studies suggest that performance on intelligence tests may be linked to survival duration. Often, participants who show decline across successive testings are closer to death that those with more stable performance, a phenomenon sometimes referred to as terminal drop or decline (Kleemeier, 1961; Riegel & Riegel, 1972; Siegler, 1975).

A long-term investigation of aging twins provides an example of these trends (see Jarvik & Bank, 1983, for a review). Psychological tests (including a vocabulary test, a tapping test of psychomotor speed, and several subtests from the Wechsler-Bellevue) were administered in the late 1940s to 134 pairs of twins who were all over the age of 60 years when the study began. Survivors of this initial sample were retested several times, and changes in psychological performance were examined in relation to survival. On each of several retest occasions, individuals who showed decline on certain "critical loss" tests (Vocabulary, Similarities, and Digit Symbol) were significantly more likely to die within five years of testing than those without such cognitive losses. Even stronger evidence was obtained when monozygotic twin pairs discordant for critical loss were compared: in 10 out of 11 such pairs, the partner with the critical loss died first (Jarvik

& Blum, 1971). In the remaining pair, both survived for many years, but the partner who had earlier shown critical loss developed a severely disabling dementia, while his twin continued to live in good health in the community.

None of the participants in this study were acutely ill at the time of assessment. However, many had chronic medical conditions, such as arteriosclerotic disease. Mild cognitive losses noted years prior to death may be mirroring subclinical cerebral dysfunction produced by medical disease, corresponding, perhaps, to cerebral blood flow declines found in people with hypertension, heart disease, or diabetes (see Chapter 2, Figure 2.3).

The last analysis of terminal decline in the twin study (Steuer, La Rue, Blum, & Jarvik, 1980) focused on a small group of very-old subjects (aged 83 to 99 years). In these individuals, changes in cognitive test scores over a six-year test–retest interval no longer predicted survival duration, a finding suggesting that the link between cognitive changes and death may not hold for very-old people (cf. Riegel & Riegel, 1972; White & Cunningham, 1988).

The terminal decline literature suggests that a drop in cognitive performance may be an early signal of failing health, especially in young-old individuals. It also supports the possibility that cognitive losses in later life may be the result of secondary aging, reflecting illness instead of intrinsic late-life development (cf. Jarvik, 1988).

A Descriptive Synthesis

Several years ago, Botwinick (1977) presented a number of useful generalizations about the literature on intelligence and aging. His summary statement was as follows:

> after reviewing the available literature, both recent and old, the conclusion here is that decline in intellectual ability is clearly part of the aging picture. The more recent literature, however, is bringing attention to what has been underemphasized in the older literature, namely [*sic*], these declines may start later in life than heretofore thought and they may be smaller in magnitude; they may also include fewer functions. (p. 580)

Several additional points were made that are useful for interpreting inconsistencies in results and for achieving perspective on the magnitude of aging changes.

1. In the literature on normal aging, proponents of decline tend to emphasize performance abilities as observed in the last years of life, whereas proponents of minimal decline stress findings on verbal abilities in the middle years of life.
2. Negative age patterns tend to be less apparent in longitudinal research than in cross-sectional research.
3. The classic verbal–performance split with advancing age is a "robust" pattern. Moreover, "the performance decrement part of the classic aging pattern is not be attributed to peripheral, non-intellective factors, but to intellective ones" (p. 588).
4. Chronological age accounts for only about 20% of the variance in full-scale IQ scores.

These generalizations still apply to the rapidly growing literature on intellectual abilities and aging. In addition, recent studies demonstrate the need to adjust our picture of normative aging for background factors such as education and occupation, and for age-related changes in the contextual demands of everyday life. The terminal decline literature suggests that some of the losses now attributed to normal aging may result from subclinical illness, placing a premium on research that will help to differentiate the cognitive changes associated with healthy aging from those caused by various illnesses. It is also becoming increasingly clear that intellectual declines in old age can be modified by practice and training.

ATTENTION

Although adequate attention is recognized as a prerequisite for optimal performance on cognitive tasks, relationships between attention and other facets of cognition are unclear. Part of the problem in studying attention is that specific terms such as *vigilance* and *flexibility* are often used in varying ways; there is also no accepted taxonomy for different types of attentional processes. As discussed by Stankov (1988), there are at least six different types of attention that have been examined in various studies:

1. Concentration (or sustained attention)—the ability to apply mental effort in a sustained way.
2. Search (or perceptual/clerical speed)—the ability to find a given signal within a larger array of similar signals.
3. Divided attention—the ability to do two different tasks at the same time.
4. Selective attention—the ability to attend to a particular signal and to ignore other potentially intrusive signals.
5. Attention switching (or attentional flexibility)—the ability to shift attention from one set of stimuli in a demanding task to another set of relevant stimuli.
6. Vigilance—the ability to detect rarely occurring signals over a prolonged period of time.

These varying aspects of attention may be affected by aging in different ways. Also, while a number of researchers (e.g., Botwinick & Storandt, 1974a; Hasher & Zacks, 1979; Layton, 1975; Rabbitt, 1979) have proposed that attentional changes may contribute to other cognitive losses in old age, specific interpretations vary, and conclusions have often been based on unfamiliar laboratory tests.

Stankov (1988) recently provided a more comprehensive study of attention and age. A sample of 100 subjects, with at least 20 in each age-decade interval from 20 to 70 years, were given a very extensive battery of psychometric and experimental measures, including the WAIS-R, 9 additional tests believed to tap Gc or Gf, and 11 tests of attention. Factor analyses were used to address the question of the relationship between different aspects of attention and components of intelligence. Eight first-order factors were identified, of which three were the expected Gc, Gf, and short-term acquisition and retrieval (SAR) dimensions of intelligence, and three (search, concentration, and attentional flexibility) were clearly interpretable attentional dimensions. When second-order analysis of factor intercorrelations was performed, the two factors to emerge were Gc and a broad factor defined by a combination of the attentional constructs, Gf, and SAR. Thus, at the first-order level of analysis, three attentional factors were identified that were clearly distinct from well-established psychometric abilities; at the second-order level of analysis, attentional tasks were identified as belonging to the fluid intelligence domain.

As expected, Gf exhibited a negative correlation ($r = -.31$) with age, whereas Gc and age were positively correlated ($r = .27$). Negative associations with age were observed on all three attentional factors, with the magnitude of correlations ranging from .43 to .48. To examine how attentional changes may have affected different intelligence factors, part correlations were used. Partialing out the effect of the three attentional factors, especially the flexibility component, virtually eliminated the age-related decline in Gf. With Gc, partialing out the effects of attentional factors led to an estimated improved rate of increase in Gc with age. The author commented, "if Attentional Flexibility . . . were to remain the same throughout the life span, we could expect the increase in crystallized intelligence to be close to 5.0 IQ points, rather than 2.7 IQ points per decade" (p. 71).

Stankov interpreted his results as a strong indication that age-related changes in fluid and crystallized intelligence are dependent on changes in attentional processes, especially attentional flexibility, concentration, and search. In effect, these data suggest that if older individuals could attend as well as the young, then many of the aging declines we have come to anticipate on intelligence testing would be eliminated.

These outcomes illustrate the importance of being specific when assessing attentional functions and in interpreting the effects of attentional changes on other aspects of cognitive performance. Unfortunately, clinical tests of attention are not well developed, and as a result, this area of cognitive function is often evaluated in a superficial way (see Chapter 4).

Changes in attentional flexibility with age are similar to, but less severe than, those observed in depression and Parkinson's disease (see Chapters 8 and 11). Biochemical factors, such as altered catecholamines, may contribute to attentional problems, including those noted in normal old age (see Chapter 2). However, much more work is needed to clarify neurobiological correlates of attention and to determine if training or medication improves attentional skills.

MEMORY

When older people complain about their cognitive abilities, it is most often problems with memory that are mentioned (Williams, Denney, & Schadler, 1983). Gerontologists have studied memory more thoroughly than any other aspect of cognitive function, and there is now an extensive experimental literature examining the effects of subject characteristics, task specifics, and instructional and training interventions. Detailed summaries can be found in Botwinick (1984), Kausler (1982), and Poon (1986).

A Model of Learning and Memory

Many reviews of the literature on memory and aging have summarized findings with reference to information-processing models in which to-be-learned material is assumed to undergo a series of transformations (processing steps or stages) between sensory registration and storage in long-term memory. Each step in the process may be affected differently by age, and in fact, evidence suggests selective age-related impairments.

Table 3.1 outlines the different stages of one information-processing model and summarizes findings with regard to age-related decline at each stage. Age changes are discussed in more detail below. At this point, however, it is interesting to note that if speed of response is used to measure function, virtually all aspects of information processing appear to be diminished by age (see Table 3.1C). By contrast, when accuracy of response is measured (see Table 3.1B), there is less evidence for decline with age, except in the area of secondary (long-term) memory.

TABLE 3.1. Age-Related Changes in Information Processing[a]

	Memory process			
	Sensory	Primary	Secondary	Tertiary
	A. Examples of different memory processes			
	Register letters of new name.	Recall new name just after hearing it.	Recall new name after meeting several other people.	Recall names of family members.
	B. Evidence for decline in memory capacity[b]			
Cross-sectional				
Anecdotal		+	+	+
Psychometric		−	+	?
Experimental	+	−	+	−
Longitudinal				
Psychometric		−	+	−
Experimental			+	
	C. Evidence for slowing of memory processes[c]			
Perceptual motor	+	+	+	+
Decision making		+	+	−

[a]From Fozard (1980, pp. 274–275). Copyright 1980 by the American Psychological Association, Inc. Adapted by permission.
[b]A plus sign indicates decline; a minus sign indicates no decline; a question mark denotes conflicting findings.
[c]All data are from experimental cross-sectional studies.

Age Effects on Processing Stages

Sensory Memory

Sensory memory is assumed to provide a short-lived, relatively complete representation of an external stimulus. In the visual modality, sensory memory may be thought of as a photographic image, and in the auditory modality as an echo. As soon as information is registered in sensory memory, it quickly begins to decay, so that in less than a second, most or all of the information is lost unless it is transferred to primary memory, the next stage in the information-processing sequence.

Experimental investigations, using tachistoscopic presentation of multiattribute stimuli, indicate that there are age-related deficits in the operation of sensory memory (e.g., Cerella, Poon, & Fozard, 1982; Walsh, Till, & Williams, 1978). In practical terms, this finding implies that older adults require a longer exposure time to adequately register a given amount of information.

Primary Memory

Primary (short-term) memory is conceptualized as a temporary, capacity-limited store, the contents of which are usually maintained through rehearsal or conscious mental effort. One everyday use of this aspect of memory is holding a telephone number in one's awareness for the duration of time it takes to dial.

Older people often report subjective declines in short-term memory. However, the research literature is only partially supportive of this complaint. On relatively simple tasks such as forward digit span, where only accuracy of response is measured, most studies report an absence of age differences, at least through the seventh decade (for reviews, see Botwinick, 1977; Craik, 1977). On tests that measure how quickly an individual can access information from the primary store, older people are sometimes reported to perform more poorly than younger adults (Craik, 1977). In general, however, age effects on primary memory appear to be minimal.

Secondary Memory

Secondary memory is assumed to be a relatively permanent, unconscious repository of acquired information that is not restricted in capacity; from a practical standpoint, information can be said to have been learned when it has entered secondary memory. Age differences in this aspect of memory have been reported in numerous studies using a wide range of methods (see Table 3.1B).

Encoding Operations. The problems that older people have with secondary memory have been interpreted in several ways. Craik (1977) championed a depth-of-processing interpretation, in which normal aged subjects are described as engaging in less extensive and less efficient initial processing of to-be-learned material. Less extensive processing results in a degraded engram, or memory trace, that is subsequently more difficult to retrieve.

There is an extensive experimental literature that supports the notion of shallower or less efficient spontaneous encoding activities in old age. For example, Hulicka and Grossman (1967) asked younger and older subjects to describe how they attempted to learn a list of verbal paired associates; while most of the young adults reported that they had used some type of verbal or visual association strategy, a majority of the healthy, community-resident elderly did not describe spontaneous mnemonic strategies. Other studies have measured memory following activities that indirectly encourage different depths of processing. For example, subjects might be asked to sort a list of words according to the initial letter or according to semantic category; semantic encoding is assumed to result in a more retrievable memory trace, and therefore, sorting by category would be expected to preferentially enhance recall. Perlmutter and Mitchell (1982) found that older adults benefit more from such categorization activities than younger adults, presumably because younger people already employ organizational strategies in learning new information. Most of the encoding-enhancement studies have used verbal memory measures, but Sharps and Gollin (1988) found that recall of objects can also be enhanced if distinctive cues are provided at the time of learning (e.g, placing the objects on a colored map).

Effects of Training. Experimental training studies (e.g., Canestrari, 1968; Hulicka & Grossman, 1967; Treat, Poon, & Fozard, 1981) have demonstrated marked short-term benefits from instructing older subjects in the use of mnemonic strategies for encoding such as visual imagery and verbal associations or the method of loci (Robertson-Tchabo, Hausman, & Arenberg, 1976). Encouraged by the success of these investigations, several more extensive memory-training programs have been developed for older people with memory complaints (e.g., Scogin, Storandt, & Lott, 1985; Yesavage, Rose, & Bower, 1983b; Zarit, Cole, & Guider, 1981). Despite initial benefits, follow-up outcomes of these programs have been disappointing. For example, two recent studies with three-year follow-up data have found no long-term benefits of training on memory test scores (Anschutz, Camp, Markley, & Kramer, 1987; Scogin & Bienias, 1988). In both cases, investigators noted that subjects had stopped applying the techniques they had learned.

The reasons for discontinuing helpful techniques are unclear. Using mnemonics over a long period of time may require a greater expenditure of effort than most older people can afford (see discussion below). Or mnemonics may be viewed more as a game than a practical, everyday tool (Anschutz *et al.*, 1987).

Memory training may be perceived as beneficial even if objective benefits are not maintained (Anschutz *et al.*, 1987). For example, training may help to convince people that occasional memory lapses are normal or may enhance their sense of control over memory problems.

Retrieval Operations. Age-related secondary-memory deficits may stem from problems with retrieval as well as encoding. The major evidence for retrieval deficits comes from comparisons of performance on "supported-retrieval" tasks (e.g., recognition) as opposed to "unsupported-retrieval" tasks (e.g., recall). Recognition memory exceeds free recall at all ages, but the magnitude of difference appears to be reliably greater for the old than for the young (e.g., Craik & McDowd, 1987; Kaszniak, Poon, & Reige, 1986). However, even on recognition tasks, age differences (favoring the young) are often observed. Signal detection analyses suggest that some of this difference results from a reduction in sensitivity instead of a conservative response bias (Le Breck & Baron, 1987; Poon & Fozard, 1980).

The Role of Limited Effort. Recent studies have begun to ask *why* older subjects seem to engage in less effective encoding and retrieval activities. One hypothesis is that older people have more limited resources in terms of energy and attention; therefore, they encounter the greatest problems on tasks that require a substantial outlay of effort (e.g., Craik, 1983; Craik & Byrd, 1982; Craik & McDowd, 1987; Hasher & Zacks, 1979, 1984; Rabinowitz, Craik, & Ackerman, 1982). Free recall of specific details is an effortful process, requiring the subject to engage in self-initiated activity during both the learning and the retrieval phases; by contrast, in a recognition test, appropriate mental operations are cued by the re-presentation of the external stimuli (Craik & McDowd, 1987).

The differential effort hypothesis receives some support from studies in which subjects are asked to perform a secondary task (generally, choice reaction time) at the same time that they are attempting to recognize or recall a list of words (Craik & McDowd, 1987; Macht & Buschke, 1983). Reaction times are slower for both young and old during recall as opposed to recognition, but disproportionate slowing during recall is noted for older subjects, a finding suggesting greater "energy costs" of recall in old age.

Everyday Memory Tasks. Young and middle-aged adults routinely encounter situations that require learning and retention of facts and details; formal education makes heavy demands on these skills, as do many jobs. By contrast, many of the things that retired older people try to remember are action- or activity-based; for example, they may have eaten breakfast, gone shopping, or visited a museum and may later attempt to recall these activities in conversation with relatives or friends. Investigators concerned about the validity of laboratory tests have hypothesized that memory of activities may be a more natural task for elderly subjects and that their recall of activities may be superior to their recall of other types of information.

The first studies to examine this possibility reported an absence of age differences on free recall of simple subject-performed activities (Backman, 1985; Backman & Nilsson, 1985). This finding generated great interest in the field, because it was one of the few demonstrations of equality of memory for young and old adults. On longer lists of actions, however, age-related deficits have subsequently been observed (Cohen, Sandler, & Schroeder, 1987; Guttentag & Hunt, 1988); also, young adults appear to be better able than the old to use the logical structure inherent in a series of actions as a basis for recall (Padgett & Ratner, 1987).

This type of research is only one aspect of a broader line of investigation focusing on everyday memory and aging (for reviews, see Poon, Rubin, & Wilson, 1989; West, 1986). Many different approaches have been taken to try to bring memory testing into closer alignment with naturalistic learning and memory demands. Some researchers have replaced arbitrary laboratory stimuli with more familiar or meaningful stimuli (e.g., testing recall of medication information rather than lists of unrelated words; Morrell, Park, & Poon, 1989); others have used arbitrary stimuli but have tried to alter the conditions of learning or retrieval to approximate natural situations. The variability in approaches and tasks limits the generalizations that can be drawn from these studies (West, 1986). It is safe to state, however, that on many everyday tasks as well as many artificial ones, older subjects often perform worse than younger comparison groups. Even in areas of expertise, age-related deficits in recall have been observed, although consequences are often offset by compensatory strategies (e.g., Charness, 1981).

Subgroup Differences. A final important aspect of research concerns subgroup differences in secondary-memory performance. Craik *et al.* (1987) found that age differences in word generation, paired-associate learning, and verbal free recall were strongly modulated by characteristics of the participants. Older volunteers (mean age = 74 years) from affluent retirement communities generally performed as well as a comparison group of young college undergraduates; these older subjects had an average of 13 years of education and a mean vocabulary score equal to that of the younger subjects. By contrast, another group of aged volunteers (mean age = 78 years), consisting of low-income individuals participating in a federally funded seniors program, obtained lower scores than the young adults on each of the memory tests. Because the average educational level in this group was only slightly lower than that of the college students, the investigators hypothesized that reduced activity or poorer health may have been key factors in explaining age differences.

Arbuckle, Gold, and Andres (1986) took a different approach to the individual-differences issue, examining interrelations between memory test performance (digit span, free recall of a word list, and prose memory), and social, personality, adjustment, and lifestyle measures. Education and intellectual activity were found to be the best predictors of performance on memory tests. Among personality measures, extraversion, neuroticism, and lie scores were all significant negative predictors of performance, but measures of locus of control, emotional state, and life stress were unrelated. With regard to age effects, the investigators concluded:

> in a healthy population over age 65, age differences in memory after adjustment for relevant background variables are relatively small. Despite the large age range used, age was the last main effect to enter significantly, and it accounted for only a small proportion of the variance. To the extent that age is an index of biological change, it would appear that biological aging may be of lesser importance with respect to memory measures than the background variables considered here, at least for relatively healthy older subjects. (p. 60)

These results reinforce earlier reports of individual differences (e.g., Costa & Fozard, 1978) and suggest that models of aging and memory need to be flexible enough to explain how some individuals retain secondary-memory skills in old age. In the area of subjective complaints as well, important individual differences are being reported; for example, in national survey of nearly 15,000 older adults, Cutler and Grams (1988) found that 25% of people aged 55 and older, and 20% who were 85 or older, reported that they had had *no* memory problems in the preceding year. Those reporting frequent problems were more likely to be in poor physical health or to have hearing or visual impairments than their age-peers without complaints about memory.

Tertiary Memory

Anecdotally, the ability of older adults to recall people and events from early in their lives is often very impressive. When asked to describe how their memories operate, many older people comment on the clarity of remote memories in contrast to their memory of events of the last few days or weeks.

Literature on tertiary (remote) memory is mixed with respect to the question of age-related change, in part because this aspect of memory is very difficult to measure. On tests of recall of faces or names of famous people, or important historical events, it is impossible to control for degree of initial exposure to the material, or for subsequent rehearsal (Craik, 1977).

Using the best public events questionnaire devised to date, Howes and Katz (1988) reported significant age differences between young, middle-aged, and elderly groups. The elderly subjects had a fairly constant level of recall across all of the time periods (spanning an interval of 50 years), but they performed worse than middle-aged subjects for remote time periods during which both age groups had lived. The constancy of recall in older groups for different historical periods agrees with previous findings by Squire (1974) but disagrees with results of Warrington and Sanders (1971), who found that memory for news events decreased with the passage of time. Poorer recall ability of elderly people compared to that of middle-aged adults has also been previously reported (Squire, 1974; Warrington & Sanders, 1971), but again, not invariably (Botwinick & Storandt, 1980).

Bahrick, Bahrick, and Wittlinger (1975) took a more personal approach to the study of tertiary memory, examining recall and recognition of high-school graduating classmates over intervals of 3 to nearly 50 years. On recognition and matching tasks, for either names or pictures of faces, approximately 90% accuracy was observed for at least 15 years after graduation, and performance on picture recognition remained high through 35 years after graduation. A significant drop in performance was noted after 48 years, but even the oldest subjects were able to recognize the names and photos of about 70% of their former classmates.

Overall, the research on tertiary memory suggests the presence of age effects, but the reliability of this finding varies, most likely because of differences in the methods used to measure remote remembering.

Summary of Memory Changes

A great deal of research has focused on age differences in memory performance. Most has been conducted in laboratory settings, focusing on learning and retention of arbitrary facts and details.

The magnitude of age deficits is found to vary at different information-processing stages. Sensory memory declines slightly with age, a finding suggesting that older adults require more time than younger people to register external stimuli. Primary memory is minimally affected by age, at least until the eighth decade. Studies of tertiary memory have had variable outcomes, but most suggest some age-related decline. Often, however, the absolute level of recognition memory for remote events is impressively high, even in the oldest groups.

Pronounced age-related deficits are noted on many secondary-memory tasks. It seems unlikely that these decrements are an artifact of using laboratory memory tasks, since age differences have also been noted on many everyday memory measures. Secondary-memory problems may arise because older adults do not use efficient encoding and retrieval strategies. If normal older people are encouraged to organize information during learning or are taught specific mnemonics, their performance on tests of secondary memory improves considerably. However, they generally stop spontaneously using these techniques shortly after training, perhaps because efficient encoding of new information requires effort, and older people may be unable, or unwilling, to apply such effort on a daily basis.

Research has provided a thorough description of age differences in memory performance, but there are no clear explanations of why these differences occur. The hypothesis of decreased effort has some commonsense appeal, but the reasons why effort should be decreased are only vaguely addressed. Catecholaminergic changes have been implicated in performance deficits on effortful memory tasks in depression and Parkinson's disease (see Chapters 8 and 11), but it is not known whether a similar link holds for normal aging (see Chapter 2). Associations between cholinergic system changes and memory loss have also been proposed, but most of the pertinent research has focused on patients with Alzheimer's disease instead of normal older adults (see Chapters 2 and 7).

Despite the general trend toward poorer memory with advancing age, there are marked individual differences in memory performance among older adults; in fact, healthy and socially advantaged people in their 60s or 70s may do as well as younger adults on many memory tests. Because such wide variability exists, it is particularly important to choose appropriate normative standards in clinical memory evaluation (see Chapter 4).

Careful attention to memory testing is also required because the memory changes of normal aging overlap with those observed in dementing disorders such as Alzheimer's disease or multi-infarct dementia (see Chapters 7 and 9). In dementia, memory losses are more severe and generalized than those seen in normal aging, but in the beginning stages of illness, clinical distinction is not an easy matter (see Chapters 7 and 9).

LANGUAGE

Both research and everyday experience suggest that language abilities are well maintained in later life. Like attention and memory, however, language is not a unitary function, and there is evidence from experimental investigations that specific language skills age in different ways.

The Mechanics of Communication

In their review of linguistic communication in normal aging, Bayles and Kaszniak (1987) emphasized that the most likely causes of impaired communication in old age are mechanical problems and that such problems are more important than changes in semantic memory or linguistic knowledge. One of the most important mechanical problems is age-related hearing loss, which has been estimated to affect about 30% of people aged 65 years and older (see Chapter 1). Diminished hearing sensitivity (presbycusis) is the most common hearing impairment in older adults. Visual losses often limit reading and writing and can also affect aural communication by making analysis of lip movements and facial expressions more difficult.

Linguistic Knowledge

Age does not appear to erode knowledge of the sounds of language and rules for their combination (phonological knowledge). Syntactic knowledge (i.e., knowing how to combine words meaningfully) is also not greatly influenced by age, although there are some studies that report age differences in the correct use of grammar and syntax (Bayles & Kaszniak, 1987).

Older and younger adults are alike in finding certain sentence forms easier to comprehend than others, such as single negative or active as opposed to double negative or passive (Obler, Fein, Nicholas, & Albert, 1981a). Also, when young and elderly subjects were given pairs of nouns and asked to construct sentences which included these words, no differences were observed in correct use of grammar (Nebes & Andrews-Kulis, 1976). By contrast, when 20-minute speech samples were analyzed, Kynette and Kemper (1986) observed a reduction in the variability and accuracy of syntactic structures, verb tenses, and forms of grammar across an age range of 50 to 90 years. The oldest subjects (in their 70s and 80s) avoided the use of grammatical forms and syntactic structures that placed a heavy demand on memory (Kynette & Kemper, 1986). Memory may also have played a role in a later study by Kemper (1986) where elderly subjects had more trouble than young adults in imitating complex sentences with embedded clauses.

Lexical Knowledge

Word knowledge, as indicated by vocabulary testing, is another area of comparative strength for older adults. On a recognition test of vocabulary, no age differences were found across the third through eighth decades when younger and older subjects were matched for intelligence and education (Bayles, Tomoeda, & Boone, 1985). Scores on WAIS or WAIS-R Vocabulary also remain fairly constant across the adult age span, although qualitative analysis suggests declining use of synonyms as definitions in old age (e.g., Botwinick & Storandt, 1974b, discussed earlier in this chapter).

Bowles and Poon (1985) used lexical decision tasks to assess age effects on word knowledge. First, young and old subjects were presented with strings of letters and asked to decide if they were actual words. No age differences were observed in either accuracy or speed; that is, the oldest participants were clearly able to make efficient decisions about what constitutes a proper English word. In a second study, young and old subjects were given definitions of target words and asked to supply the names; in this case, the young performed more accurately and more quickly than the old, a finding suggesting that there may be a breakdown with age in ready *access* to lexical knowledge, even though the knowledge base itself is well preserved.

Naming

As Bayles and Kaszniak (1987) pointed out, problems in accessing the lexical network (the "tip-of-the-tongue" phenomenon) are experienced by adults of all ages and are often seen in young adults in test situations. However, data from studies of confrontation naming concur with those of Bowles and Poon (1985) in suggesting that this phenomenon is likely to be a greater problem for older adults.

Borod, Goodglass, and Kaplan (1980) studied performance on the Boston Naming Test (Kaplan, Goodglass, & Weintraub, 1978), where the task is to provide the names of pictured objects. Scores were stable between the ages of 30 and 50 years, declined slightly in the 60s, and clearly decreased among people aged 70 years or older. In a similar study, Obler, Albert, and Goodglass (1981b) compared responses of younger and older adults on both the Boston Naming Test and a related task requiring the naming of verbs for pictured activities. In both tasks the age trends were the same, with older adults producing fewer correct responses and requiring greater time for completion than younger adults; again, however, differences did not become statistically significant until the eighth decade. Similar outcomes were observed by Albert, Heller, and Milberg (1988) in a study with optimally healthy adults using the Boston Naming Test (see Chapter 4 for specific norms).

Qualitative changes in the nature of naming responses have also been reported. Each of the following types of errors appear to increase with age (Albert *et al.*, 1988; Bowles, Obler, & Albert, 1987; Obler *et al.*, 1981b):

1. Circumlocutions—multiword responses providing accurate information.
2. Nominalizations—words describing the function of the pictured object (e.g., *swinger* for pendulum).
3. Perceptual errors—misidentifications of the stimulus (e.g., *speedometer* for protractor).
4. Semantic association errors—responses that name a conative associate of the pictured object (e.g., *dice* for dominoes).

These errors indicate that older people possess correct information about the pictured objects. However, they may have difficulty retrieving precise words within a general semantic field. In effect, these data confirm what older patients frequently report during testing, that is, that they know the item but just can't think of its name.

Problems with naming may have multiple determinants. Limited intelligence, poor memory, or diminished fluency may all result in naming difficulties. Therefore, before a naming problem can be interpreted as suggesting a deficit in the language system, each of these other factors must be taken into account.

Albert *et al.* (1988) studied interrelations between performance on the Boston Naming Test and several other cognitive functions, including verbal intelligence (Vocabulary), memory (digit span and paragraph recall), and verbal fluency. Subjects were optimally healthy adults in the age range of 30 to 80 years. In multiple regression analyses, the only variables that were found to contribute significantly to naming scores were age and Vocabulary test performance. Thus, this study did not support the notion that age-related naming deficits are the direct result of memory problems. Also, while Vocabulary ability was important as a predictor of naming performance, covarying Vocabulary scores did not eliminate the age-related naming effects.

Verbal Fluency

Compared to younger adults, older people generally produce fewer words in a limited time when asked to generate items beginning with specific letters (e.g., Albert *et al.*, 1988; Benton & Hamsher, 1976; Obler & Albert, 1981) or words within specific categories (e.g., Borod *et al.*, 1980). Age effects are generally small in absolute magnitude, but the downward trend with increasing age is quite consistently observed, particularly for people aged 70 years and above (see Chapter 4 for pertinent age norms). When more time is given to respond, more words are usually produced, but age differences in productivity remain (Obler & Albert, 1985).

Rosen (1980) provided a careful contrast of performance on letter and category fluency tasks for a small sample of old-old adults (mean age = 83.6 years) with well-preserved mental status. Although performance was highly correlated between the different measures ($r = .94$), these subjects were able to name more animals in one minute than words beginning with specified letters (mean scores = 11.3 vs. 9.2, respectively). With letters, subjects presumably had to enter into semantic or phonemic subsets to retrieve appropriate words, whereas for animals, there may have been more clear exemplars of the general category that could be retrieved without subset search.

Discourse: Production and Comprehension

Studies of sentence and story production indicate that older adults are likely to produce more verbose, elaborate responses than middle-aged individuals. Obler (1980) found that, when asked to write a description of a complex picture (the Cookie-Theft picture from the Boston Diagnostic Aphasia Examination), 70- and 80-year-olds produced more complex, embedded sentences; in oral description, there was more evidence of personalization, repetition of items, redundancy, and use of indefinite terms such as *something* in the speech of older adults. Interestingly, young adults were also found to be more verbose and elaborate in their responses to these tasks than middle-aged participants.

Comprehension of discourse has also been studied in relation to age. Taub (1979) asked young and older women to read prose passages and to answer multiple-choice questions about their content. Some of the probe questions were presented simultaneously with the passage; others were presented after it had been removed and, therefore, involved recall as well as comprehension. A negative age effect was found for both types of comprehension scores, but only among subjects with average (as opposed to superior) verbal intelligence. Ulatowska, Hayashi, Cannito, and Fleming (1986) compared the abilities of older and younger subjects to retell a story and answer probe questions about it. Participants were from a relatively homogeneous linguistic environment and were subdivided into young-old (64 to 76 years), old-old ($\geq$ 76 years), and middle-aged (27 to 55 years) groups. The oldest group performed more poorly than the middle-aged group on most of the comprehension questions, but in the young-old group, problems were noted only when questions required the drawing of an abstract inference from the story. Cohen (1979) also found that older people had greater difficulty than the young in drawing inferences from facts presented in spoken discourse; she noted, further, that when recounting a story, older subjects often failed to make clear reference to a protagonist or attributed characteristics or actions to the wrong protagonist. The latter outcomes may have been due to problems with memory, but the difficulties in inferential processes did not appear to be due to memory problems.

Summary of Language Changes

Although some aspects of language are well maintained in later life, decremental changes in other aspects may be observed with normal aging. Normal older adults are likely to have a well-preserved functional knowledge of syntax and grammar, although they may find complex grammatical constructions difficult to process and may avoid such constructions in their spontaneous speech. Word knowledge is well maintained, but older people may not define words as succinctly as younger adults. Generation of words, names, and ideas on command may be reduced in older adults, even though spontaneous discourse tends to be more elaborate (as well as more repetitive, personalized, and nonreferential). Finally, there may be mild reductions in the ability to form associations among verbal concepts or to draw inferences from information presented in written or oral passages.

Bayles and Kaszniak's review of the literature (1987) led to the conclusion that the ability to communicate diminishes with age; however, they described age effects as "generally subtle" and most likely to be observed "when information to be comprehended is new, complex, and implied, and the time allowed for processing is short" (pp. 152–153). They interpreted language changes as secondary to declines in sensory acuity and in other cognitive processes, such as memory, the processing of new information, or inferential reasoning. Obler and Albert (1985) emphasized the great diversity of language behavior with age and underscored how task and subject selection can influence the picture of normative language changes.

Because communication skills are generally well preserved in normal aging, noticeable problems with speech or language should raise a question of cerebral dysfunction. Naming and verbal fluency impairments are usually much more severe in Alzheimer's disease than in normal aging (see Chapter 7), but because of overlap in these areas, careful attention to norms and qualitative features of response is required. In multi-infarct dementia, a wide range of speech and language changes may be noted (see Chapter 9), and in Parkinson's disease, slowed, dysarthric speech is characteristic (see Chapter 8).

VISUOSPATIAL ABILITIES

Age-related declines in visuospatial abilities are suggested by normative studies of intelligence test data (e.g., WAIS-R), where older adults routinely perform worse than young people on subtests such as Block Design, Object Assembly, and Picture Completion (see "Intelligence," above). Studies using other nonverbal tasks generally corroborate the intelligence test findings.

Simple tests of visual perception, such as judging the spatial orientation of lines relative to a standard, are influenced by age through middle adulthood (Benton, Varney, & Hamsher, 1978b), but in one study of healthy and well-educated older adults, most people in their 80s (92%) scored within two standard deviations of the mean for people in their 50s (Benton, Eslinger, & Damasio, 1981).

Complex visual perception tasks produce larger age effects. Older adults perform worse than middle-aged or young adults on visual-closure tests that require the identification of figures from incomplete drawings (Danziger & Salthouse, 1978; Read, 1988), and on embedded-figure tasks, where a simple geometric pattern must be identified within a more complex random design (Axelrod & Cohen, 1961; Capitani, Sala, Lucchelli, Soave, & Spinnler, 1988). Advanced age also has a negative influence on a person's ability to match pictures of unfamiliar faces (Benton, Van Allen, Hamsher, & Levin, 1978a; Benton *et al.*, 1981).

Age-related visuoconstructive deficits have been consistently observed on tasks such as Block Design. In addition, Plude, Milberg, and Cerella (1986) found significant age differences when young and old adults (mean ages = 21 and 67 years, respectively) were asked to judge the accuracy of drawings of cubes and to try to draw a cube on command. The older subjects performed less well than the young on both the judgment and the production tasks.

Differences between younger and older subjects have also been found on Raven's Progressive Matrices (Raven, 1960), a multiple-choice task in which the person selects one of six puzzle pieces to complete a larger visual pattern. On the easier series of stimuli, judgments can be based on perceptual matching alone, whereas more difficult series entail conjunctive or disjunctive reasoning. Wilson, DeFries, McClearn, Vandenberg, Johnson, and Rashad (1975) and Burke (1972) found that performance on this task decreases from the decade of the 20s onward. Other nonverbal reasoning tasks, such as Figural Relations (Thurstone & Thurstone, 1949), also show age-related declines (e.g., Hertzog & Schaie, 1988; Schaie, 1983).

Performance on visuospatial tasks is influenced by many individual difference parameters other than age. For example, judgments of line orientation (Benton *et al.*, 1978b), embedded figures (Capitani *et al.*, 1988), matrices (Guttman, 1981; Vincent & Cox, 1974), and facial recognition (Benton *et al.*, 1978a) are all influenced by education. In addition, since many of the studies that report age differences have not evaluated visual acuity, some outcomes may have been confounded by visual sensory changes. Finally, a very important characteristic of most of these tests is the unfamiliarity of procedures; it may be this aspect of the testing, rather than the visual and perceptual demands *per se*, that places the old at a disadvantage.

Because visuospatial performance is an area of comparative weakness for older adults, it is sometimes difficult to differentiate normal aging changes in visuospatial ability from those caused by brain disorders. However, most normal old people do not find it difficult to copy two-dimensional designs, and performance on Block Design is typically free of blatant errors such as stacking of blocks (see Chapters 4 and 5 for further discussion).

PROBLEM SOLVING AND EXECUTIVE FUNCTIONS

In the literature on normal aging, tasks that assess a person's ability to identify concepts and rules, to reason logically and abstractly, and to apply reasoning skills in the solution of hypothetical or real-life tasks are often discussed under the general heading of *problem solving*. Neuropsychologists have focused on a related, but somewhat broader, set of abilities termed *executive functions*. Executive functions have been defined as "those capacities that enable a person to engage in independent, purposive, self-serving behavior successfully" (Lezak, 1983, p. 38), including initiating and terminating activities, making shifts in attention and ongoing behavior, and planning and implementing series of actions related to goals; emotional self-control and maintenance of socially appropriate behavior are also classified under the heading of executive functions by some investigators.

A diverse set of tasks has been used to study problem solving and executive functions, so that it is difficult to summarize age trends or to develop theories to organize the results. This book focuses on a few of the most commonly used measures, including concept identification tasks, tests of abstract reasoning, and measures of cognitive flexibility. This section examines how normal older adults perform on these types of tasks, while Chapter 4 discusses age trends on related tests used in clinical application.

Problem Solving in the Laboratory

Concept Identification

Experimental studies suggest that there are pronounced age differences in the manner in which people form and infer concepts. When asked to classify or categorize objects, elderly subjects are more likely than young adults to group stimuli on the basis of functional relationships (e.g., a knife slicing an orange) as opposed to more abstract semantic relationships (e.g., orange and banana grouped as fruits). Or when instructed to ask questions that will help them identify which of several pictures an examiner has in mind (the "Twenty Questions" game), older people ask more questions that eliminate a single alternative as opposed to those that remove a whole category of alternatives (Denney & Denney, 1982). Similarly, when presented with a series of stimuli that differ in multiple dimensions (e.g., shape, color, size) and asked to infer a particular dimension as "correct" based on feedback from the examiner, older people have been reported to perform very poorly; many appear to respond randomly on such tasks and seemingly receive no benefit from feedback provided across the trials (Offenbach, 1974).

Inquiry and Organization

Older individuals make many repetitious selections on concept identification tasks (Arenberg, 1982a). Many seem to have problems reviewing their past selections and planning future steps, even when demands on memory are kept to a minimum by aids such as written notes. Redundant inquiry has also been observed on other types of reasoning tasks. For example, Welford (1958) presented young and old adults with a problem simulating the servicing of radios. While attempting to discover the correspondence between terminals on a box (the "radio") and those drawn on a circuit diagram, the older adults took many more redundant meter readings, a finding suggesting to Welford that they had difficulty attaching meaning to the results of their inquiry.

Concrete Approach

Without explicit instruction to the contrary, older people often approach reasoning tasks in a concrete way. On classification tasks, as noted above, they may group objects according to functional connections or may arrange them to form a pattern, rather than sort them on the basis of more abstract semantic categories. On WAIS or WAIS-R Similarities, older people are more likely than young adults to name specific concrete resemblances (e.g., "You can eat them both" or "Both have four legs"), and on proverb interpretation, choice of concrete responses increases with age (Bromley, 1957).

Longitudinal Trends

Almost all information about problem solving and aging has been provided by cross-sectional studies. However, longitudinal data are available for concept identification tasks from the Baltimore Longitudinal Study of Aging (Arenberg, 1982a). Most of the 376 participants were well educated and were either employed in or retired from managerial, scientific, or other professional positions. Initial and retest evaluations were completed at varying intervals between 1967 and 1979.

Cross-sectional findings from both the first and the second tests showed monotonic declines with age in the number of problems correctly solved; for example, at initial testing, men in their 20s solved an average of 10.4 of 12 tasks, whereas men in their 70s completed an average of 6.6 tasks correctly.

Longitudinal changes with age were less noticeable. For example, on the four simplest tasks, the correlation between age and problem-solving change score was very small ($r = -.07$). Also, regression analyses for separate age cohorts indicated that the slope of change over time was significantly less than zero only for the oldest cohort (i.e., subjects who were in their 70s at the beginning of the study).

These data provide more support for maintenance of problem solving in old age than most cross-sectional studies. However, Arenberg (1982a) cautioned that they probably underestimate the extent of age change. Findings may have been enhanced by the high educational and occupational backgrounds of participants and by selective attrition of ill or less able subjects. Also, while the longitudinal trends were generally negative for older age groups, they were positive for young and middle-aged men.

Modifying Variables

Education and Health. Cross-sectional studies of problem solving have often used lax criteria for subject selection; as a result, some of the reported age declines may be due to differences in health, education, or other confounded factors.

Using tasks adapted from Piaget and Inhelder's studies of the development of reasoning abilities (La Rue & D'Elia, 1985), La Rue and Waldbaum (1980) addressed this issue with middle-aged (40- to 59-year-old) and elderly (60- to 79-year-old) volunteers. Three reasoning tasks were presented: the pendulum problem, where the task was to identify factors affecting oscillation rate; a combinations task requiring identification of all combinations of six elements; and a proportional reasoning task which involved converting units of measurement to a different scale. Younger and older samples were matched for educational level as well as for physical health (based on physician examination, laboratory tests, and review of medical records).

No differences were observed between the age groups in terms of their use of concrete versus abstract (formal operational) reasoning (cf. Blackburn, 1984). By contrast, education effects were significant, as was the effect of health. People with a high-school education or less, and those with mild to moderate health problems, produced more concrete solutions than college-educated, optimally healthy subjects (La Rue & Waldbaum, 1980). Among older adults who had attended college, those majoring in physical and natural sciences tended to do better on these types of reasoning tasks than social science or humanities majors (Blackburn, 1984).

Performance Anxiety. In high-pressure situations, people often report anxious blocking that precludes their providing sensible responses to difficult questions. Experimental problem-solving tasks may elicit such anxiety since they tend to be quite demanding; however, relationships between age and performance anxiety are unclear.

In our study with middle-aged and older adults (La Rue & Waldbaum, 1980, described above), scores on the State Anxiety Inventory (Spielberger, Gorusch, & Lushene, 1970) were correlated with performance on Piagetian problem-solving tasks as well as WAIS Similarities and Progressive Matrices. Heightened performance anxiety had an adverse affect on all of the reasoning tasks, but the degree of disruption was similar in both the middle-aged and the elderly groups (La Rue & D'Elia, 1985). Also, we did not find our older volunteers to be more test-anxious overall than the younger subjects.

Familiarity of Stimuli. Older people sometimes perform better on reasoning tasks that involve familiar stimuli. For example, Arenberg (1968) presented two versions of concept identification tasks, one involving abstract categories such as shape and the other involving concrete food categories. In the latter task, subjects were presented with a series of meals (combinations of specific beverages, meats, and vegetables) and told that one food item was poisoned; they were to infer the poisoned item from "died/lived" feedback given across a series of meals. Older subjects (aged 60 to 77 years) still performed worse than young adults (aged 17 to 22 years) on the poisoned-food problem, but their performance on this task was much superior to their performance on the abstract version.

Other research suggests that familiarity sometimes produces paradoxical effects. In our Piagetian problem-solving study (La Rue & D'Elia, 1985; La Rue & Waldbaum, 1980), familiar analogues were constructed to the pendulum problem (pushing a child in a tire swing), combinatorial task (combining brands of tobacco to make new blends), and the metric conversion task (adjusting ingredients in a cake recipe). There were few significant differences in reasoning observed for the familiar versus traditional tasks. However, for some individuals, the familiar tasks produced a diminished reliance on logic and greater emphasis on aesthetic approaches or past experience (e.g., revising the cake recipe to match personal taste).

Training and Practice. Older adults' performance on reasoning tasks can be altered quite easily with training in the use of logical rules (e.g., Plemons *et al.*, 1978; Sanders, Sterns, Smith, & Saunders, 1975). On some tasks, unaided practice may produce more improvement than training. On figural relation tasks or letter series, for example, self-guided practice results in a more durable gain in solution rate than explicit tutoring (e.g., Baltes *et al.*, 1989; Blackburn, Papalia-Finlay, Foye, & Serlin, 1988; Labouvie-Vief & Gonda, 1976).

Everyday Problem Solving

Denney and Palmer (1981) asked older adults to indicate how they thought their abilities to reason, think, and solve problems had changed across adulthood. Most (76%) reported improvement in these abilities with age, 20% reported no change, and a small minority (4%) indicated age-related decline.

The research summarized above does not agree with this self-appraisal. Part of the discrepancy appears to stem from the fact that older people and researchers have different things in mind when they refer to problem solving (cf. Arenberg, 1982a; Botwinick, 1984; Poon *et al.*, 1989). When queried about what they meant by problem solving, older people indicated everyday problems such as personal or financial difficulties (Denney & Palmer, 1981). By contrast, most laboratory studies have focused on tasks requiring specific forms of logical reasoning, often in abstract form.

Cornelius and Caspi (1987) constructed an Everyday Problem Solving Inventory assessing approaches to consumer issues, technical information, home management, and interpersonal conflicts. For each situation, different modes of solution were rated for effectiveness by both psychologists and lay raters. Volunteers (aged 20 to 78 years) then completed this inventory in addition to tests of verbal intelligence and logical reasoning. Results showed a linear increase with age in effectiveness of everyday problem solving, despite declines in logical reasoning. This study suggests that knowledge about practical problem solving may be an area of strength for older people (cf. Demming & Pressey, 1957; Denney, Pearce, & Palmer, 1982). However, it did not assess how people actually behave in problem situations, where emotional factors may influence outcomes. For example, studies of medical decision making suggest there may be certain problem-solving domains where older people do not feel confident to make decisions and may tend to defer to others (see Chapter 1).

Cognitive Flexibility

Age-related declines in attentional flexibility discussed earlier in the chapter (see "Attention" above), combined with evidence for redundant inquiry and difficulties in utilizing feedback in problem solving (see "Inquiry and Organization" above), suggest a relatively pervasive change in cognitive flexibility at older ages. This impression is supported by cross-sectional findings for clinical tasks that require switching from one concept to another (e.g., the Category Test or Wisconsin Card Sort), alternating between two sequences (e.g., the Trail Making Test), or inhibiting overlearned responses (e.g., the Color-Word Test; see Chapter 4 for additional discussion). Loss of cognitive flexibility may also contribute to declining scores on WAIS or WAIS-R performance subtests, where the novelty of the tasks is combined with an emphasis on speed of response (Stankov, 1988).

Although the trend toward decreased mental flexibility in old age is quite consistent, the significance of these findings in everyday function is less clear. On familiar tasks, or in situations where rapid changes in behavior are not required, the gradual, mild flexibility changes that characterize normal aging would be expected to have minimal impact.

Summary of Changes in Problem Solving and Executive Functions

Old people generally have greater difficulty with logical problem solving than young adults, at least on those tasks developed for research. However, as in other areas of cognition, performance can be modified by practice and training, and some of the apparent age-related decline can be attributed to poor health or limited education.

Botwinick (1984) is highly critical of the relevance of laboratory tasks to the understanding of problem solving in older adults. He stated, "The types of tasks used in the problem-solving laboratory just are not suited to what many older people can do" (p. 288), and also, "There is reason to believe that if studies were carried out with tasks based on personal aptitudes and occupational specialization, the results would be otherwise" (p. 291). Research on everyday problem solving provides some support for these assertions, although the link between practical knowledge and behavior remains to be established.

Because clinical tests of problem solving and executive functions usually involve abstract concepts, many normal old people obtain low scores (see Chapter 4). Information gained from such tests should be supplemented with interviews evaluating everyday judgment, adaptability, and practical problem solving before conclusions are drawn about reasoning and executive abilities.

NEUROPSYCHOLOGICAL INTERPRETATIONS OF NORMAL AGING CHANGES

Historically, the principal data base in human neuropsychology has been obtained by studying individuals with acquired brain injury and, in particular, those with discrete brain lesions. The value of this literature for understanding normal brain function has long been a matter of debate. In aging, where changes develop slowly across a broad range of neurobiological measures, it may be particularly difficult to extrapolate from lesion investigations (see Chapter 2). Despite these concerns, there have been occasional attempts to interpret age changes in cognition by comparison to brain-damaged patients.

The Right-Hemisphere Hypothesis

A right-hemisphere hypothesis has been advanced (e.g., Klisz, 1978; Schaie & Schaie, 1977) based on similarities in cognitive performance between normal older people and patients with right-hemisphere lesions. There are several problems with this interpretation. The data base for this comparison was limited to studies using the WAIS and the Halstead-Reitan Neuropsychological Battery (Reitan & Davison, 1974), neither of which adequately evaluates learning and memory (see Chapter 4). In addition, the Wechsler scales are not well suited to inferring hemispheric differences since Verbal and Performance scales differ in many ways (e.g., confounding speed requirements and novelty with differences in stimuli and cognitive processing demands); as a result, bilateral brain impairment often yields a Verbal–Performance discrepancy (Matarazzo, 1972). Finally, in neurobiological studies, there is little evidence that age changes are lateralized to the right hemisphere (see Chapter 2).

The Frontal Deficit Hypothesis

A frontal deficit hypothesis of normal aging changes has also been advanced (e.g., Albert & Kaplan, 1980; Hochanadel & Kaplan, 1984; Mittenberg, Seidenberg, O'Leary, & DiGiulio, 1989). Older people often perform poorly on measures of cognitive flexibility—a hallmark of frontal lobe impairment—and make some of the same types of errors on neuropsychological tests as patients with frontal lesions (Albert & Kaplan, 1980; Hochanadel & Kaplan, 1984). In an investigation comparing performance of younger and older subjects on tests of frontal, temporal, and parietal functions, the strongest correlations were observed between age and frontal measures (Mittenberg *et al.*, 1989); in addition, there are occasional findings in the neurobiological literature suggesting prominent frontal lobe aging (e.g., neuronal loss in the superior frontal cortex and scattered reports of frontal glucose hypometabolism in older individuals). As discussed in Chapter 2, however, findings such as neuronal loss, plaques and tangles, and neurotransmitter changes occur in many other brain regions as well. Furthermore, relationships between the frontal lobes and behavioral functions are exceedingly complex and difficult to evaluate with a few psychometric measures. For example, there is little indication that people routinely become emotionally labile or socially inappropriate as they age, although such changes might be expected if significant frontal lobe impairments were occurring.

Comment on Neuropsychological Interpretations

Neuropsychological accounts of cognitive aging are in a very rudimentary stage of development. Although the frontal hypothesis appears more tenable than the right-hemisphere hypothesis, neurobiological indications of selective frontal changes are scattered at best. Much more research will be required to constructively integrate the complex cognitive changes summarized in this chapter with the knowledge base on neurobiological aging changes. Also, future neuropsychological models will need to move away from the current emphasis on brain impairment to incorporate evidence for compensation, adaptation, and cognitive plasticity in normal aging.

ENHANCING COGNITIVE PERFORMANCE

Frequent reference has been made throughout this chapter to benefits of practice and training and to differences in cognitive function between healthy and active old people and those with medical problems. Clinicians are just beginning to learn how to apply this information in designing programs for cognitive enhancement. The amount of practical benefit that can be gained from specific interventions is currently unclear, and we do not know which approaches are best for different individuals. However, in reviewing available options with an older client, it is helpful to discuss a variety of approaches, as outlined briefly below.

Biological Approaches

Medications and Nutrition

Various medications and nutritional supplements have been proposed for improving cognitive performance. These treatments have usually been aimed at counteracting neurotransmitter changes that occur in aging or disease (see Chapter 2), and much of the pertinent research has involved dementia patients instead of normal old people. To date, no drugs have been identified that consistently improve cognitive performance to a degree that is likely to influence everyday function (see Chapter 7 for further discussion); nutritional supplements have also not shown major benefits (Lieberman & Abou-Nader, 1986). However, many new medications for cognitive enhancement are currently in the development phase (Pharmaceutical Manufacturers Association, 1989).

Improving Cardiovascular Fitness

Exercise programs can improve cardiovascular and respiratory function in older people, and in some studies (see Stones & Kozma, 1988, for a review), gains in cognitive function have also been observed. Other well-controlled investigations find only subjective improvements in cognitive function from increased amounts of exercise, with no demonstrable gain on tests of memory or psychomotor speed (e.g., Blumenthal, Emery, Madden, George, Coleman, Riddle, McKee, Reasoner, & Williams, 1989). Studies of chronic or long-term exercise are more consistent in showing that older people who participate regularly in aerobic activities perform better on tests of reasoning, memory, and reaction time than medically healthy older adults who are sedentary (Clarkson-Smith & Hartley, 1989).

Psychological Approaches

Mood Disturbance and Anxiety

Subjective complaints about memory are often more closely linked to depression than to objective memory performance (e.g., Zarit *et al.*, 1981). Therefore, when an older client complains about cognitive problems, the possibility of mood disturbance should be carefully evaluated (see Chapter 11).

Anxiety can amplify cognitive problems at any age, particularly on tasks that are novel or demanding. Desensitization or relaxation techniques may be helpful for people who are unusually anxious about their performance; those with milder concerns may benefit from reassurance that their problems are normal or from group discussions where everyday problems with memory are aired.

Training and Self-Help Techniques

Although training in specific mnemonics usually does not produce long-term objective improvements (see "Memory," above), a few people benefit greatly from this training (see Anschutz *et al.*, 1987). Many others show short-term gains that may be enough to relieve anxiety and to improve self-confidence. In fact, one of the major benefits of memory-training programs is that they may help a person to put minor cognitive problems into better perspective. Self-help books written for older adults (e.g., Gose & Levi, 1985; Lapp, 1987; West, 1985) are another source of reassurance and practical memory aids.

Social Approaches

Old people with active, socially demanding lives often do better on cognitive tests than those who are less active (for a detailed analysis, see Lawton, 1986). Cause and effect are usually hard to disentangle in these comparisons, and often, active people also have other advantages (e.g., better physical health or higher education). However, examining the social context of a person's cognitive complaints may identify interpersonal factors (e.g., loneliness, intimidation, or dependency) that contribute to cognitive problems. In addition, new friendships or recreational activities can increase self-confidence and provide a positive challenge to cognitive abilities.

SUMMARY AND CONCLUSIONS

Decline is clearly a part of normal cognitive aging (see Table 3.2). Areas showing relatively pronounced age decrements include fluid intellectual abilities, complex attentional processes, secondary memory, accessing of word knowledge, visuospatial abilities, and some forms of abstract reasoning and problem solving. These declines emerge gradually, allowing time for compensation, and changes are usually of minimal functional significance until very advanced old age.

Preservation of ability and cognitive growth are also present in normal aging (see Table 3.2). Areas of preservation include simple attention, primary and tertiary memory, and everyday communication through language. Crystallized verbal intelligence continues to grow throughout adulthood, and the knowledge of everyday problem solving may also increase.

There are marked individual differences in rates of cognitive aging. These are related in part to psychosocial parameters such as level of education. Physical health is another crucial mediator: even persons with subclinical medical conditions may show more pronounced aging decrements than optimally healthy people.

Another distinctive feature of normal older-adult cognition is plasticity. In areas where age-related decrements occur, improvements result from cueing, training, or even unstructured practice. Often, benefits are observed after only a few training sessions, a finding that raises doubts about the permanence or seriousness of age-related declines.

The growing literature on individual differences and plasticity in cognitive aging is prompting gerontologists to develop new models of adult development. For example, a three-tiered model of cognition has been proposed by Perlmutter (1988). Tiers 1 and 2 correspond to fluid and crystallized intellectual abilities as described in the Horn/Cattell

TABLE 3.2. Summary of Age Differences in Cognitive Performance[a]

Cognitive function	Direction of change	Comments
Intelligence		
Crystallized	Stable or improved	May decline slightly in advanced old age.
Fluid	Decreased	Decline begins between age 55 and 70; onset varies for cohorts and individuals.
Attention		
Attention span	Stable	May decline slightly in advanced old age.
Selective attention, concentration, and flexibility	Decreased	
Language		
Everyday communication	Stable	Sensory deficits may cause decline.
Phonological and syntactic knowledge	Stable	May be decreased use of complex syntax.
Lexical knowledge	Stable	
Naming	Decreased	Suggests problems in accessing the lexicon.
Word fluency	Decreased	
Discourse comprehension	Stable	Some decline if complex.
Discourse production	Variable	Speech may be more verbose, repetitive, and imprecise.
Learning and memory		
Sensory memory	Decreased	
Primary memory	Stable	May decline slightly in advanced old age.
Secondary memory	Decreased	Less optimal encoding; retrieval problems.
Tertiary memory	Variable	
Visuospatial ability		
Simple visual perception	Stable	May decline slightly in advanced old age.
Complex visual perception	Decreased	
Design copying	Decreased	
Visuoconstruction	Decreased	
Problem solving and executive functions		
Self-rated ability	Increased	
Concept identification	Decreased	Decline less pronounced for practical concepts.
Inquiry	Decreased	Redundant questions.
Logical analysis	Decreased	
Solving everyday problems	Variable	May improve with age for some types of problems.

[a]From Spar and La Rue (1990, pp. 14–15). Copyright 1990 by American Psychiatric Press, Inc. Adapted by permission.

model. However, a third tier has been added which includes strategies that derive from a person's self-awareness of cognitive activity. These self-generated aspects of cognition are predicted to increase throughout life and to be relatively immune from deterioration due to neurobiological aging and routine medical problems. Therefore, Tier 3 reflects potential for adaptive modification of cognition in old age.

Increasing numbers of healthy old people are seeking clinical advice about cognitive problems. Some want reassurance that occasional forgetfulness is not a sign of Alzheimer's disease; others want to find ways to enhance everyday abilities. To be of assistance to these clients, it is helpful to keep models like Perlmutter's in mind, since they emphasize growth and compensation in aging as well as decline. Appreciation of the full range of normal aging trends can help to offset the deficit-oriented approach of the clinical neuropsychological literature, where the emphasis has traditionally been on detection of brain impairment. Knowledge about normal aging is also crucial for selection of appropriate tests and norms (see Chapter 4) and for integrating specific test outcomes with informal observation and historical information (see Chapter 5).

4

Neuropsychological Assessment Procedures

There are three general aims of clinical neuropsychological assessment: (1) to document strengths and weaknesses in cognition and related behaviors; (2) to interpret outcomes diagnostically; and (3) to make recommendations for treatment and management of problem behaviors. In diagnostic interpretation, contributions of suspected brain impairment must be integrated with a variety of nonorganic factors (e.g., decreased motivation, psychiatric disturbance, educational limitations) to explain performance deficits, and with elderly patients, special attention must be given to the possibility that these deficits are age-consistent.

Clinical assessment of older adults is complicated by several factors. Very few tests have been normed for patients aged 80 years and older. The heterogeneity of normal older adults presents additional problems. Since average scores vary widely for different subgroups of older people (see Chapter 3), different norms may be needed for individuals with particular health or education characteristics. Decreased stamina, sensory impairments, and lack of familiarity with formal testing can further restrict the range of suitable measures.

This chapter reviews neuropsychological test options for older patients. Priority is given to clinical studies that include old-old individuals, and when normative data are summarized, other sample characteristics are also described. Guidelines for qualitative analysis are provided to supplement norm-referenced interpretation. Tests are evaluated for their ease of administration to different types of older patients, and recommendations are provided for designing brief and extended test batteries.

COMPREHENSIVE NEUROPSYCHOLOGICAL BATTERIES

Neuropsychologists who work with older adults use a wide range of formal and informal assessment techniques. Training and tradition play a role in test selection, since many practitioners prefer familiar instruments, even if they were not designed for use with older adults. An examiner's implicit and explicit assumptions about older people are also important; for example, a clinician who perceives the elderly as a distinct group, with unique abilities and needs, is likely to place a premium on using geropsychological tests, or on developing such tests if none are available. The purpose of the evaluation, the general intellectual and functional level of the individual, and the practical constraints of the testing situation further shape the process of test selection.

One approach to assessing older adults is to use the same comprehensive neuropsychological batteries developed for use with younger adults. There are several potential advantages to this approach. Often, more extensive data exist on reliability and validity for these batteries than for lesser known neuropsychological or geropsychological measures. In addition, the comprehensive nature of these batteries helps to insure that many pertinent functions are evaluated. Test materials and norms can be purchased through commercial sources, and continuing-education workshops are available for learning the test procedures.

It is also important to be aware of the limitations of traditional neuropsychological batteries, especially for elderly clients. The most serious problem concerns the adequacy of normative reference points for upper age ranges; manuals must be carefully examined to determine the number of older people included in the normative sample and their characteristics (e.g., patient vs. nonpatient status). In addition, because these batteries were developed to detect brain damage in general, norms often pertain only to gross categories such as *brain-damaged* versus *psychiatric*; usually, there is no information provided about total scores or subscore profiles for old-age neuropsychiatric disorders. Other limitations are practical. Administration of the complete battery may exceed the attention and energy capabilities of most older patients, certain subtests appropriate for younger adults may be too difficult for the aged, and there may be no information regarding the relevance of test scores to everyday functioning in later life. A final general concern is that standardized batteries may be liable to misuse by examiners who lack training or experience in neuropsychology.

The Halstead-Reitan Neuropsychological Battery

The best known neuropsychological battery in the United States is the Halstead-Reitan Neuropsychological Battery (HRNB). The HRNB was developed empirically, beginning with tests that Halstead (1947) used in his attempts to quantify "biological intelligence" in patients with frontal lobe damage. The goal of the battery is to accurately predict organic disturbance, by using standardized testing procedures and quantitative interpretation.

Reitan and Davison (1974) provided descriptions and data summaries for the 10 original Halstead measures and several additional tests that have been added over the years (cf. Reitan, 1986; Reitan & Wolfson, 1985). The complete HRNB provides brief examinations of language and sensory functions, as well as extensive evaluations of psychomotor, visuospatial, and abstract reasoning abilities, but relatively little information about learning and memory. Some of the best known measures from the HRNB are the Aphasia Screening Test (see "Language," below); the Category and Trail Making tests (see "Problem Solving and Executive Functions," below); the Tactual Performance Test, a measure of tactile, spatial, and memory functions which entails placement of forms on a puzzle board under blindfolded conditions, followed by drawing of the forms and their locations from memory; and Finger Tapping, a measure of motor speed and lateralization which requires depression of a key as rapidly as possible for brief periods of time.

Cutting scores have been designated for each scale, identifying "impaired" versus "unimpaired" ranges, and scores on several of the scales can be combined to form overall impairment indices. For example, on the Halstead Impairment Index (defined as the proportion of selected tests yielding scores in the impaired range), scores of .40 or above are traditionally interpreted as indicating brain damage.

Age Differences in Performance

A recent study has provided contemporary normative data on the HRNB for young, middle-aged, and young-old groups (Heaton *et al.*, 1986; cf. Heaton, Grant, and Matthews, 1991). Subjects (n = 553) were tested at the neuropsychological laboratories of three university medical centers; only those who were without neurological signs and symptoms and whose histories were negative for neurological illness, traumatic brain injury, or substance abuse were included. Participants ranged in age from 15 to 81 years and were grouped into three age categories: 20 to 39 years, 40 to 59 years, and 60 years and older.

Age was found to account for 20% to 35% of the variance in scores from the Category Test, Tactual Performance Test, and Trail Making Test; by contrast, only one of the Wechsler Adult Intelligence Scale (WAIS) subtests, Digit Symbol, was affected to this extent by age. Figure 4.1 shows mean scores on an overall impairment index and percentages of subjects classified as normal for nine different age/education subgroups. Fewer elderly subjects were classified as normal than young or middle-aged adults; this effect was most pronounced among poorly educated older individuals. The age trend is particularly noteworthy because the older subjects were still quite young (mean age = 68 years).

Moehle and Long (1989) corroborated these results. They found a nearly linear increase with age in an HRNB impairment index in a medically ill sample with an average of about 12 years of education; the mean impairment index for patients aged 65 years and older was .79, compared to .39 for 25- to 34 year-olds and .56 for 45- to 54 year-olds. Earlier validation studies also demonstrated age-sensitivity of the HRNB (e.g., Klisz, 1978; Price, Fein, & Feinberg, 1980; Reed & Reitan, 1963; Reitan, 1955).

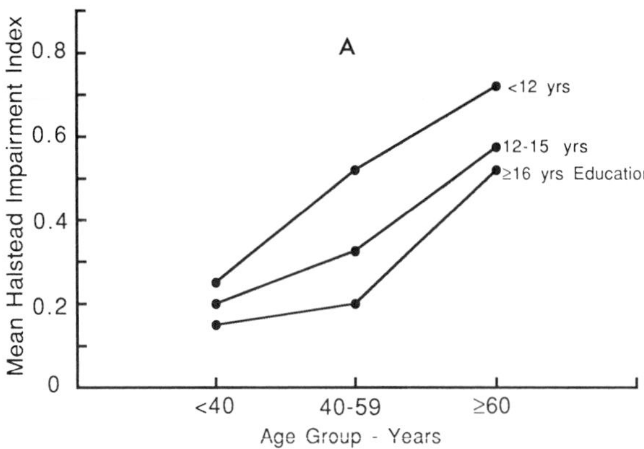

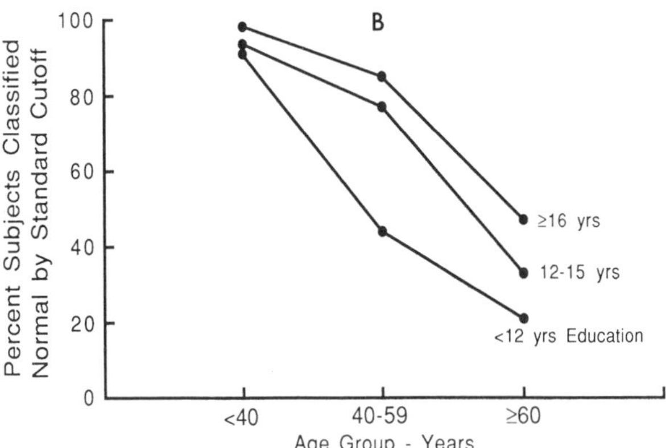

FIGURE 4.1. A. Mean scores on the Halstead Impairment Index for nine age/education groups. B. Percentage of each group classified as normal on the Halstead Impairment Index. (From Heaton, Grant, and Matthews, 1986, p. 112. Copyright 1986 by Oxford University Press. Reprinted by permission.)

These outcomes clearly indicate that, at least as operationalized in the HRNB, normal aging appears to produce many of the same performance impairments as acquired brain damage. However, these trends require careful interpretation. Should 40% to 60% of normal older people be classified as brain-damaged? From social and clinical perspectives, this seems potentially damaging. When the HRNB findings are examined in light of the experimental literature on cognition and aging (see Chapter 3), it is apparent that many of the measures tap areas of comparative weakness in older adults. Fluid intellectual abilities are more heavily assessed than crystallized skills, a premium is placed on speed of response, and the stimuli and procedures are unlikely to be encountered in the everyday activities of older adults. In clinical assessments of older patients, therefore, it would seem important to balance HRNB findings against other clinical and functional assessments before drawing conclusions about brain impairment.

Diagnostic Utility

The general sensitivity of the HRNB to brain impairment is well established; however, several studies raise doubts about the diagnostic specificity of the HRNB, at least when interpretations are based on objective findings alone. In a representative investigation, Anthony, Heaton, and Lehman (1980) examined the accuracy of the Halstead Impairment Index and two computerized actuarial systems based on the HRNB in distinguishing brain-damaged patients from controls and in identifying specific types of lesions. Subjects were 150 patients with clinically diagnosed brain lesions substantiated by neurosurgical postoperative reports, pneumoencephalogram, cerebral angiograms, or computerized tomography (CT); 42% of the patients had tumors, 25% cerebrovascular accidents, and 21% head trauma. Mean ages for the brain-damaged and control groups were 43 years and 39 years, respectively, and both groups had an average of 12 years of education. The Halstead Impairment Index correctly identified 79% of the brain-injured patients and 85% of the controls. The best of the actuarial programs (incorporating the "key" approach of Russell, Neuringer, & Goldstein, 1970) correctly identified 69% of the right-hemisphere lesions, 61% of the left-hemisphere lesions, and 32% of the diffuse lesions; 76% of the static lesions were correctly identified, but only 35% of the acute lesions. Negative outcomes were attributed to the inclusion of many difficult-to-diagnose cases and to the absence of corrections for age and education in quantitative impairment computations (misclassified control subjects tended to be older and less well educated than the rest of the sample).

Reviews of additional studies have reported that, in general, neuropsychological tests have a median accuracy of about 75% for making binary classifications of brain-damaged patients versus controls (Heaton, Baade, & Johnson, 1978; Spreen & Benton, 1965). Because many briefer and less costly examinations produce such classification rates, routine use of lengthy batteries such as the HRNB may not be justifiable. In younger patients, administration of the complete HRNB requires between five and eight hours of testing, depending on the extent of impairment; in geriatric patients, administration times are likely to be longer.

It is important to note that a comprehensive battery such as the HRNB may be useful for developing a more complete understanding of preservations and impairments in a specific individual; this can be helpful in certain difficult diagnostic assessments, in legally contested cases, and in planning for rehabilitation. In addition, performance on certain HRNB measures has been found to correlate with practical occupational, social, and self-care abilities in several different clinical populations (see Heaton & Pendleton, 1981, for a review), including medically ill older adults (McSweeny, Grant, Heaton, Prigatano, & Adams, 1985).

Conclusions Regarding the HRNB and Older Patients

Because so many clinically normal older individuals perform in the brain-damaged range on the HRNB, and because of the time-consuming and demanding nature of many of the tests, the complete HRNB is not recommended for routine geropsychological assessment.

However, selected subtests of the HRNB can be applied with good effect in screening for organic impairment or in evaluating certain complex perceptual and motor functions. The Trail Making Test has frequently been included in geriatric studies and is discussed in detail below (see "Problem Solving and Executive Functions"). The Finger Tapping Test can be used to measure simple motor speed and to screen for lateralized brain impairments. The Aphasia Screening Test provides a quick check of a wide range of speech and language functions (see "Language," below), and the Category Test provides one of the few clinically standardized measures of logical problem solving (see "Problem Solving and Executive Functions").

Research is continuing to extend the data base on the HRNB in directions that may increase its utility for geriatric evaluations. Procedures for making age and education corrections have been described (e.g., Alekoumbides, Charter, Adkins, & Seacat, 1987; cf. Heaton *et al.*, 1991), and abbreviated test batteries, more suitable for geropsychological assessment, have been proposed (see Schear, 1984, for an excellent example). There are also an increasing number of studies describing HRNB performance in older patients with neuropsychiatric disorders, including Alzheimer-type and multi-infarct dementia.

The Luria-Nebraska Neuropsychological Battery

Many neuropsychologists have taken issue with the actuarial, atheoretical nature of the Halstead-Reitan battery, preferring the more clinical approach exemplified by the work of Aleksandr Luria (e.g., Luria, 1974, 1980; Luria & Majovski, 1977). Luria's descriptions of his work with brain-damaged patients present an individualized, qualitative approach to neuropsychological assessment. The initial aim is to develop a detailed knowledge of the psychological (i.e., behavioral) disturbance, followed by formulation of a hypothesis as to the symptom's "structure" and its relationship to a local brain lesion. Behavior is assumed to proceed from the participation of all parts and levels of the brain, and a tripartite system of brain–behavior relations is offered to describe brain organization.

In reading Luria's work, one quickly realizes how difficult it would be to reliably implement this approach without extensive training. Christensen (1975) developed a set of examination materials and questions based on her studies with Luria that represented a step toward operationalizing the clinical techniques. Golden and colleagues have taken this approach further, developing the Luria-Nebraska Neuropsychological Battery (LNNB; Golden, Hammeke, & Purisch, 1980; Hammeke, Golden, & Purisch, 1978; Purisch & Sbordone, 1986). In the LNNB, many of the specific questions and tasks included in Luria's works have been preserved; however, the flexible approach to evaluation has been replaced by a set battery.

The LNNB, Form I, consists of 269 items organized into several scales (e.g., Motor, Rhythm, Tactile, Visual, Receptive Speech, Expressive Speech, Writing, Reading, Arithmetic, Memory, Intellectual, Pathognomonic, Left Hemisphere, and Right Hemisphere). It takes about 1½ hours to administer to an alert younger adult (perhaps 3 hours with an elderly patient), so that it is considerably more practical for routine use than the HRNB. Each item is scored on a 3-point continuum (0, 1, or 2), with 2-point scores indicating clear impairment. Raw scores on each of the scales are converted to *T* scores, and a performance profile is charted. An age- and education-adjusted baseline is computed with which individual subscale scores are compared (Golden *et al.*, 1980; Marvel, Golden, Hammeke, Purisch, & Osman, 1979). A general interpretive guideline is that any individual with three or more scores above baseline "will almost always have brain dysfunction" (Golden *et al.*, 1980, p. 104).

Age Differences in Performance

Relatively few investigations have examined LNNB performance of normal older adults. In a representative study (McInnes, Gillen, Golden, Graber, Cole, Uhl, & Greenhouse, 1983), healthy elderly volunteers were found to score below the critical level on all scales, in contrast to older brain-damaged patients, who scored in the impaired range on all measures. The normal subjects in this research were highly selected (e.g., financially independent and with no cardiovascular disease) and the brain-damaged patients were a heterogeneous group (including neoplasms, cerebrovascular accidents, and various types of degenerative disorder).

A short form of the LNNB has been developed which reduces the number of items from 269 to 141 (McCue, Shelly, & Goldstein, 1985). This form has been recommended for use with impaired older adults, since it substantially reduces the time and effort required for completion. Scaled scores obtained with this form correlate quite strongly (r's = .80 to .90) with those obtained from the full administration (McCue *et al.*, 1985).

Diagnostic Utility

The validation data presented in the original LNNB test manual were obtained from 146 neurological patients, 83 psychiatric patients, and 103 normal controls. The neurological patients were a heterogeneous group, cerebrovascular disorders, head trauma, and tumor being the most frequent diagnoses; the psychiatric patients were primarily chronic schizophrenics, although some with more acute disorders were included. Control subjects were individuals hospitalized on internal medicine wards. An overall hit rate of 93% was reported for differentiation of neurological patients and controls and 88% for neurological patients versus psychiatric patients. Hit rates for individual scales were lower, particularly for the psychiatric group. For example, scores on the Pathognomonic Scale correctly identified 82%, 62%, and 81% of the neurological, psychiatric, and control subjects, respectively; for the Memory Scale, the corresponding hit rates were 83%, 40%, and 78%, respectively.

Scores on LNNB scales correlate fairly highly with HRNB measures (e.g., Vicente, Kennelly, Golden, Kane, Sweet, Moses, Cardellino, Templeton, & Graber, 1980). In addition, experienced neuropsychologists have been reported to be as accurate in judging the presence of brain damage using the LNNB as they are with the HRNB (Kane, Parsons, Goldstein, & Moses, 1987). Sizable correlations (r's = .53 to .84) have also been observed between WAIS IQ and LNNB subscales (McKay, Golden, Moses, Fishburne, & Wisniewski, 1981) and between subscales from the Wechsler Memory Scale and LNNB memory measures (McKay & Ramsey, 1983).

The LNNB has often been criticized because of the composition of its scales. Like WAIS subtests, LNNB scales do not provide clean estimates of specific functions (e.g., the Receptive Speech scale appears to measure more than receptive language) and do not always relate in predictable ways to the loci of brain lesions (e.g., Crosson & Warren, 1982; Delis & Kaplan, 1982, 1983; Spiers, 1981). The battery may still have clinical utility in spite of these limitations. However, too literal an interpretation of subscale patterns could lead to diagnostic errors. In a revised version of the battery (Form 2; see Purisch & Sbordone, 1986), scales have not been given content-related names; this may help to reduce oversimplified applications.

Conclusions Regarding the LNNB and Older Patients

The LNNB may be useful for evaluating elderly patients, particularly in light of its brief administration time and its mix of relatively simple and difficult items. However, caution is recommended in applying this test until a broader base of validation studies is available for older patients. Using the short form of the LNNB, McCue, Goldstein, and Shelly (1989) reported 83.5% correct classification of elderly depressed and demented patients (see Chapter 11 for additional discussion). Other studies of this type are needed, particularly for groups that are at high risk for misdiagnosis of dementia (e.g., medically ill elderly, old-old individuals, or pseudodementia patients).

It is important to recognize that the LNNB, with its set battery and quantitative norms, is quite distinct from the clinical, qualitative evaluations that characterized Luria's work. Interpreting findings from this battery with respect to Luria's models of brain and behavior requires a thorough knowledge of Luria's work and of the general field of neuropsychology.

INDIVIDUALIZED BATTERIES

Many neuropsychologists use an individualized, hypothesis-testing approach in clinical assessment. Most begin with a core battery composed of traditional intellectual assessment measures, specialized neuropsychological tests, and observational or interview scales. Modifications in the core may be made for different referral questions, and measures may be added or subtracted as the examiner develops a sense of the patient's performance level, and as additional hypotheses are formulated about the nature of the problem. This approach is used by the Boston neuropsychological group (see Milberg, Hebben, & Kaplan, 1986, for an excellent description) and many others (e.g., Lezak, 1983, 1984; McKenna & Warrington, 1986); it is also employed in the case examples presented in this book.

The hypothesis-testing approach lends itself well to differential diagnosis, enabling the examiner to select measures that will help to rule out competing explanations for impairment, and can be used so as to encourage consideration of both organic and nonorganic hypotheses. An individualized approach is sometimes the only feasible one with patients who have limited tolerance for testing (e.g., because of fatigue, distractibility, or emotional distress) or who have special cultural, language, or sensory limitations. This approach can also help the examiner to avoid redundancy in an evaluation, reducing costs and preventing unnecessary distress or anxiety.

One disadvantage of an individualized approach is the danger of overlooking an important aspect of a patient's behavior. A judgment of diffuse impairment based on too few tests may leave significant areas of preservation undiscovered; on the other hand, important deficits may not be identified if pertinent measures are omitted (e.g., mild frontal impairment may be overlooked if the battery does not assess initiation and cessation of complex behaviors). Students who are new to the field are often uncomfortable about these possibilities—with good reason. As an examiner gains more experience in neuropsychological testing, however, the likelihood of significant oversights is reduced.

Albert (1981) identified five areas that should normally be evaluated in neuropsychological assessment of older patients: attention, memory, language, visuospatial abilities, and cognitive flexibility/abstraction. General intelligence, mood, and personality should also be examined in most clinical geriatric assessments. If each of these areas is assessed, a broad but relevant sample of behavior is obtained. Many different measures can be used to tap each area, as discussed in detail below.

The process of matching tests to individuals requires an appreciation of the available options for assessing specific functions. The following discussion reviews some of the measures that have been recommended for geropsychological testing. It is not a comprehensive survey; instead, it focuses on instruments that the author has found to be particularly useful. Familiarity with standard intellectual and psychodiagnostic tests (e.g., the WAIS-R and the Minnesota Multiphasic Personality Inventory, or MMPI) is assumed, and with respect to these tests, only a few findings relevant to older patients are included. For certain additional measures that are widely used with younger patients (e.g., the Wechsler Memory Scale, or WMS), the reader is referred to other sources for detailed descriptions and critiques. Tests that have been developed specifically for older adults, or which may be new to many readers, are covered in greater detail, and tables of age norms are provided in the Appendix for a few of the most useful tests.

Mental Status Examinations

Clinical interview supplemented by a structured mental status exam is a useful way to begin the neuropsychological assessment of an older person. Such procedures can help to identify important subjective complaints, provide an estimate of the overall level of impairment, and suggest areas for more detailed examination. For older patients with acute medical illness or high levels of emotional distress, formal testing must sometimes be limited to these procedures.

Many different cognitive mental status exams have been developed, and several, including the Information-Memory-Concentration Test (Blessed, Tomlinson, & Roth, 1968), the Mini-Mental State Examination (MMSE; Folstein *et al.*, 1975), the Mattis Dementia Rating Scale (Mattis, 1976), the Kahn-Goldfarb Mental Status Questionnaire (Kahn, Goldfarb, Pollack, & Peck, 1960), and the Short Portable Mental Status Questionnaire (Pfeiffer, 1975), have been widely used with geriatric patients (for additional examples and critiques, see Kane & Kane, 1981; Poon, 1986; Roca, 1987). Two such instruments, the Mini-Mental State and a newer scale, the Neurobehavioral Cognitive Status Examination (NCSE; Kiernan, Mueller, Langston, & Van Dyke, 1987), are discussed in detail below.

The Mini-Mental State Examination

The MMSE was developed as "a practical guide for grading the cognitive state of patients" (Folstein *et al.*, 1975). The scale consists of 10 orientation questions, immediate and delayed recall of three words, measures of attention and calculation, several simple language items, and a single visuographic item (see Table 4.1). Errors are summed and subtracted from a maximum score of 30 points.

The original study of the MMSE (Folstein *et al.*, 1975) included 206 hospitalized patients diagnosed as having dementia syndromes, affective disorder, affective disorder with cognitive impairment ("pseudodementia"), mania, schizophrenia, and personality disorders, as well as 63 normal older subjects. The mean score for elderly normal subjects was 27.6 (*SD* = 1.7, range = 24–30), whereas the mean score of patients with dementia was only 9.6 (*SD* = 5.8, range = 0–22). Age-matched groups with affective disorder scored in between these two extremes. Those with uncomplicated depressive disorder had a mean score of 26.1 (*SD* = 4.4, range = 17–30), and those judged to have depression with cognitive impairment averaged 18.4 correct (*SD* = 5.7, range = 9–27). These preliminary data led to the recommendation that a cutoff of 23 be used to raise the question of cognitive impairment (i.e., none of the normal older adults had scored less than 24).

Subsequent studies have found that the MMSE has acceptable reliability, sensitivity, and specificity when used with general adult populations (see Roca, 1987, for a review). However, misclassification rates are increased in certain patient groups. Older and poorly educated individuals often score below the standard cutoff of 23. For example, an epidemiological investigation (Folstein, Anthony, Parhad, Duffy, & Gruen-

TABLE 4.1. Items on the Mini-Mental State Examination (MMSE)[a]

Cognitive skill	Task(s)	Score
Orientation for time	Specify year, season, month, date, and day.	0–5
Orientation for place	Specify state, county, city, building, and floor.	0–5
Registration	Repeat three words (e.g., *ball*, *flag*, *tree*, or *apple*, *table*, *penny*) immediately after presentation.	0–3
Attention/calculation	Serial subtraction of 7 from 100 or spelling of *world* backward.	0–5
Recall	Repeat three words presented earlier.	0–3
Naming	Identify pencil and watch by name.	0–2
Repetition	Repeat "No ifs, ands, or buts."	0–1
Verbal command	"Take a piece of paper in right hand, fold it in half, and place it on the floor."	0–3
Written command	Read and perform the following: "Close your eyes."	0–1
Writing	Write a spontaneous sentence.	0–1
Visuoconstruction	Copy two interlocking pentagons.	0–1
	Total score	0–30

[a]From Folstein, Folstein, and McHugh (1975, pp. 196–197). Copyright 1975 by Pergamon Press, Inc. Adapted by permission.

berg, 1985) found that 20.8% of older adults in the community obtained scores of 23 or lower on the MMSE; for a substantial proportion (33%) of these individuals, there was no indication of neurological or psychiatric disorder on clinical evaluation. In an earlier study focusing on medical inpatients (Anthony, Le Resche, Niaz, Von Korff, & Folstein, 1982), the MMSE was found to have an overall sensitivity of 87% and a specificity of 82% relative to a clinical diagnosis of dementia or delirium; however, specificity was only 63% among patients with an eighth-grade education or less and 65% for individuals aged 60 years and older. A lowering of the cutoff for impairment (from < 23 to ≤ 20) was recommended for older, poorly educated patients (see Table 4.1). Additional modifications have been proposed to minimize sociocultural artifacts for patients of Hispanic background (Escobar, Burnam, Karno, Forsythe, Landsverk, & Golding, 1986).

The opposite problem is observed in younger patients or healthy and well-educated older adults; that is, when scored and interpreted in a standard way, the MMSE is often insensitive to mild brain impairment in these cases (e.g., Galasko, Klauber, Hofstetter, Salmon, Lasker, & Thal, 1990; Jackson & Ramsdell, 1988; Schwamm, Van Dyke, Kiernan, Merrin, & Mueller, 1987). For example, in older patients with mild dementia of the Alzheimer type, who are otherwise healthy and well educated, 15% to 33% can be expected to score 24 or higher on this exam (Galasko *et al.*, 1990; Jackson & Ramsdell, 1988).

Based on a normative study of healthy volunteers, Bleecker, Bolla-Wilson, Kawas, and Agnew (1988) recommended raising cutoffs for clinical screening to a score of 28 for people between the ages of 50 and 79 and a score of 26 for 80- to 89-year-olds. These levels would be appropriate, however, only for patients who lack any significant health problems and who have a minimum of a high-school education. Others have proposed modifications of the MMSE to increase its sensitivity. Galasko *et al.* (1990) suggested replacing the current language items with a brief test of verbal fluency; Teng and Chui (1987) expanded the scoring system for several items (e.g., replacing the pass-fail scoring of the visuoconstructive item with a 10-point scale) and added some additional procedures to test the limits of performance (e.g., providing cues and multiple-choice recognition for items missed on delayed recall).

As Folstein *et al.* (1985) emphasized, the MMSE is inadequate for making a diagnosis of brain impairment; instead, a low score suggests a need for further assessment. As a screening test for older adults, the primary advantages of the MMSE are twofold: it probes a broad range of cognitive functions in a brief and reliable manner, and it is sensitive to generalized impairments in cognitive state. In addition, because the MMSE is now commonly used in clinical settings where geriatric patients are treated, findings are interpretable by a relatively wide audience of health care professionals. However, the insensitivity of the scale to mild brain impairment is an important limitation; also, because of the high risk of false positive errors, caution must be used in interpreting scores for patients with serious medical illness, low levels of education, or very advanced age.

The Neurobehavioral Cognitive Status Examination

Several new screening tests have been developed that provide a differentiated index of various cognitive domains while still retaining brevity. One of the most recent of these measures is the NCSE, designed by Kiernan *et al.* (1987) based on their experience with patients in a general medical hospital.

In administering the NCSE, an examiner first rates a patient's consciousness, attention, and orientation. Then a graded series of questions is asked in each of five areas: language (assessing fluency, comprehension, repetition, and naming); constructional ability; memory (recall of four words at 10 minutes with category prompts, followed by multiple choices); calculation; and verbal reasoning (similarities and comprehension items). Each of the sections begins with a difficult item (called the *screen*); if the subject passes this item, no other questions of this type are given. If the screen is failed, the remaining items in that section (the *metric*) are administered. Because normal subjects often need to be given only the screens for most sections, the test is said to take less than 5 minutes to administer to these individuals. For patients with impairment, administration time ranges from 10 to 20 minutes. Results are summarized in profile format, with separate points plotted for alertness, orientation, and attention, and for language, memory, calculation, visuoconstruction, and reasoning performance. Preliminary standardization data have been reported for several groups, including older adult volunteers (70 to 92 years). Lower mean scores were observed in the older group in three areas (constructions, memory, and similarities), and cutoffs for clinical interpretation are adjusted downward on these scales for elderly patients.

The NCSE shows some promise as a screening instrument for older patients. The profile of outcomes is potentially useful, since a single summary score may mask important individual areas of weakness. However, no independent validation studies have been published as yet, and there are no data on reliability. It will be important for performance on this test to be studied in medically ill elderly patients, and in those with psychiatric disorder, before abnormal scores are considered suggestive of neurological impairment.

In a preliminary examination with an geropsychiatric sample (Osato, La Rue, & Yang, 1989), we found that the NCSE was more effective than the MMSE in distinguishing individuals with organic brain disorders from those with affective disorder, based on the number of clinical subscales yielding scores in the impaired range. However, even in depressed patients with no indication of neurological disorder, only a small proportion (5 out of 20) scored completely within the limits recommended for normal older adults. At present, therefore, a reasonable procedure would be to use the NCSE in conjunction with some more established mental status measure or more complete neuropsychological testing.

Intelligence Testing

Despite criticisms concerning factor structure and external validity, the WAIS and WAIS-R remain the instruments of choice for clinical evaluation of intellectual ability in both younger and older adults (Lubin, Larsen, & Matarazzo, 1984). Chapter 3 discusses the general effects of age on verbal and performance subtests, and the test manuals (Wechsler, 1955, 1981) summarize age adjustments in subtest and IQ scores.

There is an extensive literature on the use of the WAIS in neuropsychological evaluations (for discussions, see Lezak, 1983; McFie, 1975). The WAIS-R generally yields lower IQ scores (from 4 to 8 points) than those produced by the WAIS, in both normal volunteers and patients referred for neuropsychological testing (e.g., Wechsler, 1981; Zarantonello, 1988), and in a recent study with normal older adults (Quereshi & Erstad, 1990), even larger discrepancies were reported. However, summary IQs and subtest scores are highly correlated for the two tests, and the factor structures have been shown to be comparable (e.g., Parker, 1983; Silverstein, 1982). Whether WAIS and WAIS-R subtest patterns can be treated as interchangeable for inferring brain impairment is a matter of some debate.

Individual WAIS or WAIS-R subtests are frequently used to estimate specific functions or skills (Lezak, 1983). For example, Digit Span is often given as a measure of attention and short-term memory, Similarities as an index of verbal abstraction, and Block Design as a visuospatial measure (see "Assessing Specific Cognitive Areas," below). Summary IQ scores are important for estimating the presence or absence of intellectual decline and for interpreting performance on many other neuropsychological measures (e.g., tests of learning and memory).

These applications of intelligence testing are as important for geropsychological assessment as for evaluation of younger adults. However, certain complicating issues are likely to arise in testing of older patients. The first concerns limitations in patients' attention and energy which may necessitate the use of short forms or abbreviated administrations. Some examiners administer only selected subtests and estimate summary IQ scores from these measures. A two-test form (Vocabulary and Block Design) has been recommended, and several four-test combinations have been proposed (Silverstein, 1982; Wechsler, 1981). Intercorrelations between IQs estimated from these forms and those obtained from complete administration have been found to be quite high, both in general adult populations and in geriatric samples (e.g., Ryan, Georgemiller, & McKinney, 1984), although brief forms may lead to overestimates of IQ and to poorer discrimination of diagnostic groups (Thompson, 1987). Another approach is to administer subsets of items from each of the subtests. A screen-and-metric technique has been used (Vincent, 1979) in which questioning begins at higher starting points on various subtests, with easier items administered only if the patient fails the starting item. An alternate technique (Satz & Mogel, 1962) is to administer every third item on several of the subtests. Both techniques have been found to yield good estimates of summary IQ scores in geriatric samples (e.g., Burns, Elias, Hitchcock, & St. Germain, 1980; Cargnello & Gurekas, 1987), but subscale profiles appear less reliable.

Geropsychological assessments also frequently call for reexamination in six months to a year; this is especially likely for patients with questionable deficits who may be in early stages of a dementing illness. Data summarized in the WAIS-R manual and several subsequent studies (Atkinson, Bowman, Dickens, Blackwell, Vasarhelyi, Szep, Dunleavy, MacIntyre, & Bury, 1990; Shuerger & Witt, 1989) indicate that there is high short-term test–retest reliability for IQ summary scores, but most of this research has focused on younger adults. Therefore, expectations for normal retest performance in older adults over longer time intervals have been dubious at best. Fortunately, some relevant data have recently been reported for normal older volunteers (n = 101; mean age = 67 years) who were retested with the WAIS-R approximately one year after their initial evaluation (Snow, Tierney, Zorzitto, Fisher, & Reid, 1989). Relatively high test–retest correlations were observed for each of the IQ summary scores (.86, .85, and .90, for Verbal, Performance, and Full-Scale IQs, respectively), and for individual subtests, all but one of the correlations were greater than or equal to .65. More subjects improved on retest than declined (60% versus 33% on FIQ). Only about 1% of patients showed changes of more than 10 points on VIQ and FIQ, and 5% had PIQ changes of this magnitude. However, more than 30% declined by 1 to 10 points on each of these scales. Discrepancies between VIQ and PIQ were less reliable than other summary scores; for example, of 21 individuals whose VIQs were initially at least 15 points higher than their PIQs, only 12 still had discrepancies of this magnitude at retest.

These findings suggest that WAIS-R summary scores are reliable for normal older people over retest intervals of about a year. Large declines in scores are highly unusual in a normal sample, but smaller declines (e.g., 5 or 6 points) are unlikely to be of clinical significance; also, VIQ-PIQ discrepancies based on a single testing should be interpreted with caution. Slightly lower one-year retest reliabilities (r's = .70 to .83) have been reported for IQs obtained with the Satz-Mogel short-form of the WAIS-R (Mitrushina & Satz, in press).

A final common problem in geropsychological testing concerns evaluation of patients who are older than 74 years of age (the upper limit in the WAIS-R norms). The WAIS-R manual states that "many people who are older than 74 may be tested using the norms for ages 70–74" (Wechsler, 1981, p. 51). However, since continued aging decrement can be expected beyond age 74 in many of the functions tapped by the WAIS-R (see Chapter 3), this procedure is likely to inflate the estimated rate of impairment in very-old adults. An alternative, and probably preferable, procedure is to extrapolate from the age trends reflected in the WAIS-R norms. For example, on age-sensitive subtests such as Digit Symbol, linear extrapolation suggests that normal 84-year-olds may perform at least a standard deviation lower than 74-year-olds; therefore, an age-scaled score of 7 (based on norms for age 70 to 74) could be considered normal for an 84-year-old. This interpretation may still underestimate true age differences, since rates of normal aging change often accelerate at very advanced ages (see Chapter 3).

Two recent studies provide the beginnings of a normative data base for the WAIS-R in individuals over the age of 75. One (Ryan, Paolo, & Brungardt, 1990) described findings for two age groups (75 to 79 years and 80+ years) based on a study of 130 volunteers (mean age = 81 years; mean education = 9.5 years), and the other (Ivnik, Malec, Smith, Tangalos, Petersen, & Kurland, 1992) reported outcomes for successive five-year age brackets based on data from over 500 volunteers (age range = 56 to 97 years, 86% with a high-school education or more). Both studies excluded individuals with neurological or psychiatric disease but included subjects with chronic, well-controlled medical conditions common in the elderly (e.g., hypertension and adult-onset diabetes). Both document a continued lowering of performance beyond age 74 on many subscales and on each of the standard summary scores. Ryan *et al.* provided tables for estimating VIQ, PIQ, and FIQ from different sums of scaled scores, but since their sample was small and limited in its educational, geographic, and ethnic diversity, caution should be used in applying these estimates clinically. Ivnik and colleagues attempted to correct for sampling differences between the WAIS-R standardization data and their normative study, but they stated explicitly that their IQ estimates should not be considered a direct equivalent of WAIS-R scores. In general, therefore, a "benefit-of-the-doubt" approach is warranted in interpreting intelligence test performance of very-old individuals (see Chapter 5 for examples) until further normative information becomes available.

Assessing Specific Cognitive Areas

Attention

Although diminished attention can affect many aspects of cognitive performance (see Chapter 3), clinical procedures for assessing attention are not well developed. Examiners often rely on subjective impressions of a patient's ability to direct and sustain attention and frequently intervene to redirect attention. Formal assessment of attention is usually limited to a few simple procedures (see Table 4.2), none of which provides a pure measure of the attentional process it is designed to assess.

TABLE 4.2. Clinical Tests of Attention[a]

Measure	Description	Comments
Digit Span (WAIS or WAIS-R)[b]	Repetition of strings of numbers, forward and backward.	*Pros*: Brief; age norms available. *Cons*: Insensitive to mild impairment; confounds attention and primary memory.
Mental Control (WMS or WMS-R)[c]	Counting backwards from 20, reciting alphabet, counting forward by 3's.	*Pros*: Brief; age norms available. *Cons*: Same as for Digit Span; also requires skill in calculation.
Attention/Concentration Index (WMS-R)	Combination of Digit Span, Mental Control, and Visual Memory Span (repetition of block-tapping sequences).	*Pros*: Measures both verbal and nonverbal attention; age norms available. *Cons*: Same as for Mental Control; also requires intact visual perception.
Digit or Letter Cancellation[d]	Crossing off of specified digits or letters on printed pages; number of targets and total response time varies for different versions.	*Pros*: Provides a clinical index of vigilance; easy and difficult versions available. *Cons*: Age norms limited; requires intact visual perception.
The "A" Test[e]	Patient indicates each occurrence of a specified letter in a random series of spoken letters.	*Pros*: Oral analogue of digit cancellation. *Cons*: Age norms limited; lack of standardization.

[a]See text for additional references.
[b]Wechsler (1955, 1981).
[c]Wechsler (1945, 1987).
[d]Lezak (1983); Moran & Mefferd (1959); Ruff, Evans, & Light (1986).
[e]Strub and Black (1977).

The simplest and most commonly used test is Digit Span. Forward digit span remains constant across most of the adult life span (Chapter 3), but slight declines in mean scores for older age groups have been observed in some normative studies. Albert *et al.*, (1988), examining optimally healthy and well-educated subjects, found a mean forward digit span of 7.38 ± 0.89 for 30- to 39-year-olds compared to 7.14 ± 0.96 for 60- to 69-year-olds and 6.78 ± 1.04 for 70- to 80-year-olds. Benton *et al.* (1981), who also studied healthy volunteers, found that 8% of 80- to 84-year-olds scored significantly below the median level of 55- to 64-year-olds on WAIS Digit Span (cf. Klonoff & Kennedy, 1966).

The Mental Control subscale from the WMS can also be used as a rough indicator of attention. Cross-sectional age differences in Mental Control scores appear to be quite small (e.g., Hulicka, 1966; Margolis & Scialfa, 1984), but reduced scores are not uncommon in very-old subjects. For example, Klonoff and Kennedy (1966), studying male veterans aged 80 years and older, reported a mean WMS Mental Control score of 5.72 ± 2.07 for community-residing subjects and 4.69 ± 2.17 for residents in custodial care. These can be contrasted with the mean of 6.61 ± 1.90 reported for 40- to 49-year-olds in the WMS manual (Wechsler, 1945).

The WMS-R includes an Attention/Concentration Index composed of scores on three tests: Digit Span, Mental Control, and Visual Memory Span (repetition of block-tapping sequences). Although mean differences across the range of 16 to 74 years are quite small, age declines on the composite index are reported to be statistically significant (Wechsler, 1987).

Letter or digit cancellation tasks are commonly used to estimate vigilance or sustained attention. Several different forms of these tests have been developed (see Lezak, 1983, for descriptions), but most lack adequate norms for older patients. The simplest version instructs the subject to mark a single target digit every time it occurs on a page of randomly ordered typed digits. Because of the simplicity of this task, even one or two errors may suggest problems with sustained attention in patients with good visual acuity. In the absence of generalized motor slowing, very lengthy completion times (exceeding three or four minutes) may suggest an abnormal reduction in speed of mental processing; however, strict guidelines for interpreting speed scores are not available in older age ranges.

Ruff, Evans, and Light (1986) provided normative data for a related measure in which the task was to mark occurrences of two different target digits (see Table 4.2 for a description). A relatively large sample (n = 259) varying in age (16 to 70 years), education, and gender was studied, but no information was provided about health status or method of recruitment. A steady decline in the rate of crossing out targets was observed with increasing age, and subjects who had attended college worked more quickly than those with a high-school education or less. Test–retest correlations over an interval of six months were quite high in all age groups (r's ranged from .84 to .97).

Several other interesting vigilance measures have been described in the clinical literature. The Perceptual Speed test (Moran & Mefferd, 1959; cf. Lezak, 1983) is a digit cancellation measure in which the target digit changes randomly from line to line, placing a greater demand on flexibility of attention than most cancellation tasks. An auditory vigilance task (the "A" Test; Strub & Black, 1977) has also been developed, in which the subject listens to a series of spoken letters and indicates when a target letter occurs. Both of these tests may be useful for a given individual, the former when problems with attentional switching are suspected, and the latter for patients with visual impairment. However, both must be interpreted qualitatively, since speed and accuracy norms are lacking for elderly patients.

The Picture Completion subtest from the WAIS or WAIS-R is sometimes used as a measure of attention to detail, but visual sensory, perceptual, and conceptual skills must be intact before inferences can be drawn about attention. The Trail Making Test also involves important attentional components (concentration, search, and flexibility), but as with Picture Completion, performance is clearly affected by other cognitive processes.

Learning and Memory

Memory testing is one of the most important procedures to include in clinical assessment of older patients. Memory tests can provide an objective basis for reassuring older people who are concerned about normal forgetfulness (see Chapter 3); they are also very sensitive to distinctions between normal aging and beginning dementia.

Verbal Memory: Story recall. There are many options for assessing verbal learning and memory in older adults (see Table 4.3), including traditional measures such as the Logical Memory subtest from the WMS or WMS-R (Wechsler, 1945, 1987). At least two research groups (Storandt, Botwinick, Danziger, Berg & Hughes, 1984; Tierney, Snow, Reid, Zorzitto & Fisher, 1987) have reported that Logical Memory is sensitive to the distinction between early dementia and normal aging (cf. Christensen, Hadzi-Pavlovic, and Jacomb, 1991). This subscale also has high face validity; most older people recognize it as a test of memory and can see how their ability to perform on it may relate to everyday situations.

Table A.1 in the Appendix illustrates some of the findings that have been reported for older adult samples on Logical Memory. The table pertains only to immediate recall of the paragraphs used in Form I. Mean scores from the WMS manual (Wechsler, 1945) are summarized first, followed by the results from three studies (Albert *et al.*, 1988; Haaland, Linn, Hunt, & Goodwin, 1983; Van Gorp, Satz, & Mitrushina, 1990) of very exceptional older adults. The next two studies (Abikoff, Alvir, Hong, Sukoff, Orazio, Solomon, & Saravay, 1987; Hulicka, 1966) examined more heterogeneous groups, and the Klonoff and Kennedy (1966) investigation focused on very-old, socially disadvantaged subjects. Benton's old-age normative study (Benton *et al.*, 1981), which also used exceptional subjects, is listed last because the findings are not reported in terms of mean scores.

Outcomes for the studies with superior samples compare favorably with the mean score reported in the WMS manual for the 40- to 49-year-old standardization group; in fact, these studies illustrate that exceptional old people may do *better* on Logical Memory than average younger adults. Fairly high mean scores were also noted in the two heterogeneous samples (Abikoff *et al.*, 1987; Hulicka, 1966), although the standard deviations are larger. In the Klonoff and Kennedy (1966) investigation, mean scores are decidedly lower than what one would expect for younger groups. This study examined very-old subjects, all male and all veterans, most of whom had unskilled or semiskilled occupational backgrounds; nonetheless, those who were living in the community scored considerably higher than those in long-term care, and in both residential groups, activity level was significantly related to memory performance.

High variability and low mean scores can limit the clinical utility of Logical Memory for certain older patients. For example, in order to score two or more standard deviations below most of the relevant means shown in the table, a very-old or poorly educated patient would have to recall next to nothing of either of the paragraphs!

Revised scoring techniques and education corrections can help to increase the sensitivity of Logical Memory (cf. Loring & Papanicolaou, 1987). Abikoff and colleagues (1987) reported means and standard deviations on Logical Memory for different education groups as well as for age groups and provided age- and education-adjusted equations for both gist and verbatim recall. In general, they observed much higher gist than verbatim recall and much stronger education than age effects. Scoring for gist, then, may increase diagnostic sensitivity by curtailing floor effects; adjusting for education may narrow the confidence intervals for making judgments about impairment.

Testing of delayed recall can further enhance the utility of Logical Memory (Loring

TABLE 4.3. Tests of Verbal Learning and Memory[a]

Measure	Description	Comments
Logical Memory (WMS or WMS-R)[b]	Two stories presented orally; recall tested immediately (WMS) and after 30-minute delay (Russell revision of WMS; WMS-R).	*Pros*: High face validity; old-age norms available. *Cons*: Low scores expected for old-old and poorly educated subjects; scoring unclear for WMS.
Associate Learning (WMS or WMS-R)[b]	Ten pairs of words presented for a minimum of 3 trials; recall tested immediately (WMS) and after 30-minute delay (WMS-R).	*Pros*: Old-age norms available; errors may be informative. *Cons*: Little learning on hard pairs for old-old or poorly educated patients.
Paired Associate Learning Test (PALT)[c]	Only 3 pairs of words presented at a time; easy, intermediate, and hard pairs available.	*Pros*: Developed for elderly patients; brief; errors may be informative. *Cons*: Norms very limited.
Selective Reminding Test (SRT)[d]	List of 10 or 12 words presented for 6 to 12 trials; recall tested after each trial and, optionally, after delay; subjects reminded only of items forgotten on a given trial.	*Pros*: Separate subscores for different memory processes. *Cons*: Old-age norms limited; too difficult or frustrating for some older patients.
Object Memory Evaluation (OME)[e]	Set of 10 objects identified by touch, sight, and name prior to recall; 5 recall trials separated by 30 or 60 seconds of distraction (naming within categories); 5-minute delayed recall and recognition testing.	*Pros*: Developed for elderly patients; separate subscores for different memory processes; unaffected by low education. *Cons*: No norms for patients under age 70.
Auditory Verbal Learning Test (AVLT)[f]	List of 15 words presented for 5 trials; recall tested after each trial and after presentation of a second (interference) list; optional recognition testing.	*Pros*: Can evaluate primacy, recency, semantic clustering, proactive inhibition. *Cons*: Few norms for healthy elderly.
California Verbal Learning Test (CVLT)[g]	Similar to AVLT with more detailed instructions for administration and scoring; both free and cued recall tested following inteference list; 15-minute delayed recall and recognition.	*Pros*: Same as for AVLT; preliminary norms for ages 17 to 80 years. *Cons*: Limited data for pathological groups.
Shopping List Test[h]	List of 10 names of grocery items presented for 5 trials; 15-minute delayed recall and recognition.	*Pros*: Can evaluate primacy, recency; high face validity. *Cons*: Norms are very limited; may be too easy for well-educated patients.
Controlled Learning with Cued Recall[i]	Set of 16 labeled pictures presented 4 at a time; patient given category cue and asked to point to and name the item representing that category; after all items presented, 3 trials of free and cued recall, followed by recognition.	*Pros*: Evaluates ability to benefit from encoding and retrieval support. *Cons*: New test; norms very limited.
Delayed Word Recall Test (DWRT)[j]	Patient asked to make up sentences about each item on a 10-word list; after 5-minute delay, tested for free recall of items.	*Pros*: Tests recall under conditions that enhance encoding; brief; designed for older patients. *Cons*: New test; norms very limited.

[a]See text for additional references.
[b]Wechsler (1945, 1987).
[c]Inglis (1959).
[d]Buschke & Fuld (1974).
[e]Fuld (1981).
[f]Rey (1964); cf. Lezak (1983).
[g]Delis, Kramer, Kaplan, & Ober (1987).
[h]McCarthy, Ferris, Clark, & Crook (1981).
[i]Grober & Buschke (1987).
[j]Knopman & Ryberg (1989).

& Papanicolaou, 1987). Several studies indicate that normal older adults retain a high percentage of the information that they immediately report following delays of 20 to 30 minutes. Russell (1988) reported new norms for his revision of the WMS, which includes both immediate and 30-minute delayed recall of Logical Memory. Although there was a modest decline with increasing age in the percentage of information retained on delayed recall, retention scores were still quite high for the older age groups (69.5% to 74.2% for 70- to 79-year-olds and 65.8% to 70.6% for 80- to 89-year-olds). Haaland *et al.* (1983) found 30-minute retention scores ranging from 56.3% to 65.7% for healthy volunteers aged 65 years and older, and Abikoff *et al.* (1987) reported similarly high scores for 20-minute delayed recall.

Qualitative analysis of Logical Memory responses may also be clinically useful. One study (Butters, Granholm, Salmon, Grant, & Wolfe, 1987; cf. Chapter 7) found that it was very rare for normal elderly to confuse details of the different stories during their recall; by contrast, among patients with Alzheimer-type dementia, a substantial proportion of responses (approximately 25%) consisted of this type of error. Extrastory intrusions were somewhat less discriminating, comprising 20% of the responses of normal old subjects compared to 40% for dementia patients. Overall, the ratio of accurately recalled information to errors was much higher for healthy elderly than for patients with dementia.

On the WMS-R, which uses gist scoring for Logical Memory, relatively small age differences in mean scores are reported across the range of 17 to 74 years for the standardization sample (Wechsler, 1987); norms are also provided for 30-minute delayed recall. Independent validation studies of WMS-R are only beginning to be reported, and few have focused on older adults; however, the revised Logical Memory subtest clearly has good potential for geriatric applications.

Paired-associate learning. Table A.2 in the Appendix summarizes results of several old-age normative investigations using the Associate Learning subtest of the WMS. Fairly good performance is noted in young-old adults, but reduced mean scores are typical at age 80 years and older. Almost all of the age-related decline in Associate Learning results from decreasing performance on the less meaningful pairs (des Rosiers & Ivison, 1986; McCarty, Siegler, & Logue, 1982).

An alterative to the WMS Associate Learning test that has been used fairly often in geropsychological studies is the Paired Associate Learning Test developed by Inglis (1959; cf. Erickson & Scott, 1977). This measure entails presentation of only three pairs of words at a time; three different sets of words, varying in strength of association, are available. Our procedure in using this test (cf. La Rue, D'Elia, Clark, Spar, & Jarvik, 1986a) has been to first present the Mediate Pairs, consisting of items with modest associative strength (*cat-milk*, *cup-plate*, *gold-lead*). If a patient learns these items quickly (within five or six presentations), the more difficult New Pairs (*cabbage-pen*, *sponge-trumpet*, *knife-chimney*) are then presented; otherwise, testing ends with the easier Old Pairs (*east-west*, *hand-foot*, *knife-fork*). This approach helps to minimize the frustration that can result from attempting to learn lengthy or excessively difficult lists. However, normative data are very limited for nonclinical samples and for middle-aged and young-old adults. In a small sample of healthy older adults (mean age = 73 years; mean education = 13 years), average correct responses in five trials were 14.10 ± 1.10 and 10.50 ± 4.14 for the Mediate and New Pairs, respectively (La Rue *et al.*, 1986a).

Monitoring of error types during paired-associate learning can be helpful in deciding whether performance is age-consistent. Intrusion errors (irrelevant responses or interjection of old, overlearned associations) are very rare in normal aged samples and in geriatric depression (La Rue *et al.*, 1986a; Whitehead, 1973); therefore, the occurrence of such errors is sufficient to raise a question of organic impairment. Omissions ("don't know" answers or no response) are the most common type of error observed in normal aging, although transpositions (mispairing of response items) also occur fairly often. For example, on the Paired Associate Learning Test, New Pairs, healthy elderly subjects averaged 2.11 ± 2.09 omission errors and 1.50 ± 2.51 transpositions, but only 0.12 ± 0.35 intrusion errors, in five learning trials (La Rue *et al.*, 1986a).

List-learning tests. WMS or WMS-R subscales have been criticized for their failure to identify the components of learning and memory that are responsible for poor performance. As a result, many neuropsychologists supplement these measures with tests that attempt to isolate different information-processing skills.

The Selective Reminding Test (SRT; Buschke & Fuld, 1974; cf. Table 4.3) has been included in many drug studies of memory and in several studies comparing normal, demented, and depressed elderly subjects (e.g., Hart, Kwentus, Hamer, & Taylor, 1987a; Masur, Fuld, Blau, Levin, & Aronson, 1989). The SRT is a free-recall test in which the person is asked to learn and remember a set of common words, usually 10 to 16 nouns; after each recall attempt, the person is reminded only of the items that he or she failed to remember (selective reminding procedure). Several subscores can be derived that measure retrieval from short-term memory, retrieval from long-term memory, long-term memory storage, consistency of retrieval, and reminding failures. Therefore, one advantage of this test is that it may help to identify a memory problem more precisely; for example, a person may be able to store information in long-term memory (i.e., to learn) but may have difficulty retrieving it consistently.

Ruff, Light, and Quayhagen (1988) reported normative data on the SRT for a large sample (n = 392) of volunteers screened for neurological or psychiatric illness. The age range included young, middle-aged, and young-old adults, and education varied from less than a high-school degree to 16 years or more. The stimuli consisted of a list of 12 nouns (*bowl*, *passion*, *dawn*, *judgment*, *grant*, *bee*, *plane*, *county*, *choice*, *seed*, *wool*, and *meat*; Form I; Hannay & Levin, 1985) presented for a series of 12 trials with use of the selective reminding procedure. Table A.3 in the Appendix summarizes findings on the Long-Term Storage index (cumulative recall across all trials) and on Consistent Long-Term Retrieval (instances in which a given word was recalled two or more consecutive times). Women generally performed better than men on this test. Scores tended to be higher for well-educated subjects and for younger individuals, but neither age nor education effects were as pronounced on this test as on other clinical memory measures. Test–retest reliability, based on two different forms of the test administered six months apart, was statistically significant but of modest strength (*r*'s = .66 to .73).

Additional norms for the same form of the SRT were reported by Banks, Dickson, and Plasay (1987) for healthy and well-educated 65- to 75-year-olds (see Table A.3 in the Appendix). Masur *et al.* (1989) provided norms for a six-trial administration of the SRT for 70- to 85-year-olds with a lower level of education (see Table A.3 in the Appendix). This study suggests that very old adults with limited education may find the SRT a difficult test; on the average, subjects retrieved only three to four words consistently across trials. This performance was still much better, however, than that of patients with dementia, a finding suggesting that a six-trial version of the SRT may be sufficient for diagnostic purposes.

Recently, the SRT has been shown to be of modest utility in predicting the development of dementia in very-old (mean age = 80 years) individuals (Masur, Fuld, Blau, Crystal, & Aronson, 1990). Sums of recall and delayed-recall scores were the most useful measures in this respect, with specificities of 86% and 88%, respectively. However, sensitivities were low (47% and 46%, respectively), indicating that individuals who will develop dementia may still perform normally on the SRT a year or two before the cognitive loss becomes clinically apparent.

For patients with limited verbal intelligence or reduced ability to tolerate testing, an alternative for evaluating components of verbal learning and memory is the Object Memory Evaluation (OME; Fuld, 1981). This test was developed for people in their 70s and 80s and was designed to be useful with nursing-home residents as well as community elderly. It is similar in format and scoring to the verbal SRT but uses 10 common objects as stimuli. The patient touches, sees, and labels the objects prior to recall and, therefore, has several possible ways to learn them; after the initial presentation, however, recall and reminding are verbal. Five learning trials are presented, separated by 60 or 30 seconds of distraction (naming within common categories). Delayed-recall and recognition testing is performed after a five-minute interval. As with the SRT, several different subscores can be computed for the initial learning and recall trials. Outcome measures include Storage (cumulative tally of items recalled on any trial), Retrieval (simple sum of items recalled), Repeated Retrieval (items recalled on two consecutive trials), and Ineffective Reminders (items forgotten on consecutive trials, despite reminding).

Preliminary normative data were provided by Fuld (1981) for small groups of community residents and nursing-home patients aged 70 to 79 years and 80 to 89 years. For community residents, mean Storage scores (maximum = 50) were 45.73 ± 2.08 and 40.82 ± 6.02 for the younger and older groups, respectively; nearly all subjects stored at least 9 of the 10 items by the fifth recall trial. Mean Repeated Retrieval scores (maximum = 40) were 25.87 ± 4.96 and 21.00 ± 5.69 for younger and older groups; by the fifth recall trial, both groups were consistently retrieving an average of five to seven items. In a separate study (La Rue *et al.*, 1986a), the OME was found to be more useful for differentiating both dementia and depression from healthy aging than either verbal paired-associate learning or a visual memory test (La Rue *et al.*, 1986a). Also, outcomes do not appear to be affected by differences in education (Fuld, 1981; La Rue *et al.*, 1986a) or ethnic or cultural differences (Fuld, Muramoto, Blau, Westbrook, & Katzman, 1988).

A short form of the OME, using only the first recall trial and delayed recall and recognition, has been developed and normed with 75- to 85-year-olds (Fuld, Masur, Blau, Crystal, & Aronson, 1990). This version has utility comparable to that of the SRT in predicting the development of dementia over a span of one to two years.

The SRT and related measures such as the OME have been criticized on a number of grounds, including relatively poor test–retest reliability, nonequivalence of alternate forms, and lack of validation for the distinctions drawn between component memory processes (cf. Loring & Papanicolaou, 1987). Nonetheless, these measures are often more effective than traditional tests in distinguishing the memory impairments observed in normal aging from those seen in dementia and depression (see Chapters 7 and 11), and as a result, they are being increasingly used by clinical neuropsychologists. At present, these tests should not provide the sole basis for inferring impairments in specific memory processes, and examiners must be alert to the variable procedures that have been used in normative studies (e.g., differing stimulus lists and numbers of trials).

There are several other list-learning measures that are appropriate for older adults (see Table 4.3), including the Auditory Verbal Learning Test (AVLT; Rey, 1964; for a detailed description, see Lezak, 1983), the California Verbal Learning Test (CVLT; Delis, Kramer, Kaplan, & Ober, 1987; Delis, Kramer, Freeland, & Kaplan, 1988), and the Shopping List Test (McCarthy, Ferris, Clark, & Crook, 1981). The original norms for the AVLT included mean scores for two groups of older adults (Rey, 1964; cf. Lezak, 1983), but these were based on small samples of French-speaking subjects. However, several subsequent studies have reported data for English-speaking samples (Ivnik, Malec, Tangalos, Petersen, Kokmen, & Kurland, 1990; Mitrushina, Satz, Chervinsky, & D'Elia, 1991; Montgomery, 1982; Query & Megran, 1983; Van Gorp *et al.*, 1990; Wiens, McMinn, & Crossen, 1988). The CVLT is adapted from the AVLT but provides more detailed instructions for test administration and scoring and normative data for a more diverse age span. This test is currently available only in a research edition (Delis *et al.*, 1987), but it offers promise as an instrument that can help to distinguish normal and pathological aging changes. The Shopping List Test (McCarthy *et al.*, 1981) follows a simple free-recall format with grocery-shopping items as stimuli; more than 80% of a sample of healthy, well-educated old people (mean age = 69 years; 68% with some college) met criterion on this test within five trials. Because of its relative simplicity, the Shopping List Test may be insensitive to mild learning and memory impairments, especially in young-old or well-educated patients; however, it can be useful with old-old or less sophisticated patients and is well suited to qualitative analysis (e.g., detection of primacy and recency effects, screening for errors of intrusion).

Newer measures with potential clinical utility are the Delayed Word Recall Test (DWRT; Knopman & Ryberg, 1989) and the Controlled Learning with Cued Recall procedure (Grober & Buschke, 1987; Grober, Buschke, Crystal, Bang, & Dresner, 1988). The DWRT (see Table 4.3 for a description) is predicated on the ability of normal older adults to benefit from procedures that encourage effective encoding (see Chapter 3). In an initial validation study, healthy elderly performed much better on this test than a comparison group of dementia patients (mean recall = 6.0 ± 1.8 and 0.8 ± 1.0, respectively), a finding suggesting that this measure may have utility as a screening instrument. The Controlled Learning with Cued Recall procedure (see Table 4.3 for a description) also evaluates ability to benefit from encoding- and retrieval-enhancement. In an initial investigation (Grober & Buschke, 1987), normal elderly volunteers obtained near-perfect scores on cued recall, and in a larger investigation (Grober *et al.*, 1988), the cued-recall procedure distinguished healthy elderly from dementia patients more accurately than either free recall or recognition testing. Both of these measures are interesting for theoretical reasons since they help to focus on processes that characterize memory in healthy aging (Chapter 3); however, because normative data are very limited, it would be best to use these measures in conjunction with other more established tests.

Nonverbal Memory: Copying tasks. Memory for designs, pictures, and places is a problem area for older adults (see Chapter 3), and clinical tests of these abilities (see Table 4.4) tend to show large age differences in normative levels of performance.

Table A.4 in the Appendix summarizes findings from old-age normative studies using the WMS Visual Reproduction subscale. Some studies report that very exceptional older adults perform as well as Wechsler's (1945) 40- to 49-year-old standardization group (see Van Gorp *et al.*, 1990, for ages 58 through 75), but others show reduced scores even for superior aged subgroups (see Haaland *et al.*, 1983, all ages). Older or less advantaged subjects clearly perform poorly on this measure (see Hulicka, 1966; Klonoff & Kennedy, 1966).

The Visual Retention Test (VRT; Benton, 1974) has been used in many studies with older adults and provides a good alternative to WMS Visual Reproduction. However, on this test, too, there are clear decremental age differences and problems with floor effects in many old-age subgroups.

The standard memory version of the VRT uses Form C, Administration A, where the subject studies a design for 10 seconds and then immediately attempts to draw the figure from memory. Normative data for this administration were obtained from more than 600 medical patients, excluding individuals with psychosis, cerebral injury or disease, or "serious physical depletion" (Benton, 1974). Findings from this sample were used to develop expected scores for various age and IQ subgroups.

The oldest age bracket in the norms for total correct scores is 55 to 64 years. At that age, superior-IQ, average-IQ, and low-average-IQ subjects are expected to correctly copy seven, six, and five designs, respectively. A score that is 2 points below the expected score is said to "raise the question" of acquired brain impairment, and a score of 4 or more below the norm provides a "strong indication" of brain impairment. Norms are also provided for total errors.

This version of the VRT was used by Benton *et al.* (1981) in their old-age normative study with healthy, well-educated subjects. The rate of defective performances ($\geqslant 2$ *SD*'s below the norm for ages 60 to 64 years) increased sharply within old age, from 7% at

TABLE 4.4. Tests of Nonverbal Learning and Memory[a]

Measure	Description	Comments
Visual Reproduction (WMS or WMS-R)[b]	3 or 4 geometric designs studied for 5 seconds each; patient attempts to copy each design from memory immediately (WMS) and after a 30-minute delay (Russell revision of WMS and WMS-R).	*Pros*: Widely used; age norms available. *Cons*: Old-old and poorly-educated patients may obtain very low scores; memory and visuographic abilities confounded.
Visual Retention Test (VRT)[c]	Series of 10 geometric designs presented for 10 seconds each; task is to copy each design from memory immediately after study.	*Pros*: Age norms available; errors may be informative. *Cons*: Same as for Visual Reproduction.
Rey-Osterrieth Complex Figure Test[d]	Complex geometric design is first copied and, after variable delays, drawn from memory.	*Pros*: Taps storage and retrieval of complex visuospatial information. *Cons*: Limited old-age norms; too difficult for many older patients.
Visual Retention Test, Multiple Choice (VRT-MC)[e]	Multiple-choice recognition of 16 designs, either immediately after study or following a 15-second delay.	*Pros*: Does not require visuographic ability; errors may be informative. *Cons*: Norms very limited for older patients.
Continuous Recognition Test[f]	Stimuli consist of line drawings of flowers and animals; task is to identify repeated items within a series of pictures.	*Pros*: Same as for VRT-MC; use of meaningful stimuli may help to maintain attention. *Cons*: Although age norms are available, there are few comparative data for pathological groups.
Continuous Visual Memory Test[g]	Stimuli are geometric designs that are difficult to label; task is to identify repeated items within a series of designs.	*Pros*: Same as for VRT-MC; may be sensitive to mild impairment. *Cons*: May be too difficult for many patients.
Nonverbal List Learning[h]	Series of 10 designs presented for 5 trials; task is to draw as many designs as possible after each trial; recognition tested after last recall trial; delayed recall and recognition after 20 minutes.	*Pros*: Nonverbal analogue of verbal list-learning tests; measures several aspects of memory. *Cons*: New test; norms very limited.

[a]See text for additional references.
[b]Wechsler (1945, 1987).
[c]Benton (1974).
[d]Rey (1941) and Osterrieth (1944); cf. Lezak (1983).
[e]Benton, Hamsher, and Stone (1977).
[f]Hannay, Levin, and Grossman (1979).
[g]Trahan and Larrabee (1988).
[h]Glosser, Goodglass, and Biber (1989).

65 to 69 years, to 16% at 70 to 74 years, 40% at 75 to 79 years, and 38% at 80 to 84 years. Klonoff and Kennedy (1966) also reported very poor performances for aged veterans (mean correct = 3.76 ± 2.70 and 2.78 ± 2.37, for community and custodial-care groups, respectively). In addition, age-related decline on the VRT has been documented longitudinally, with the sharpest rates of decline observed in the highest age brackets (Arenberg, 1978, 1982b).

In elderly patients, therefore, scores on the VRT are most informative when they are higher than expected, serving as a contraindication of nonverbal memory impairment. This test also lends itself to qualitative analysis, with low frequencies of perseverations, rotations, and size errors expected in normal aging (Eslinger, Pepin, & Benton, 1988; La Rue *et al.*, 1986a).

For very exceptional older adults, an alternative to either WMS Visual Reproduction or the VRT is the Rey-Osterrieth Complex Figure Test (Osterrieth, 1944; Rey, 1941; see, also, Lezak, 1983). Van Gorp *et al.* (1990) included this test in their normative study of superior older adults, using a three-minute delayed-recall procedure. Even in this advantaged group, however, relatively poor performance was observed; out of a maximum of 36 points, the mean score for 76- to 85-year-olds was only 8.41 ± 5.86.

Nonverbal memory tests that require the copying of designs correlate strongly with Performance IQ (Benton, 1974; Wechsler, 1987) and with measures of visuoconstructive ability (Van Gorp *et al.*, 1992). Therefore, part of the age-related decline on these tests may be due to nonverbal intellectual changes rather than to memory *per se*. Correlations with visuospatial measures tend to be higher for immediate reproduction than for delayed (20 or more minutes) reproduction (see Loring & Papanicolaou, 1987). Therefore, whenever possible, delayed administrations of copying tasks should also be administered. For WMS Visual Reproduction, Russell (1988) reported 30-minute retention scores of approximately 79% for normal 70- to 79-year-olds and 75% for 80- to 89-year-olds. Haaland *et al.* (1983) reported even higher retention scores (89% to 92%) for healthy, well-educated subjects aged 65 years and older.

Recognition measures. Nonverbal recognition tests have been recommended in order to minimize the demands placed on visuomotor abilities. A multiple-choice version of the VRT has been developed (Benton, Hamsher, & Stone, 1977) in which the patient studies a design for several seconds and then selects a matching design from one of four alternatives (see Table 4.4). Montgomery (1982) reported relatively good performance on this test for healthy 65- to 85-year-olds (community volunteers, mean education = 12.42 years); mean correct scores (maximum = 15) were 10.80 ± 1.89 and 12.98 ± 2.01 for immediate and delayed administrations, respectively.

The Continuous Recognition Test (Hannay, Levin, & Grossman, 1979; Trahan, Larrabee, & Levin, 1986) provides another option for multiple-choice testing (see Table 4.4). Trahan *et al.* (1986) conducted a normative study of this measure with community-resident volunteers ranging in age from 10 to 89 years who were screened for visual acuity and for history of psychiatric or neurological illness. A significant decrease in hits (i.e., correct detections of target drawings) was observed for elderly volunteers compared to middle-aged and young adults, a finding suggesting a decline in sensitivity in recognition (see Chapter 3). However, age differences tended to be small; for example, out of a maximum of 40 hits, the mean score for 78- to 89-year-olds was 36.79 ± 3.43 compared to 38.63 ± 1.48 for 30- to 41-year-olds. The rate of false alarms (i.e., incorrectly identifying a distractor as a target drawing) showed a more pronounced increase with age; for example, 78- to 89-year-olds had an average of 18.68 ± 7.46 false alarms compared to 9.32 ± 5.87 for 30- to 41-year-olds. Nearly all of the false alarms produced by older subjects involved within-class errors (i.e., inaccurate recognitions of items that were from the same semantic class as the target, but different in detail); therefore, gross misrecognitions on this test would be inconsistent with normal aging.

The Continuous Visual Memory Test (Trahan & Larrabee, 1988) is another multiple-choice task that has been normed across a broad age range (18 to 91 years). Procedures are similar to those of the Continuous Recognition Test, but the stimuli are abstract shapes that are difficult to label. In this author's experience, this measure is most likely to be useful with motivated, high-functioning patients whose attention is well preserved; patients with effort or attentional problems, or more than a mild degree of dementia, may complain that the task is lengthy and excessively difficult.

Nonverbal list learning. Glosser, Goodglass, and Biber (1989) recently introduced a list-learning test (adapted from Rey, 1968) that uses geometric designs as stimuli (see Table 4.4). Normal volunteers (aged 40 to 79 years), screened for psychiatric or neurological illness, were included in an initial study using this measure. On the initial free-recall trials, normal 60- to 79-year-olds had a slower rate of learning than 40- to 59-year-olds; however, in all other respects (e.g., shape of the learning curve, recognition performance, and delayed free recall), older subjects performed as well as middle-aged individuals. Since this is a new test, further validation and normative studies are clearly needed. However, this measure offers promise as a nonverbal counterpart to verbal list-learning tests and may prove useful in distinguishing different aspects of nonverbal memory (e.g., recall versus recognition, immediate versus delayed retention).

Memory Batteries for Older Adults. The WMS and WMS-R are the best known memory batteries and are frequently used with geriatric patients as well as younger adults. However, since the WMS was not initially standardized for older adults, interpretation of findings has presented problems. Also, while some of the subtests have been included in old-age normative studies, as discussed above, few studies have administered the complete battery to older samples. For the WMS-R, norms are available through age 74, and other changes have been made (e.g., adding a nonverbal recognition test and delayed-recall indices) that increase the utility of the battery for older patients. Butters, Salmon, Cullum, Cairns, Troster, Jacobs, Moss, and Cermack (1988) found the WMS-R to be sensitive to both dementia and amnesia. However, additional validation studies are needed, particularly with old-old samples.

A few batteries of memory tests have been developed specifically for older adults. One example is the New York University Memory Test (Osborne, Brown, & Randt, 1982; Randt, Brown, & Osborne, 1980), which consists of brief scales assessing general information, verbal list learning, digit span, paired associates, story recall, picture recognition, and incidental learning. Several of these components are reassessed after delays of several minutes or 24 hours. This battery was intended for use in longitudinal assessments, and it has been normed with subjects between the ages of 20 and 80. Comparative data have been reported for normal elderly and patients with dementia (Osborne *et al.*, 1982), but there have been few independent validation studies.

Crook and colleagues have also developed clinical memory measures for older adults (e.g., Crook, Ferris, & McCarthy, 1979; Crook, Ferris, McCarthy, & Rae, 1980). These tests examine aspects of memory that have been studied in the laboratory but use stimuli that more closely mirror everyday memory tasks. Specific measures include the Shopping List Test described above, a misplaced-objects test (Crook *et al.*, 1979), and a digit span task that entails repetition of telephone numbers (Crook *et al.*, 1980). Computerized versions of these and related tasks have been developed (Crook, Salama, & Gobert, 1986; Larrabee & Crook, 1989). An extensive normative data base has been collected for the computerized battery, but this version is not available for clinical use. There are less extensive norms for the pencil-and-paper versions of these tests, and there have been few independent validation studies reported with these measures.

The Rivermead Behavioral Memory Test (Wilson, Cockburn, & Baddeley, 1985; Wilson, Cockburn, Baddeley, & Hiorns, 1989) is another battery that focuses on everyday memory problems. Tasks include remembering a name, an appointment, and a newspaper article; finding a hidden object; recognizing faces; and remembering a route. Normative data are available from a mixed age sample (16 through 69 years), and within this range, no significant age differences were reported. However, the authors caution that subjects 70 years or older may show some deficits on these measures, and they are currently collecting normative data for elderly adults.

Remote and Subjective Memory Measures. There are occasional clinical situations in which tests of remote memory or surveys of subjective memory complaints may be required. Lezak (1983) reviewed some of the options for assessing old memories, including public events questionnaires (Squire, 1974) and tests of recall or recognition of famous people (e.g., Albert, Butters, & Brandt, 1981). A newer public events scale, developed by Howes and Katz (1988), attempts to address some of the methodological problems associated with these measures (see Chapter 3). Gilewski and Zelinski (1986) provided a thorough review of self-report memory scales, including their own Metamemory Questionnaire (cf. Zelinski, Gilewski, & Anthony-Bergstone, 1990); the recently developed Memory Assessment Clinics Self-Rating Scale (Crook & Larrabee, 1990) is an additional promising measure.

Language

Aphasia Examinations. Because many language functions are well preserved in old age (see Chapter 3), neuropsychological evaluations of older adults often include only brief evaluations of speech and language. Tests of confrontation naming and verbal fluency are usually administered, but other language functions may not be formally tested in patients who clearly comprehend test instructions and communicate effectively.

When more complete language assessment is indicated, appropriate options include the Boston Diagnostic Aphasia Examination (BDAE; Goodglass & Kaplan, 1972, 1983) and the Multilingual Aphasia Examination (MAE; Benton & Hamsher, 1976). The Aphasia Screening Test (Halstead & Wepman, 1959; Reitan & Davison, 1974) provides a quick survey of language and visuographic abilities, and the Token Test (Boller & Vignolo, 1966) is useful in screening for receptive language impairments, especially in the short form developed by Benton and Hamsher (1976). Table 4.5 provides brief descriptions of these measures (cf. Lezak, 1983).

Borod *et al.* (1980) summarized age and education effects for several measures from the Boston Diagnostic Aphasia Examination. No consistent age trends were noted from 25 to 85 years for Body Part Identification, Commands, Complex Ideational Material, Verbal Agility, Automatized Sequences, Rhythm, Repetition of Words or High Probability Phrases, Oral Sentence Reading, Comprehension of Oral Spelling, or Spelling to Dictation. However, poorer performance in the older subgroups was observed on a few measures, including Repeating of Low Probability Phrases, Animal Naming, Reading Sentences and Paragraphs, and Narrative Writing. Suggested cutoff scores for inferring impairment were provided for each of the measures, together with indications of tests that may yield low scores in older or poorly educated patients.

Naming. Table A.4 in the Appendix summarizes findings on the Boston Naming Test (BNT; Kaplan *et al.*, 1978; Kaplan, Goodglass, & Weintraub, 1983) for older age groups. In general, subjects who are 70 years or older have lower mean scores than those in younger age groups, although the magnitude of the age difference varies from study to study. Albert *et al.* (1988) used the most stringent screening procedures, including only optimally healthy men who were experienced participants in a longitudinal aging study. This investigation yielded high levels of performance, with the oldest age group providing correct answers for nearly 88% of the test items (cf. Van Gorp *et al.*, 1990). Borod *et al.* (1980) reported much lower mean scores and markedly increased variability. The oldest subjects in this investigation were not well educated (68% had a high-school education or less) and may have had physical health problems.

Errors made on the BNT are also important in clinical interpretation. As discussed in Chapter 3, normal older adults generally make errors that suggest knowledge of the to-be-named items. Nicholas, Obler, Albert, and Goodglass (1985) found that semantic errors accounted for nearly 30% of all naming mistakes made by healthy people in their 70s; imprecise comments, circumlocutions, and perceptual errors comprised an additional 23%, 14%, and 8%, respectively. Perseverations, responses unrelated to the pictured items, or paraphasic errors are rarely observed in normal aging.

Fluency. The most commonly used measure of verbal fluency is the Controlled Oral Word Association Test (Benton & Hamsher, 1976), in which the subject is asked to name

TABLE 4.5. Clinical Tests of Language[a]

Measure	Description	Comments
Boston Diagnostic Aphasia Examination (BDAE)[b]	Thorough battery of tests of receptive and expressive language; additional scales for musical and visuographic abilities.	*Pros*: Thorough clinical survey of language; useful for diagnosis of aphasic disorders. *Cons*: Time-consuming; age norms limited for many subtests.
Multilingual Aphasia Examination (MAE)[c]	Eight-part battery assessing expressive and receptive language and immediate memory.	*Pros*: Same as for BDAE; multiple forms on most subtests; education and age corrections. *Cons*: Time-consuming; normed only to age 64.
Aphasia Screening Test[d]	Brief survey of language and visuographic skills; 51- and 32-item versions available.	*Pros*: Useful in screening for aphasia. *Cons*: Qualitative scoring; limited age norms.
Token Test[e]	Task is to manipulate colored tokens in response to oral commands of increasing complexity; long and short forms (ranging from 100 to 22 items) available.	*Pros*: Brief but sensitive test of receptive language. *Cons*: Age norms limited, especially for old-old patients; affected by deficits in attention and memory.
Boston Naming Test (BNT)[f]	Task is to name line drawings of objects; 85-item and 60-item forms most commonly used.	*Pros*: Sensitive test of naming for high and low-frequency items; age norms available. *Cons*: Poorly educated patients may have reduced scores.
Controlled Oral Word Association Test[c]	Patient names items beginning with specified letters; typical procedure is to use 3 different letters with a 60-second report interval for each.	*Pros*: Sensitive test of verbal fluency and retrieval from semantic memory; age and education corrections through 64 years. *Cons*: Limited age norms for old-old patients.

[a]See text for additional references.
[b]Goodglass and Kaplan (1972, 1983).
[c]Benton and Hamsher (1976).
[d]Halstead and Wepman (1959); Reitan and Davison (1974).
[e]Boller and Vignolo (1966); Benton and Hamsher (1976).
[f]Kaplan, Goodglass, and Weintraub (1978); Goodglass and Kaplan (1983).

as many words as possible beginning with a specific letter. Three 60-second trials are given, each with a different letter; standard letter combinations include *FAS*, *CFL*, and *PRW*.

Benton and Hamsher (1976) provided ranges of scores for superior to severely impaired performance together with formulas for making age, education, and gender adjustments; however, the oldest age group included in the manual is 60 to 64 years. Table A.6 in the Appendix summarizes results of verbal fluency studies with older age groups. Mild declines in verbal fluency can be expected at advanced ages, even when subjects are healthy and well educated (Albert *et al.*, 1988). However, severe impairment is quite rare, even in advanced old age (Benton *et al.*, 1981).

Visuospatial Abilities

Visuospatial functioning, like secondary memory, is an area in which relatively pronounced age decrements can be expected with normal aging (see Chapter 3); however, qualitative analysis of performance can often distinguish normal and pathological visuospatial problems. Table 4.6 describes a few of the clinical visuospatial tests that have been used with older adults.

A Parietal Lobe Battery. The Boston Diagnostic Aphasia Examination (Goodglass & Kaplan, 1972) includes a series of brief tests designed to evaluate parietal lobe functions. Most involve some form of visuospatial processing, although several entail other cognitive operations as well. Specific tasks include drawing to command and copying of two- and three-dimensional figures, construction of designs using blocks and sticks, finger naming and identification, tests of right–left orientation, calculations, drawing of clock settings, and a test of topographical orientation.

Borod *et al.* (1980) observed decremental age differences across the span of 25 to 85 years on most tests from the Parietal Lobe Battery, including drawing to command, copying drawings, right–left orientation, and clock settings. Farver and Farver (1982) reported age declines from 40 to 89 years, with pronounced decrements in older age groups on clock settings and block constructions based on photographs. Samples for both of these studies were small and only briefly described. Although attempts were made to exclude individuals with neurological and psychiatric illnesses, little detail is provided about screening procedures; also, the oldest groups had relatively low levels of education (means $\leq$ 11 years).

WAIS or WAIS-R Performance Subtests. Performance subtests from the WAIS or WAIS-R are often used to evaluate visuospatial abilities. These subtests are complex measures, requiring the application of many different cognitive skills; therefore, deficits in other areas (e.g., attention) must be ruled out before inferences can be drawn about visuospatial preservations or impairments.

Block Design is one of the most informative Performance subtests for neuropsychological evaluation, although relatively pronounced age declines can be expected. This test examines both visuoperceptual and visuoconstructive ability; to perform well, the person must adapt to the novelty of the task, organize a series of responses, and monitor each step for accuracy. To achieve an age-scaled score of 10 on Block Design, a 70-year-old needs to obtain a total of only 16 points, compared to 32 points required for a 20-year-old and 25 points for a 45-year-old (Wechsler, 1981). A 70-year-old who completes only the first design correctly earns an age-scaled score of 5.

Attending to qualitative features of performance can increase the clinical utility of

TABLE 4.6. Tests of Visuospatial Abilities[a]

Measure	Description	Comments
Parietal Lobe Battery[b]	Subtests entail copying of designs and drawing to command, construction of figures using blocks and sticks, clock drawings, finger identification, right–left orientation, topographical location.	*Pros*: Survey of visuospatial and visuoconceptual skills; some age norms available. *Cons*: Time-consuming.
Performance subtests (WAIS or WAIS-R)[c]	5 subtests which require processing of visuospatial stimuli; 4 require motor responses; scoring based on time and accuracy.	*Pros*: Wide range of abilities assessed; age norms available; qualitative analysis informative. *Cons*: Complex tests that confound a variety of cognitive skills.
Visual Retention Test, Copy Administration (VRT-Copy)[d]	Subject copies 10 designs composed of 1 or more geometric figures.	*Pros*: Explicit scoring criteria; useful supplement to memory version of VRT. *Cons*: Age norms limited.
Rey-Osterrieth Complex Figure, Copy Administration[e]	Subject copies a complex design.	*Pros*: Can assess planning, attention to visuospatial detail. *Cons*: Age norms limited.
Judgment of Line Orientation[f]	Task is to match lines differing in angular orientation.	*Pros*: Relatively pure test of spatial perception; simple response required; some age norms available. *Cons*: Measures a single, restricted function.
Facial Recognition Test[g]	Task is to match pictures of faces presented from different orientations.	*Pros*: Relevant to everyday function; some age norms available. *Cons*: Requires good visual acuity; may be too difficult for some older patients.

[a]See text for additional references.
[b]Goodglass and Kaplan (1972, 1983).
[c]Wechsler (1955, 1981).
[d]Benton (1974).
[e]Rey (1941); Osterrieth (1944).
[f]Benton, Varney, and Hamsher (1978b).
[g]Benton, Van Allen, Hamsher, and Levin (1978a).

Block Design. Normal older adults often work slowly on this test and may resort to a trial-and-error method for placing individual blocks; some older patients refuse to attempt the most difficult items. On the simpler, four-block designs, errors usually involve relatively minor misplacements (e.g., incorrect orientation of a single block), whereas the more severe types of errors associated with right parietal brain lesions (e.g., stacking of blocks or failure to produce a square design) are rare in normal old people.

Drawing and Copying Tasks. Copying of two-dimensional designs can be evaluated by means of Administration C of the VRT (Benton, 1974) or the copy version of the Rey-

Osterrieth Complex Figure Test (Osterrieth, 1944; Rey, 1941; see, also, Lezak, 1983). Benton (1974) did not provide age norms for copying the VRT designs, so outcomes for older patients must be interpreted cautiously. However, when the memory version (Administration A) of the VRT is given, it is helpful to follow this with copying of designs to assess the contributions of visuospatial difficulties to performance on the memory task. For the Rey-Osterrieth Complex Figure Test, copying precedes reproduction of the figure from memory. In a healthy and well-educated sample, Van Gorp *et al.* (1990) found minimal age decline across the range of 57 to 85 years in Rey-Osterrieth copying performance.

Qualitative analysis of design copying may provide useful information, although there are few data available on error distributions in older samples. Farver and Farver (1982) noted a variety of errors in older adults' drawings from the Parietal Lobe Battery, including size errors, poor reproduction of angles, loss of perspective, rotations, errors in spatial relations, overscoring, and asymmetry. However, no information was provided about the frequency of these errors. In the author's experience, omissions of detail and minor distortions are the most common errors produced by normal older adults on simple design-copying tasks. On the interlocking pentagons of the MMSE, for example, a normal 80-year-old may "round" one or more of the angles, fail to close one of the angles, or slightly misplace the point of intersection. Similarly, on Administration C of the VRT, errors are likely to be limited to misplacement of an internal detail, minor distortions, or occasionally, omission of a peripheral figure. Gross distortions, omissions of major elements of a design, substitution of figures, or perseveration are rarely observed.

Other Visuospatial Measures. Benton *et al.* (1981) provided old-age normative data for Judgment of Line Orientation, a relatively simple test that is closely associated with right-hemisphere function (Benton *et al.*, 1978b). Young-old subjects (65 to 74 years) did not differ significantly from a 50- to 59-year-old standard group on this test, but there were slightly increased rates of defective performances among 75- to 84-year-olds (8% to 11%). On the Facial Recognition Test (Benton *et al.*, 1978a), in which the subject must match pictures of unfamiliar faces presented in different orientations, no deficits were observed among 65- to 69-year-olds, but 10% to 14% of 70- to 84-year-olds scored significantly below a 56- to 65-year-old normative group. Additional measures that tend to yield large decremental age differences include the Visual Organization Test (Hooper, 1958), in which the task is to identify pictures of cut-up objects by name (for age effects, see Farver & Farver, 1982; Mason & Ganzler, 1964; Montgomery, 1982), and picture recognition tests in which visually degraded or embedded items must be identified (see Chapter 3).

Problem Solving and Executive Functions

Table 4.7 describes tests that evaluate logical reasoning and problem solving and the ability to shift attention or action from one concept to another. As discussed in

TABLE 4.7. Tests of Reasoning, Problem Solving, and Executive Functions[a]

Measure	Description	Comments
WAIS or WAIS-R subtests[b]	Useful options include Similarities, Comprehension, Picture Arrangement, and Digit Symbol.	*Pros*: Potentially relevant to everyday function; age norms available. *Cons*: Influenced by education, social sophistication.
Progressive Matrices[c]	Task is to identify missing pieces of geometric patterns; advanced, standard, and colored versions available; latter version usually used with older adults.	*Pros*: Evaluates abstraction in a nonverbal mode; age norms available for colored version. *Cons*: Colored form insensitive to mild reasoning deficits, especially in well-educated patients.
Category Test[d]	Series of geometric figures presented; task is to infer "correct" attribute based on feedback from examiner; slide and booklet administrations available.	*Pros*: Sensitive test of abstract concept identification; some age norms available. *Cons*: Norms limited for old-old patients; too difficult and frustrating for many older adults.
Wisconsin Card Sort Test[e]	Patient sorts pictures of geometric figures and attempts to infer rule for classification based on feedback from examiner; once initial concept is established, classification rule is changed, and patient must identify new concept.	*Pros*: Same as for Category Test; also measures ability to shift from one concept to another. *Cons*: Same as for Category Test.
Stroop Color-Word Interference Test[f]	Series of three tasks: naming of color words, patches of color, and an interference task; in the latter, a list of color words is presented that has been printed in conflicting colors (e.g., *red* printed in green ink); the patient is told to name the colors of ink, ignoring the printed words.	*Pros*: Sensitive test of ability to inhibit a response; some age norms available. *Cons*: Measures a single, discrete skill; premium placed on speed.
Trail Making Test[g]	In Form A, task is to draw a line connecting a series of numbers scattered across a page, keeping correct numerical sequence; in Form B, the task is to alternate between numbers and letters, keeping both in correct sequence.	*Pros*: Brief test of sequencing, shifting between sequences; some age norms available. *Cons*: Confounds cognitive flexibility with scanning and motor speed.

[a]See text for additional references.
[b]Wechsler (1955, 1981).
[c]Raven (1960, 1965).
[d]DeFillipis, McCampbell, and Rogers (1979); Halstead (1947); Reitan and Davison (1974).
[e]Berg (1948); Heaton (1981).
[f]Stroop (1935); Golden (1978).
[g]Reitan (1958); Reitan and Davison (1974).

Chapter 3, formal tests of these abilities may seriously underestimate practical coping and problem-solving ability; therefore, it is important to supplement test information with other indicators of reasoning ability (e.g., observation of the patient in medical decision-making situations or interviews with family members).

Intelligence Subtests. Several subtests from the WAIS or WAIS-R provide a rough indication of reasoning abilities. Comprehension and Similarities estimate practical reasoning and verbal abstraction, respectively. Block Design and Object Assembly provide opportunities to observe how a person plans, evaluates, and modifies a series of responses. Picture Arrangement taps social and sequential reasoning in a nonverbal format, and Digit Symbol can be used to screen for problems with sequencing and inhibition (see below).

Tests of Concept Identification. A test of nonverbal reasoning that has been used fairly often with older adults is Progressive Matrices (Raven, 1965). Initial items require only simple visual matching, but more difficult items require identification of visual concepts (see Table 4.7 for a description). Percentile norms for the age range of 65 to 85 years are available in the test manual (Raven, 1965). These norms were based on a community-resident sample for Great Britain; health was said to be good, but educational characteristics were not specified. A more difficult version of this test, Standard Progressive Matrices (Raven, 1960), is also available (for age trends, see Burke, 1972; Guttman, 1981).

The Category Test from the HRNB and the Wisconsin Card Sort Test (WCST; Berg, 1948; Heaton, 1981) provide additional measures of concept identification. Both entail presentation of a series of geometric figures that differ in several dimensions (e.g., color and shape), and for both, the task is to infer a "correct" attribute or dimension based on feedback from the examiner. These measures are very similar to experimental tests of concept identification discussed in Chapter 3.

Several studies report large decremental age differences in performance on the Category Test. For example, Ernst (1987) found that 84% of a sample of community residents aged 65 to 75 years scored in the impaired range (i.e., 51 errors or more) on a booklet form of this test (cf. De Filippis, McCampbell, & Rogers, 1979). Most subjects performed well on the easier concepts but never learned the more complex or abstract concepts (cf. Mack & Carlson, 1978). This sample was screened to exclude individuals with a history of neurological or psychiatric disorder, but about half of the participants had chronic medical conditions (e.g., hypertension); also, the mean educational level was relatively low (10.3 years). Better educated or optimally healthy elderly adults may perform better on this measure (Heaton *et al.*, 1986; Willis, Yeo, Thomas, & Garry, 1988).

Most investigations using the WCST have also found substantial age differences (e.g., Berg, 1948; Heaton, 1981; Loranger & Misiak, 1960). However, a study of very healthy and well-educated elderly volunteers (Haaland, Vranes, Goodwin, & Garry, 1987) found relatively small age decrements compared to results from college undergraduates on a 64-card version of this test. Statistically significant decrements were limited to only two measures (number of categories attained and total errors) and to the oldest subgroup (80 to 87 years). A young-old subgroup (64 to 69 years) performed slightly better than the young adults. There were no significant differences among age groups in perseverative errors or failure to maintain a conceptual set.

Although the Category Test and the WCST may be useful for certain older patients (especially well-educated individuals when there is a question of frontal lobe deficits), they tend to be too demanding and frustrating for routine use with older adults. The abstract stimuli and arbitrary nature of these tasks can undermine motivation and may jeopardize willingness to continue with other types of tests. When administration of these measures is clinically indicated, the use of shortened forms is recommended. For the WCST, the first 64 cards can be given in lieu of the complete set of 128 (e.g., Haaland *et al.*, 1987); for short forms of the Category Test, see Sherrill (1985).

Additional Tests of Cognitive Flexibility. The Trail Making Test from the HRNB (Reitan, 1958) is a visuospatial sequencing measure that has commonly been included in geriatric studies (see Table 4.7 for a description). It requires organized visual search, motor tracking, and the ability to follow single and alternating sequences. Scores on the Trail Making Test correlate more highly with the overall impairment index from the HRNB than with any other single measure (Heaton *et al.*, 1986), and the easier version, Trails A, has been reported to distinguish between patients with early Alzheimer-type dementia and matched normal controls (Storandt *et al.*, 1984; Tierney *et al.*, 1987).

Table A.7 in the Appendix summarizes old-age normative data for the Trail Making Test. Studies with very old samples are rare; also, with the exception of the study by Van Gorp and colleagues (1990), these investigations provide very little information about sampling characteristics. The study by Davies (1968) has been the most widely cited as a normative reference because of the relatively large sample sizes and the inclusion of multiple age groups; however, almost no information was given in this study about subject characteristics. In the other investigations, the very large standard deviations are noteworthy, particularly on Part B in the oldest age brackets.

Because of the limitations in norms, the Trail Making Test tends to be most informative when extremes of performance are observed. Rapid, error-free completion of Trails B is a relatively strong contraindication of most forms of brain impairment; by contrast, repeated sequencing errors, failure to comprehend the task, or extremely protracted completion times should raise a question of pathology.

Another important aspect of cognitive flexibility is the ability to inhibit overlearned responses. One of the best clinical measures of this skill is the Stroop Color-Word Interference Test, which entails naming of colors and reading of color words, followed by an interference task which requires ignoring of printed words (see Table 4.7 for a description). Completion times are increased in late adulthood for all components of the test, but there is a proportionally greater age handicap on the interference test (Comalli, 1965; Comalli, Krus, & Wapner, 1965). Golden (1978) provided a standardized version of this test; age corrections are given for two ranges (45 to 64 years and 65 to 80 years) based on a composite of normative data, including those of Comalli *et al.* (1965).

A final useful measure of cognitive flexibility is the Digit Symbol subtest from the WAIS or WAIS-R. This test requires that symbols be copied in a partially random sequence. Few normal older adults have problems with this aspect of the task; by contrast, patients with even mild dementia may have difficulty adhering to the specified sequence and may revert to copying symbols in consecutive numerical order. Therefore, when only brief testing can be performed, the Digit Symbol subtest can be used to screen for abnormal difficulties with sequencing and response inhibition.

Personality and Mood

Table 4.8 describes a few of the measures that can be used to evaluate personality and mood in older patients. Lawton, Whelihan, and Belsky (1980) and Hassinger, Smith, and La Rue (1989) have provided more detailed reviews.

Traditional psychodiagnostic measures, such as the MMPI (Hathaway & McKinley, 1943), Rorschach Inkblot Test (Rorschach, 1942), and the Thematic Apperception Test (TAT; Murray, 1943) can be used with good effect with older patients who have adequate cognitive function and sufficient attention and motivation. Contemporary age norms have been provided for the MMPI by Colligan, Osborne, Swenson, and Offord (1984). The MMPI-2 (Butcher, Dahlstrom, Graham, Tellegen, & Kaemmer, 1989) does not provide separate norms for older patients; however, elderly volunteers were included in the standardization sample. For patients who cannot complete the full inventory, several MMPI short forms have been developed (e.g., Kincannon, 1968; Overall & Gomez-Mont, 1974), including a 168-item orally administered version designed for patients with mild cognitive impairment (Sbordone & Caldwell, 1979); these abbreviated versions may be useful for identifying salient symptoms and concerns but should not be viewed as interchangeable with the standard MMPI. Of the various options for projective testing, we have found the TAT to be most useful for older psychiatric patients (cf. Lawton *et al.*, 1980). A Geriatric Apperception Test (GAT; Wolk & Wolk, 1971) has also been developed. Findings for the Rorschach among older patients are conflicting (see discussions in Hassinger *et al.*, 1989; Lawton *et al.*, 1980), several studies reporting constricted and stereotyped answers in normal older people.

Brief symptom-rating scales can be used to screen for psychiatric illness or to provide a quantitative measure of symptom severity. Depression rating scales (see Table 4.8 for some options) are particularly useful in light of the high prevalence of depressive symptoms in older people. Chapter 11 provides further information about these scales.

For very impaired patients, examiners generally rely on relatives' accounts of behavior and emotional reactions. The Relatives' Assessment of Global Symptomatology (RAGS; Raskin & Crook, 1988) provides a brief survey of psychiatric and behavioral symptoms noted by caregivers; the Neuropsychology Behavior and Affect

TABLE 4.8. Measures of Personality, Mood, and Behavior[a]

Measure	Description	Comments
Minnesota Multiphasic Personality Inventory (MMPI, MMPI-2)[b]	True-false self-report questionnaire; items assess a wide range of emotions, thoughts, behaviors	*Pros*: Well-known and widely researched; surveys multiple symptom areas; includes an estimate of response bias; new age norms recently reported. *Cons*: Profiles do not conform to current diagnostic nosology; standard form too demanding for many older patients; short forms of questionable validity and reliability.
Thematic Apperception Test (TAT)[c]	Patient creates stories for pictures portraying people in various scenes; responses rated for emotional content and organization	*Pros*: Well known; useful for patients who deny or lack awareness of emotional problems; probes socially relevant reactions. *Cons*: Some older patients respond in a very constricted manner; lack of standard age adjustments in interpretive guidelines.
Hamilton Depression Rating Scale (HAM-D)[d]	23-item observer-rated measure of depressive symptoms	*Pros*: Well known and widely researched; surveys wide range of depressive symptoms; useful for patients who deny or lack awareness of depression. *Cons*: Scores may be inflated for older patients because of inclusion of somatic items.
Beck Depression Inventory (BDI)[e]	21-item self-report measure with multiple-choice alternatives; 13-item short-form available.	*Pros*: Well known and widely researched; good measure of subjective symptoms of depression. *Cons*: Does not adequately survey vegetative symptoms of of depression.
Geriatric Depression Scale (GDS)[f]	30-item true-false self-report scale; specifically omits somatic items; 15-item short form available.	*Pros*: Developed specifically for older patients; simple response format. *Cons*: Does not adequately survey vegetative symptoms of depression.
Relatives' Assessment of Global Symptomatology (RAGS)[g]	21-item scale assessing frequency of psychiatric and behavioral problems	*Pros*: Brief; surveys wide range of symptoms; examples given for each item to assist untrained observers. *Cons*: Norms limited.
Neuropsychology Behavior and Affect Profile[h]	106 items tapping mood and behavioral symptoms observed in brain injury; completed twice, for current and premorbid states	*Pros*: Designed specificially for use in known or suspected brain injury; preliminary age norms available. *Cons*: Lengthy; new scale requiring additional study.

[a]See text for additional references.
[b]Hathaway and McKinley (1943); Butcher, Dahlstrom, Graham, Tellegen, and Kaemmer (1989).
[c]Murray (1943); Wolk and Wolk (1971).
[d]Hamilton (1967).
[e]Beck, Ward, Mendelson, Mock, and Erbaugh (1961); Beck and Beck (1972).
[f]Yesavage, Brink, Rose, Lum, Huang, Adey, and Leirer (1983a).
[g]Raskin and Crook (1988).
[h]Nelson, Satz, Mitrushina, Van Gorp, Cicchetti, Lewis, and Van Lancker (1989).

Profile (Nelson, Satz, Mitrushina, Van Gorp, Cicchetti, Lewis, & Van Lancker, 1989) is another promising measure, particularly for patients with known or suspected brain injury (see Table 4.8 for descriptions).

BRIEF AND EXTENDED TEST BATTERIES

Table 4.9 presents a brief neuropsychological battery tailored to older patients. These tests can be administered to most older patients in about 1½ hours. A broad range of cognitive functions is probed, and in several of the areas most sensitive to brain impairment (e.g., learning and memory, speeded perceptual-motor integration), more than one score is available to be used in estimating ability.

This battery can be used for several purposes, including screening for suspected dementia, providing a pretreatment baseline for depressed patients who also have cognitive impairment, and estimating areas of strength and weakness in individuals with known brain impairment. The last column in Table 4.9 notes some of the findings which raise a question of significant cognitive impairment. These deficits exceed those typically observed in normal aging and are most commonly observed in patients with organic mental disorders; however, patients with severe psychiatric disturbance (e.g., psychotic depression) sometimes have similar problems (see Chapter 11).

Table 4.10 presents guidelines for extending the brief battery. Specific tests to be added will vary from patient to patient, depending on the overall level of performance and areas of deficit suggested in the brief evaluation.

On occasion, it may be more beneficial to repeat a particular test several times than to add different measures. This approach is useful when symptoms fluctuate markedly within a brief time period or when testing is used to evaluate treatment effects.

For both brief and extended batteries, it is important to cross-validate test outcomes with more practical sources of information. In an inpatient setting, observations of a patient's daily activities can help one to determine if there are practical correlates of deficits on memory or visuospatial tests (e.g., trouble recalling staff names, disorientation to place or time, or trouble learning room locations). For outpatients, input from relatives or friends can be used to identify everyday strengths and problems. When these practical sources of information fail to corroborate the impairments noted on testing, deficits should be interpreted cautiously, and alternative explanations of impairments should be considered.

SUMMARY AND CONCLUSIONS

Psychologists can often make a significant contribution to the well-being of an older client by making certain that normal aging changes are considered in diagnostic assessments. Neuropsychological testing provides the most thorough means of judging

TABLE 4.9. Brief Battery for Geropsychological Assessment

Recommended tests	Functions evaluated	Findings that raise a question of impairment
Mini-Mental State Examination	Cognitive mental status	Scores ≤ 23[a]
WAIS or WAIS-R		
Vocabulary	Verbal intelligence; semantic memory	Perseveration, paraphasia, marked circumlocution
Digit Span	Attention; primary memory	Forward span < 5; backward span < 3
Block Design	Nonverbal intelligence; visuospatial abilities; nonverbal problem solving	Stacking or stringing of blocks; grossly inaccurate designs
Digit Symbol	Speeded perceptual-motor integration; sequencing and cognitive flexibility	Inaccurate copies of symbols; inability to adhere to specified sequence
WMS or WMS-R		
Logical Memory	Narrative recall	Complete recall failure; confusing details from the two stories; major extrastory intrusions; marked decline on delayed recall
Visual Reproduction	Recall of designs	Complete recall failure; rotations, perseverations; gross distortions; marked decline on delayed recall
Object Memory Evaluation[b]	List learning and recall	≤ 7 items stored by Trial 5; ≤ 2 items consistently recalled per trial; multiple intrusion errors; marked decline on delayed recall
Boston Naming Test	Naming; object identification	Perseveration, paraphasia, marked circumlocution, frequent perceptual errors
Controlled Oral Word Association Test	Verbal fluency; semantic memory	Severely reduced output (≤ 7 items per letter); loss of set; perseveration or paraphasia
Trail Making Test	Speeded perceptual-motor integration; sequencing and cognitive flexibility	Severe slowing (> 2 minutes to complete Trails A, ≥ 5 minutes Trails B); any error on A, multiple errors on B

[a]Adjust for age and education (see text).
[b]For high-functioning patients, substitute the Selective Reminding Test, Auditory Verbal Learning Test, or California Verbal Learning Test; for low-functioning or uncooperative patients, the Shopping List Test or Delayed Word Recall Test can be substituted.

the age-appropriateness of cognitive performance and of detecting cognitive and behavioral problems that cannot be considered typical for the patient's age.

Procedures for assessing cognitive functions are numerous and varied, and since the early 1980s, significant progress has been made in extending norms for different tests into upper age ranges. The WAIS-R and WMS-R both include norms through age 74, the LNNB incorporates an age-adjustment procedure, and many studies of aged samples have been reported for the HRNB, Benton's neuropsychological measures, and the

TABLE 4.10. Principles for Extending the Brief Battery

General aims

1. Provide multiple indicators of each area.
2. Increase depth of assessment where deficits are suspected.

Recommended additions

Intelligence: Complete WAIS or WAIS-R.

Attention: Mental Control scale from WMS or WMS-R; digit cancellation.

Learning and memory: Associate Learning from WMS or WMS-R; nonverbal recognition memory (Visual Retention Test-Multiple Choice or Continuous Recognition Test); consider complete WMS-R so that summary indices may be calculated.

Visuospatial abilities: Rey-Osterrieth Complex Figure Test; Clock Drawings or other subtests from Parietal Lobe Battery; Facial Recognition Test.[a]

Language: Additional subtests from the Boston Diagnostic Aphasia Examination or Multilingual Aphasia Examination.[b]

Cognitive flexibility and reasoning: Progressive Matrices, Stroop Color-Word Interference Test, Wisconsin Card Sort Test.[c]

Mood and personality: MMPI, TAT, depression rating scales, relatives' ratings.[d]

[a]Include if parietal dysfunction suspected.
[b]Include if aphasic disorders other than anomia suspected.
[c]Include if frontal deficits suspected.
[d]Include if psychiatric disorder suggested by history or clinical interview.

original WMS. In addition, several specialized tests have been developed for use with older adults, particularly in the area of learning and memory.

Despite these advances, clinical assessment of older individuals remains a challenging task. There are still significant gaps in age norms for most measures, particularly for people aged 80 years and older; education and health differences are also poorly represented in the norms for many tests. Attention to qualitative features of performance can increase the information gained from many tests; however, as noted in Chapter 5, this type of interpretation entails considerable personal judgment. These technical restrictions, combined with more fundamental limitations on the understanding of brain–behavior relations, reinforce the need for cautious interpretation and for careful integration of test results with other clinical indicators (see Chapter 5).

5

Examples of Normal Performance

The first step in interpreting neuropsychological test outcomes is to determine whether performance is within normal limits for age and background. This chapter provides guidelines for making this determination and uses case examples to illustrate test selection and interpretation.

The first section presents a general framework for interpreting neuropsychological findings. Three case examples are then discussed. These examples address the most common presenting problem in geropsychological testing—that is, the question of failing memory. In each case, an argument is made that cognitive functioning was generally consistent with age and background, despite some areas of weaknesses in performance.

INTERPRETING NEUROPSYCHOLOGICAL FINDINGS

There are many differences of opinion among neuropsychologists about methods of test interpretation. Some rely almost exclusively on objective indicators of level of performance (e.g., percentile rankings or z scores); others evaluate test profiles, error patterns, or the manner in which a patient works on various tasks (for contrasting examples, see Lezak, 1983, 1984; Milberg *et al.*, 1986; Reitan, 1986; Russell, 1984). Many combine several different approaches, as recommended below.

The following sections present a series of interpretive questions that can be applied to test findings and other clinical data. By answering these questions, an examiner can usually arrive at an opinion about the overall adequacy of performance; when deficits exceed normal limits, additional questions concerning differential diagnosis can then be posed (see Chapters 7, 8, 9, and 11).

Judging Performance on Individual Tests

The simplest level of interpretation considers performance on individual tests. There are three important questions to be asked at this level.

1. *Is performance quantitatively within normal limits?*

For any measure with appropriate norms, scores that are 1½ to 2 standard deviations below the mean are sufficient to raise a question of impaired performance. Normative reference points should be selected by considering a patient's educational background, gender, and medical and residential status, in addition to chronological age (see Chapter 4). When several normative studies are available for a particular test (see Appendix), the sample that most closely approximates a given patient's characteristics should usually be selected as the standard of comparison, unless sample sizes are very small or procedures are unclear (cf. D'Elia, Satz, & Schretlen, 1989).

2. *Are qualitative aspects of performance appropriate for age and background?*

Qualitative analysis encompasses many aspects of behavior, some of which are task-specific. Monitoring of errors is often included under the heading of qualitative analysis, although the diagnostic significance attached to most errors depends on frequency of occurrence. Some of the errors that raise a question of brain impairment for older patients were discussed in Chapter 4 and summarized in Table 4.9. Many of these errors occur in low frequencies, even in patients with documented brain impairment; therefore, while the presence of certain errors may be meaningful, their absence does not rule out the possibility of brain disorder. Also, as age increases, greater overlap is seen in certain errors made by normal individuals and patients with brain impairment, so that a more lenient standard may be required in interpreting errors of older patients.

Other qualitative features that are important to monitor include comprehension of instructions, spontaneous use of strategies, and self-perceptions of performance. For example, when a very old person readily comprehends the nature of an unfamiliar task such as Wechsler Adult Intelligence Scale—Revised (WAIS-R) Digit Symbol and works methodically, although slowly, the impression of normality of performance is strengthened, even if the quantitative score is below expectations for the oldest normative group. Similarly, on verbal free-recall tasks, spontaneous application of a mnemonic strategy supports an impression of normal behavior. Accurate self-appraisal of cognitive skills suggests that judgment and self-monitoring are intact; by contrast, denial of obvious cognitive problems, or persistent self-criticism despite good performance, is rare in normal aging.

3. *How malleable are the deficits in performance?*

As discussed in Chapter 3, a hallmark of normal older people's performance on cognitive tests is that scores can improve with practice or instruction. There are many informal ways to evaluate flexibility in performance. On memory tests, it can be helpful to propose mnemonic strategies and to see if performance improves. On Block Design, suggesting a one-block-at-a-time approach or a more specific organizational strategy can help in evaluating sensitivity to increased external structure. Simply repeating tests to evaluate practice effects can also be informative. Indications that an older person can readily benefit from cues and practice tend to strengthen the impression of normal ability.

Evaluating Performance across a Battery of Tests

Comparing performance across tests is considerably more difficult than interpreting single measures. The reliability of difference scores must be taken into account, and often, too little is known about intercorrelations among tests to allow one to interpret discrepancies with confidence. The following questions are important to ask about intertest comparisons.

4. *Are the observed discrepancies in level of performance large enough to be clinically significant?*

The diagnostic importance of intertest discrepancies has been most thoroughly researched for the WAIS and WAIS-R. Traditionally, differences of 15 points or more between Verbal IQ (VIQ) and Performance IQ (PIQ) and of 3 or more points between scaled scores for different subtests have been used to raise a question of impairment (Wechsler, 1955, 1981). However, differences of this magnitude occur quite often in the normal population (e.g., Matarazzo & Prifitera, 1989; Matarazzo, Daniel, Prifitera, & Herman, 1988). In one analysis (Matarazzo & Prifitera, 1989), almost one-half (48.7%) of the WAIS-R standardization sample were shown to have differences of 7 or more points between scaled scores for their highest and lowest subtests. The reliability of various WAIS-R difference scores (e.g., VIQ-PIQ discrepancies) is also considerably lower than that of individual scores (e.g., Matarazzo & Herman, 1984; cf. Snow *et al.*, 1989, discussed in Chapter 4). Well-educated individuals and people over the age of 65 tend to exhibit greater scatter across subtests than younger adults or those with average education (McLean, Reynolds, & Kaufman, 1990).

When comparisons are made across tests that have been normed with separate samples, discrepant scores become more difficult to interpret, since sampling differences may be responsible for apparent discrepancies in levels of performance (Russell, 1984). For example, if performance on the Object Memory Evaluation (OME) and the Wechsler Memory Scale (WMS) Logical Memory were compared for a 70-year-old patient with nine years of education, memory for paragraphs might appear to be more impaired than list learning if Logical Memory scores were interpreted with norms obtained from a healthy, well-educated sample (e.g., Albert *et al.*, 1988, or Van Gorp *et al.*, 1990, in Table A.1 in the Appendix), while OME scores were compared to norms for a more average elderly group (Fuld, 1981).

Whenever possible, it is important to assess the reliability of differences between tests, either by administering additional measures designed to evaluate similar functions, or by repeating measures on a second occasion. When an aberrant score is observed, it is important to query the patient and other informants about lifelong areas of strength and weakness to better assess the possibility that the deficit is "normal" for the individual. Finally, especially when using individualized batteries, normative reference points must be chosen with care to minimize effects of sampling differences on interpretation.

5. *Does variability across tests fall within normal ranges, or does the pattern of performance suggest the presence of a specific disorder?*

When sizable intertest discrepancies are observed, it is a common clinical practice to compare the pattern of intertest scatter to profiles that are considered typical of certain psychiatric or neurological disorders. Neuropsychological profiles have been proposed for all of the major neurological and psychiatric disorders of old age, including Alzheimer-type and multi-infarct dementias, Parkinson's disease, and depression (see Chapters 7, 8, 9, and 11). These profiles are occasionally quite specific, as in Fuld's WAIS subtest formula (1984) for differentiating among dementias (see Chapter 7). Usually, however, the hypothesized patterns concern relationships among cognitive processes (e.g., attention versus memory) that may be inferred from various tests.

Despite the popularity of profile analysis, it is important to note that research has raised serious concerns about the validity of diagnostic test patterns (for recent examples, see Anthony *et al.*, 1980; Matarazzo & Prifitera, 1989; McDermott, Glutting, Jones, & Noonan, 1989; Piedmont, Sokolove, & Fleming, 1989). Very little is known about the base rates of different neuropsychological profiles in the normal population (cf. McDermott *et al.*, 1989). Further complications arise from the paucity of cross-validation research (see Chapter 2), a lack of precision in diagnosis (see Chapters 6, 7, 8, 9, and 11), and the complexity and crudeness of clinical tests (see Chapter 4). The inherent complexity of brain–behavior relationships also casts doubt on the search for simple correlations between specific tests and disorders (see Chapters 2 and 3).

In working with older patients, special consideration must be given to the possibility that discrepant performances are due to normal aging changes. For example, as discussed in Chapter 3, individuals who do well on tests of crystallized verbal intelligence and less well on those tapping fluid intellectual abilities may be exhibiting the effects of normal aging. Mild problems with secondary memory may also be age-consistent. By contrast, impairments in short-term memory or receptive language run counter to the "normal aging profile" (see Table 3.2).

In general, discrepancies among test performances are most likely to be diagnostically significant when they are large in magnitude, when they are at variance with normal aging trends, and when several tests measuring a particular function (e.g., learning and memory) yield lower scores than those assessing other abilities.

Integrating Test Results with Other Clinical Data

To be clinically useful, neuropsychological results must be integrated with other clinical data. Some of the more important areas of comparison are noted below.

6. *How does current performance compare with estimates of prior ability?*

Clinicians use a variety of methods for estimating premorbid or baseline abilities. One popular approach is to use regression equations based on demographic variables such as age, education, and occupation to estimate premorbid IQ (Barona, Reynolds, & Chastain, 1984; Wilson, Rosenbaum, Brown, Rourke, Whitman, & Gisell, 1978). However, most studies attempting to validate these equations show that correlations between actual IQ and estimates obtained by regression are too low to be of much clinical utility (Klesges & Troster, 1987; Sweet, Moberg, & Tovian, 1990). Another method of estimating premorbid ability capitalizes on the relatively good preservation of word-reading skills in dementia and many other forms of brain injury. The National Adult Reading Test developed in Great Britain (Nelson, 1982; Nelson & McKenna, 1975) provides a brief test for assessing this ability. A modified version has been developed for use in Canada and the United States, and in a preliminary evaluation (Blair & Preen, 1989), IQ estimates derived from this test showed a stronger correlation with actual IQ than did estimates derived from a demographic regression equation (r's = .75 and .47, respectively).

Interviews of the patient and family members should be used to supplement the ability estimates obtained by regression or other testing. Often, an informal discussion can help one to identify idiosyncratic problems or strengths (e.g., "never was able to remember names" or "always good with numbers") that may contribute to intertest scatter. Also, with elderly patients, it is important to estimate functioning from recent as well as early life phases, and to evaluate the time course of any suspected declines.

7. *How does test performance compare with current functioning in everyday settings?*

Functional assessment, using behavioral observations or interviews with the patient and family members, provides a rough means of validating test results. For example, some older people readily learn important features of the hospital environment (e.g., staff names, topographical routes, and medication regimes) but, when formally tested, may show pronounced impairment in learning and memory. A less common situation is when the person does well on formal testing but impresses staff and fellow patients as markedly impaired in everyday function. Searching for explanations of these differing estimates of ability can suggest new hypotheses about a patient's behavior that would not arise from test results alone. The complexity of demands imposed by everyday life can lead to significant dysfunction even when fairly good performance is observed during structured testing; alternatively, a familiar home environment may provide opportunities for compensation that are not apparent in the test situation.

8. *How do test results compare with other neurodiagnostic findings?*

In medical settings, most patients who are referred for neuropsychological testing also receive other neurodiagnostic tests such as computerized tomography (CT) scans, electroencephalography (EEG), or magnetic resonance imaging (MRI) scans. The degree of correspondence than can be expected among these measures varies with the nature of the brain disorder. In dementia of the Alzheimer type, for example, neuropsychological testing may suggest impairment, while CT or MRI scans are normal (see Chapters 2 and 7); by contrast, in normal aging, MRI scans may show periventricular lucencies when cognitive function is still intact (see Chapters 2 and 8).

In general, greater correspondence should be expected between neuropsychological and neuroradiological findings for focal brain injuries of recent origin than for diffuse degenerative conditions. Since many brain disorders of old patients fall into the latter category, neuropsychologists working in geriatric settings often cannot rely on other neurodiagnostic tests to corroborate test results.

Combining Interpretive Criteria

The use of multiple interpretive approaches provides a system of checks and balances that may help to reduce diagnostic errors. For example, if mild quantitative deficits are noted on only a few tests, the significance attached to these findings is likely to be reduced if performance is free of pathognomonic errors, if everyday function is intact, and if the low points of the performance profile are consistent with normal aging trends. By contrast, even mild problems noted on testing may be clinically important if they pertain to abilities not normally affected by aging and if there are other functional or neurodiagnostic data that also raise a question of impairment. When several different methods of interpretation lead to similar conclusions, diagnostic impressions can be stated with a high degree of confidence.

There are no fixed rules for weighing the importance of different interpretive criteria. A particular criterion may be a deciding factor in one case but of little significance in another, depending on the characteristics of the patient, the relative completeness of testing and other clinical data, and the training and experience of the examiner.

CASE EXAMPLES

A Young-Old Person with Subjective Complaints

The first example concerns a 58-year-old man (Example 5.1) whose assessment was prompted by his concerns that he might be developing Alzheimer's disease. Both his mother and a maternal aunt had developed severe and progressive dementias in their later years, with onset estimated at about age 76. These relatives died without autopsy, but Alzheimer's disease had apparently been mentioned as the most likely diagnosis during clinical evaluations.

Because Alzheimer's disease has been widely publicized in recent years, the general public, as well as many health care professionals, appears to be overestimating the prevalence of this condition in older adults (see Chapter 1). One consequence is an increase in self-referrals for assessment of memory or other cognitive complaints, usually prompted by fears of encroaching Alzheimer's disease. The man in this example had more reason to be concerned than most, in light of his close blood relationship with relatives who may have had the disease (see Chapter 7).

The patient complained primarily of learning and memory problems. For a few months preceding the evaluation, he found that he needed to study longer than in the past to learn something new. He reported having to use lists to remember things, whereas previously, especially in his 20 years as a produce supplier, he had been able to remember many details without mnemonic assists. In addition, the patient expressed dissatisfaction with his ability to control his anger. He did not provide details of specific incidents but noted that he had recently quarreled with a co-worker as well as with his wife. He indicated that this was not a new problem and that he was attempting to deal with it by suppression (e.g., "I try not to get angry; I've always had a temper, but this past year I've made a concerted effort to control it").

The patient's medical history was quite complicated. He had twice been evaluated for chest pain, about 10 years and 7 years before this testing. In neither case was a diagnosis of cardiac illness made, and in the more recent evaluation, he had been told that his symptoms were due to anxiety and was referred for psychological counseling. The patient had also been successfully treated for melanoma about 10 years before; he was regularly followed by his oncologist, and there had been no indications of recurrence of the cancer. He had been diagnosed as having mild, adult-onset diabetes, which was adequately managed through dietary restriction, and about a year before this testing, he had been in a motor vehicle accident which resulted in a cracked vertebra but no loss of consciousness or head injury.

The patient reported some joint and muscle pain, for which he occasionally took propoxyphene hydrochloride (Darvocet). His only other medical complaint concerned insomnia; his sleep problems consisted primarily of early-morning awakening and had been constant for the past 10 years.

Because the patient was paying for the assessment himself and had limited financial means, only a brief screening was performed. In selecting tests to administer, the aims were to tap intellectual ability, verbal and nonverbal learning and memory, confrontation naming and verbal fluency, and selected frontal functions, as well as personality. Naming and verbal fluency were examined because mild anomic aphasia, combined with problems with memory, are among the earliest reported signs of dementia of the Alzheimer type (see Chapter 7). Because the patient was only 58 years old and from an average educational and occupational background, standard tests (e.g., the WAIS-R and WMS-R) were considered appropriate (see Chapter 4 for descriptions and critiques of the various tests).

The patient's behavior during testing was interesting in several respects. Although he was generally cooperative, persistent, and highly motivated, there was a circumstantial and overly elaborate quality to a number of his responses. When asked to describe an average workday, he began as follows: "Up at 5:00 A.M., have breakfast, brush teeth, do the crossword puzzle," and so on. During verbal fluency testing, he paused on several occasions to indicate that a certain item should be counted twice because it had more than one meaning. On WMS-R Logical Memory, he ended both recitations by criticizing the specific content of the stories. Concerning the first story, he said that it didn't make sense for the woman to go hungry when she worked in a cafeteria; concerning the second, he stated that the person who wrote the story didn't know what he was talking about because a broken axle would never cause a truck to swerve into a ditch.

EXAMPLE 5.1

Background

Fifty-eight-year-old Caucasian man.

Has owned and operated a carpet-cleaning business for 10 years; formerly in produce supply business.

High school degree plus occasional college courses.

Married twice; conflicts with current spouse.

Medical history significant for two episodes of chest pain but no cardiac illness confirmed; successful treatment for malignant melanoma localized to left foot; mild adult-onset diabetes managed through diet; motor vehicle accident with no loss of consciousness or injury to head; chronic insomnia.

Occasionally takes propoxyphene hydrochloride (Darvocet) for joint and muscle pain.

Family history significant for dementia.

Purpose of evaluation

Sought assessment because "I'm starting not to remember what I used to remember."

Behavior during testing

Cooperative, motivated, persistent.

Occasional circumstantiality, impulsivity.

Test findings

WAIS-R:	Age-scaled score	Percentile
Vocabulatory	13	84
Digit Span	14	91
Similarities	13	84
Block Design	11	63
Digit Symbol	9	37
WMS-R:	Raw score	Percentile/rating
Verbal Memory Index	87	91–95
Logical Memory		
Immediate	34	94
Delayed	24	87
Visual Reproduction		
Immediate	19	7
Delayed	19	22
Mental Control	5	50
Verbal Paired Associates		
Immediate	19	63
Delayed	7	50
Incidental Recall (max = 9)	8	High normal
Boston Naming Test (60 items)	57	63
Controlled Oral Word Association Test	44 words	High normal

Trail Making Test—Part B:	92 seconds	50
Stroop Color-Word Interference Test (100-item interference card)	123 seconds	Normal
MMPI—Welsch code: 943651-72/80:F-K:L#		

Qualitative aspects of performance

No errors of intrusion on tests of verbal learning and recall; no perseverations, rotations, or size errors on Visual Reproduction. Somewhat careless in drawing designs and circumstantial during recall of stories.

Interpretation and recommendations

Performance on tests of language, verbal intelligence, and verbal learning and memory argues against early dementia. Lower nonverbal performance could be interpreted in several ways (normal verbal superiority, subclinical mania, mild subcortical or frontal impairment); personality was considered an important contributing factor. Marital therapy and a medical evaluation for insomnia were recommended.

He was also mildly expansive and inappropriate on occasion, particularly as the testing proceeded. For example, when he talked about the cancer surgery on his foot, he immediately asked if I would like to see the scar and reached to remove his shoe. In addition, on the WMS-R Visual Reproduction subscale, his drawings were completed very quickly and somewhat carelessly.

The patient scored above average on all tests of language ability, verbal intelligence, and verbal learning and memory. His verbal output was free of paraphasias, perseverations, and intrusions. His answers to WAIS-R Vocabulary and Similarities items were quick, succinct, and appropriate.

Performance was somewhat lower overall on nonverbal measures. On Digit Symbol, his score was at the 37th percentile for age, compared to the 84th percentile for Vocabulary and Similarities. His score on Block Design was somewhat higher (63rd percentile); however, he was unable to complete one of the simpler 4-block designs, even with extra time, and on the last three 9-block figures, there were some instances of apparent figure–ground misperception and inefficient trial-and-error. On Visual Reproduction from the WMS-R, his immediate recall score was only at the 7th percentile for age; he lost points on this test for omission of a major figure (design 4) as well as distortion and oversimplification of minor components (designs 1 and 3). It is important to note that after a 30-minute delay, he retained all of the information he had initially reproduced. This was true on incidental recall of Digit Symbol pairs as well, where he was able to reproduce eight of the nine pairs from memory; this performance is above expectations for normal older adults (Hart, Kwentus, Wade, & Hamer, 1987c).

Speed and accuracy of performance on both the Stroop Color-Word Interference Test and Trail B were also within normal limits for age (Comalli *et al.*, 1965; Davies,

1968; cf. Table A.7 in the Appendix). The patient made one sequencing error on Trail B and two naming errors on the interference portion of the Stroop, but he quickly identified and corrected these errors on his own.

On the Minnesota Multiphasic Personality Inventory (MMPI), scores on the Validity subscales suggested that the patient responded in a somewhat nonconformist or idiosyncratic manner. None of the clinical scales was elevated above 70 *T*, although scales 9 and 4 approached this level (*T* scores = 69 and 68, respectively). Assessment of individual items endorsed by the patient suggested resentment of authority figures, social imperturbability, excitability, stubbornness, and a sense of self-importance.

The general pattern of cognitive test results did not support a diagnosis of Alzheimer's disease. Specific strengths that ran counter to the early indications of this disease include above-average verbal learning and recall; fluent, accurate verbalization and confrontation naming; and good incidental learning and recall (see Chapter 7).

On nonverbal measures, performance was generally lower, although still within normal limits for the patient's age and background. A sizable percentage of normal adults exhibit large Verbal/Performance discrepancies on the WAIS-R (Matarazzo *et al.*, 1988), and therefore, this patient may have been among those normal individuals who are characteristically more adept at verbal than at nonverbal tasks. Also, since the Mania subscale was the high point on the MMPI profile, the patient could be expected to have a somewhat impulsive and disorganized style of information processing. This would rarely interfere with highly practiced tasks but could have undermined performance on the more novel nonverbal tasks. Some indications of impulsivity and poor organization were noted on Visual Reproduction and Block Design.

These behaviors could also have resulted from subcortical or frontal brain impairment. At least three etiologies for cerebral impairment were considered: fluctuating serum glucose levels resulting from diabetes; sleep apnea; and chronic low-level exposure to an environmental toxin. The patient reported normal serum glucose levels on all recent checkups, so the first possibility seemed unlikely. Second, although his insomnia was significant and of long duration, he did not suffer from excessive daytime sleepiness as might be expected with sleep apnea. Finally, the patient emphatically indicated that he used only cleaning solvents that contained no organophosphates and provided lists of their chemical contents consistent with this claim.

This evaluation did not disclose why the patient had recently become so concerned about his cognitive functions. His sister, who had cared for his mother in the later stages of her dementia, had recently visited the patient; this visit may have reminded him of his mother's condition and stimulated his concerns about everyday memory failures. It is also important to note that the patient had several significant emotional stressors, including marital and job conflicts and persistent problems with sleep. Because he had been treated successfully for medical problems in the past, he may have found it easier to focus on a problem that might have a medical basis (i.e., memory complaints) than to face his emotional or social concerns directly.

This assessment cannot rule out an incipient dementia, since personality changes have occasionally been noted as prodromal indicators in Alzheimer's disease (see

Chapter 7). However, deficits in learning and recall are by far the more common initial indications of Alzheimer-type dementia, and this patient's verbal learning and recall were well above normative expectations; even on a nonverbal memory task in which his immediate performance was poor, retention over time was not impaired. These findings, combined with normal scores on language measures, and the Stroop and Trail Making tests, failed to provide consistent or strong support for an interpretation of brain impairment. A better interpretation might be that lifelong personality traits contributed to this patient's social and emotional problems, which in turn increased his anxiety about everyday cognitive lapses.

Several recommendations were made to the patient based on assessment outcomes. Marital therapy was suggested, as was a comprehensive evaluation for sleep disturbance. The sleep evaluation would provide neuroencephalographic and neuroradiologic studies that could be useful in identifying neurological impairment, as well as provide information about his sleep disorder. The patient expressed relief that most of his test scores were in the normal range and was particularly interested in pursuing the recommended workup for his insomnia.

Fluctuations in Performance over Time

Example 5.2 uses findings from a clinical research study to illustrate mild memory problems that failed to progress when evaluated longitudinally. Participants in this project were relatives of patients with probable Alzheimer's disease who received periodic evaluations of medical, psychiatric, and neuropsychological functioning. Although they had not sought clinical advice because of cognitive or emotional problems, a majority of these participants had a high level of concern about their cognitive functioning and were anxious to gain feedback about their memory and thinking abilities by participating in research.

The woman selected for this example was 69 years old when first evaluated. Her older brother had begun to experience memory problems in his late 60s; as his cognitive problems worsened, he was diagnosed as having dementia of the Alzheimer type, which was subsequently confirmed by autopsy. Two maternal aunts were also described as having become "senile" in their old age, but medical records were too limited to determine the nature of their cognitive problems.

The subject was functioning well in her everyday activities when she enrolled in the study and did not meet clinical diagnostic criteria for dementia. She had moderate complaints related to her medical problems. She had a history of tuberculosis as a child and, in her mid-60s, had been diagnosed as having emphysema, chronic obstructive pulmonary disease, and mild congestive heart failure. She had smoked cigarettes most of her adult life but had stopped when told that she had emphysema. She had been treated with various medications for her respiratory problems, including corticosteroids (prednisone, beclomethasone) and inhalers (albuterol). At the time of her last evaluation, she was only using the inhaler. She also experienced chronic joint pain due to osteoarthritis, which she treated with aspirin. At age 50, she had undergone a hysterectomy for uterine

EXAMPLE 5.2

Background

Caucasian woman tested tree times between the ages 69 and 76 years.

Completed high school and attended two years of junior college; employed part time in sales and bookkeeping during her 30s and 40s; for the past 15 years, has been active as a volunteer in several community organizations.

Stable long-term marriage; describes relationship with husband as very satisfactory.

Medical history significant for uterine cancer and hysterectomy at age 50; emphysema, chronic obstructive pulmonary disease, and mild congestive heart failure diagnosed during her 60s; osteoarthritis for many years.

Medications at first testing consisted of albuterol (Ventolin inhaler) and acetaminophen (Tylenol); at second testing, she was also taking beclomethasone dipropionate (Vanceril) and imipramine hydrochloride (Tofranil); at the last testing, medications were limited to albuterol, a calcium supplement, and multivitamins.

Purpose of evaluation

Participant in a longitudinal aging study; sister of patient with Alzheimer's disease.

Initially described herself as "forgetful for my whole life"; at second testing, expressed mild concern over memory loss, especially for names and places of objects; at last evaluation, reported no change in her cognitive abilities.

Test findings[a]

	Age (years)			Percentile range or rating
	69	72	76	
Mini-Mental State Examination	29	29	29	Normal
WAIS:				
Information	18	18	17	63–84
Comprehension	21	18	20	84–95
Arithmetic	14	12	12	84–91
Digit Span	10	12	11	63–91
Similarities	21	16	19	91–99
Vocabulary	64	68	71	91–99
Digit Symbol	48	40	42	95–99
Picture Completion	12	13	15	75–99
Block Design	24	—	30	50–95
Picture Arrangement	26	18	18	84–95
Object Assembly	29	33	37	63–99
VIQ	120	121	129	91–98
FIQ	118	120	131	88–98
PIQ	114	116	130	82–98

Object Memory Evaluation				
Storage	44	44	45	5–37
Retrieval	41	42	44	55–88
Repeated retrieval	29	31	32	75–88
Paired Associate Learning Test				
Mediate pairs	15	13	14	16–75
New pairs	11	7	9	18–55
Visual Retention Test				
Total correct	6	5	4	16–63
Total errors	6	9	9	25–63
Visual Organization Test	26	25	25	Normal
Coloured Progressive Matrices	32	—	30	95–99
Controlled Oral Word Association Test	—	—	46	80
Boston Naming Test (60 items)	—	—	52	56
WMS Logical Memory				
Immediate	—	—	11	91
Delayed	—	—	8	84

Qualitative aspects of performance

No errors of intrusion on tests of verbal learning and recall; on the Visual Retention Test, rotations and distortions were predominant errors.

Interpretation

Results suggest normal cognitive aging in a bright-normal individual. Mild problems with secondary memory suggested by certain tests and by self-report; however, these were generally nonprogressive and, at final evaluation, did not exceed impairments expected for age and background.

[a]Values are raw scores, with the exception of IQs.

cancer, but there had been no indication of other malignancy in medical examinations since that time. Her history was generally negative for psychiatric problems. For a brief time that overlapped with the second testing, she took an antidepressant (imipramine) for mild depressive symptoms which were later attributed to her use of prednisone for emphysema.

The subject had completed high school and attended two years of junior college, majoring in clerical and business skills. She had worked briefly as a practical nurse and as a bookkeeper after college but had quit full-time work when she married later in her 20s. During her 30s and 40s, she had worked part time as a salesperson in various department stores. In later years, she had been active in volunteer work for the public school system and community agencies and, at the time of her involvement in our study, was volunteering at least once a week at the local commission on aging. At the last examination, when the subject was 76 years old, she was also responsible for picking her two grandchildren up after school each day and taking care of them until their mother returned from work.

At her first evaluation, this person described herself as having had a poor memory all of her life. Otherwise, she had no complaints about her cognitive function. On retest three years later, she noted increasing problems with remembering the names of objects and indicated that she sometimes had trouble remembering where she put things. At her last testing, after another four years had passed, she said that there had been no change in her cognitive function or her ability to perform her activities. She noted that she "might be slowing down a little" but thought that her time with her grandchildren, in which she often helped them with homework, was helping to keep her mentally sharp.

The cognitive assessment battery for the study consisted of the Mini-Mental State Examination (MMSE), the WAIS (the project began before the WAIS-R was available), three tests of learning and memory (the Object Memory Evaluation, the Visual Retention Test, and the Paired Associate Learning Test), the Visual Organization Test, and Coloured Progressive Matrices (see Chapter 4 for descriptions of these measures). At the last assessment, the Boston Naming Test, Controlled Oral Word Association Test, and WMS Logical Memory were also administered.

Example 5.2 summarizes performance for the first, second, and final evaluations; the table primarily includes raw scores, since the focus in this case was on changes in actual performance over time. The initial testing at age 69 showed her general intellectual ability to be in the "bright normal" range (approximately 90th percentile for age). Some scatter was observed in performance across subtests, but none resulted in any age-scaled score lower than 10. All other performances were also at or above the normal range for age. Although she recalled only 5 of 10 objects on the first trial of the Object Memory Evaluation, her performance quickly improved, and on the remaining trials, she recalled between 8 and 10 items; her consistency of retrieval was above average for age (75th percentile; Fuld, 1981), and she was able to benefit from reminders on the few items that she missed initially. She made no errors on the "mediate pairs" of the Paired Associate Learning Test and performed within expectations for age and intellectual level on the more difficult "new pairs"; she did not intrude old, overlearned associations; instead, she had errors of omission or transposition (mispairings). Her performance on the Visual Retention Test was also normal for age and intellectual level. Her rate of rotations (accounting for four of six errors) was higher than is usually expected for normal adults, suggesting some mild difficulties in visual perception or visuoconstruction. Other findings also suggested that these areas were comparatively weak for this individual; for example, Block Design was the low point of her WAIS profile, and her copy of the interlocking pentagons on the Mini-Mental State Examination (MMSE) was slightly distorted.

At the second testing, when the subject was 72 years old, overall WAIS performance continued to be strong; her full-scale IQ score, which was now based on norms for a higher age bracket (70 to 74 years), was 120. Nonetheless, she showed declining scores on a few of the subtests that may be sensitive to either terminal decline or early dementia (e.g., Similarities and Digit Symbol; see Chapters 3 and 7). The raw score changes on these measures were not large (5 points on Similarities, 8 points on Digit Symbol); nonetheless, they corresponded to a 2-point decline in age-scaled scores, despite an increased age correction. Slight declines were also noted on two of the three memory measures. On the difficult "new pairs" of the Paired Associate Learning Test, she responded correctly on only 7 of 15 items (5 learning trials with three word pairs). Similarly, on the Visual Retention Test, she made a total of 9 errors when copying the designs immediately from memory. Both performances were in the mild impairment range for age and overall intellectual ability.

The changes observed from the first to second testing raise a question of mild decline in cognitive function. Although the areas in which declines were observed (i.e., secondary memory, abstract reasoning, complex perceptual-motor integration) are ones in which some loss would be expected with normal aging (see Chapters 3 and 4), they are also highly sensitive to beginning dementia (see Chapter 7). Nonetheless, memory losses were not large, and on one measure (the Object Memory Evaluation), no reduction in performance was observed; on this test, all subscores were still at or above the mean for 70- to 79-year-olds at the second testing. Also, while certain WAIS subtests declined, others showed improvement on retest. These inconsistencies suggest that the second testing was tapping only normal aging changes and/or routine fluctuations in performance.

The most recent testing, when the subject was 76 years of age, tended to support this interpretation. That is, raw scores on WAIS subtests that had previously declined were now observed to improve; a slight improvement was also seen in paired-associate learning, and change on the Visual Retention Test was negligible. Subjective assessment of cognitive function was also more positive, as noted above.

This example illustrates normal fluctuations in cognitive functioning in a bright individual and shows that in normal old people, gains in test scores may be observed with repeated assessments. Practice effects may account for some of the gains in this case. Increasing everyday mental stimulation may also have played a role in the trend toward higher scores; for example, at the time of the final testing, she was more involved with her grandchildren than she had been in earlier years, and she helped them with homework several days a week. Reductions in medications may also have contributed to improved performance; at the second testing, she was taking two medications that sometimes affect cognitive performance adversely (i.e., beclomethasone, a corticosteroid, and imipramine, a tricyclic antidepressant; see Chapter 6). At the final testing, these drugs had been discontinued, and she was able to control her respiratory symptoms with only occasional use of an inhaler.

An Old-Old Individual

The final example (5.3) concerns a very old woman who had entered the hospital at the urging of family members who were concerned about her problems with memory and changes in her personal care.

EXAMPLE 5.3

Background

Ninety-seven-year-old Caucasian woman.
Seventh grade education; described herself as "not good at school."
Worked principally as a homemaker, occasionally as a sales clerk.
Married and widowed twice; has four children to whom she is very close.
Has been living in a retirement hotel for 1½ years.
Medical findings include a history of subendocardial myocardial infarction nine months prior to admission; history of hypothyroidism, tic douloureux, and sciatica; labile systolic hypertension; anemia.
Medications consist of propranolol hydrochloride (Inderal), nitroglycerin (Transderm–Nitro patch), dipyridamole (Persantine), ibuprofen (Motrin), and thyroid supplement.

Presenting problems

Family's description: Worsening memory for past 1½ years; less frequent bathing and less meticulous appearance; occasional refusal of meals or medications; in past three months, occasional incontinence and some possible delusional thoughts (e.g., complained to family that people were trying to expel her from the retirement hotel, but this had some basis in fact).

Patient's description: Admitted that her memory was worse than it used to be; she attributed this to her advanced age and stated that she can remember what she wants to. Comment: "My family wants me to be the way I was 30 years ago."

Behavior during testing

Alert, cooperative, euthymic. Effort was adequate; attention was generally good, although occasionally distracted. Comprehended test instructions.

Test findings

Mini-Mental State Examination: 16

WAIS	Raw score	Scaled score (75+ yrs)
Vocabulary	34	11
Similarities	3	7
Digit Symbol	7	7
Block Design	8	7
Paired Associate Learning Test		
Old pairs	15	
Mediate pairs	9	
New pairs	0	
Visual Retention Test		
Total correct	0	
Total errors	18	

Shopping List Test: 3 to 6 items recalled per trial
MMPI: Valid profile; no elevations on clinical scales.

Qualitative aspects of performance

Evidence of a learning curve on the Shopping List Test; no errors of intrusion. Able to suppress tendency to name old, overlearned associations when attempting to learn novel paired associates. Predominant type of error on the Visual Retention Test was omissions. Able to comprehend instructions to Digit Symbol and to follow the specified sequence. No evidence of paraphasias, cicumlocution, or word-finding deficits in spontaneous speech or on verbal intelligence tests.

Interpretation and recommendations

Findings indicate at least mild impairment of cognitive function, particularly in recent memory and visuospatial abilities. The extent and pattern of the impairment appear more consistent with normal aging than a dementia. Medications may have contributed to recent cognitive and behavioral problems. Family education was provided to explain age-related memory changes.

In view of the patient's advanced age and the nonexistence of appropriate quantitative norms, only a brief battery of tests was administered. Global mental status was assessed with the Mini-Mental State Examination, verbal and nonverbal intelligence were estimated with WAIS subtests, three tests were given to assess learning and recall (the Shopping List Test, the Paired Associate Learning Test, and the Visual Retention Test), and mood and personality were surveyed with an orally administered short form of the MMPI (see Chapter 4 for descriptions of these measures). Because the patient was alert and cooperative, it would have been possible to do more testing; however, her stamina was limited, and she thought the formal testing somewhat peculiar and inappropriate. She readily admitted to memory problems, but when asked to perform memory tests, she protested, "I'm *97* you know!"

Examination of raw scores clearly indicates that her performance was weak in absolute terms. Compared to most young adults, and probably to herself at a younger age, her scores were very low on measures of verbal abstraction, psychomotor speed and cognitive flexibility, visuoconstruction and visual memory, and learning and recall of new verbal information.

Nonetheless, several factors argue for judging her performance to be normal for age. Her WAIS Vocabulary score suggests that crystallized verbal intelligence was well preserved; on WAIS subtests measuring abstraction and fluid intellectual abilities, her performance was still good enough to earn an age-corrected score of 7 when compared to normative standards for people aged "75 and above" (Wechsler, 1955). She comprehended instructions for the Digit Symbol subtest and copied the symbols correctly, although quite slowly.

On verbal learning and memory tests, the patient demonstrated some ability to learn, evidenced some simple spontaneous strategies (subvocal rehearsal), showed awareness of the comparative difficulty of easy and hard tasks, and did not make errors of intrusion or perseveration. Still, some of her scores on these tasks were very low. Could her zero-correct performance on novel paired associates be considered within normal limits? At least two studies (Craik *et al.*, 1987; Klonoff & Kennedy, 1966) have reported floor effects on the learning of novel paired associates in very-old individuals with limited education and inactive lifestyles. Could the patient's failure to reach criterion on the simple free-recall test be normal for her age? The only norms available on this measure are for a much younger (median age = 69 years) and better educated sample (McCarthy *et al.*, 1981). However, qualitative analysis showed a normal serial position curve, with both primacy and recency apparent, suggesting that she was processing the material in a normal manner (see Chapters 3 and 4).

One of her poorest performances was on the Visual Retention Test; even here, however, one can argue that her performance was not entirely out of line with age expectations. Klonoff and Kennedy (1965) reported an average of 11.71 (± 4.64) errors on the Visual Retention Test for 80- to 92-year-old men with an average of seven years of schooling; similarly, Benton and colleagues (1981) found that 38% of a very healthy, well-educated sample of 80- to 84-year-olds had "deficient performances" on this test (see Chapter 4). Qualitatively, it is important to note that on each of the three-figure designs, the patient drew only one or two figures and often omitted the peripheral figure. Such omissions tend to be more common in brain-damaged patients than in normals and therefore suggest some problems with memory; however, throughout the testing, this patient tried to minimize errors of commission, so her omissions on the Visual Retention Test may have been affected by her cautious style of response.

Finally, regarding performance on the Mini-Mental State Examination, several studies have shown a high rate of false-positive errors with the use of the standard cutoff of ≤ 23 in older individuals with limited education (see Chapter 4). The woman in this example had had only a seventh-grade education and was very old indeed!

In calling this woman's performance normal, what I mean is normal, *considering*. Her history of myocardial infarction may well have been the cause of some of her functional memory changes; also, the geriatric medicine specialist who reviewed her case thought that medications may have contributed and recommended reducing her Inderal dosage by half and eliminating Motrin and Persantine.

Another significant factor in this case was the fact that the referral was based on the distress and concern of family members. The patient had long been a matriarchal figure in her extended family, tracking life developments of her numerous grandchildren and great-grandchildren, and offering advice as she saw fit. Of late, she had been less attentive to others and seemed less interested in family details. The family experienced this withdrawal as a loss and, in the patient's view, had problems facing the inevitability of her decline. Many of the changes in the patient's behavior, such as refusing to leave her room for meals or dressing less carefully, coincided with a disagreement with her daughter. One of her daughters had moved into a new home, and the patient had assumed that she would be invited to move in; when the invitation did not materialize, her cooperation took a turn for the worse. In the hospital, too, she was sometimes described as stubborn; she insisted on wearing shoes with elevated heels although they made her unsteady on her feet, and she refused to wear elastic support stockings because she didn't like the way they looked.

This patient was fortunate to have so many people who cared about her well-being, but she clearly had her own ideas about what it meant to be well. Her independent ideas, while troublesome to her family and to hospital staff at times, may have helped her to survive in style to a very advanced old age.

SUMMARY AND CONCLUSIONS

Interpretation of test outcomes is by far the most difficult aspect of assessment to learn. General guidelines can be provided, but clinical experience is clearly necessary for developing the judgment required to balance conflicting results.

This chapter has presented a series of questions to facilitate test interpretation for older patients and to encourage integration of test results with other clinical data. The case examples applied some of these principles to older individuals with memory complaints. None of the cases was free of performance deficits; however, impairments did not clearly exceed those expected for age and background. The first and third cases are good examples of the types of individuals who present for clinical assessment but then perform at average levels (or higher) on most appropriate measures. In effect, they come as close to being "normal" as one is likely to observe in clinical geropsychological practice. The second case provided an opportunity—rare in clinical practice—to observe the normal waxing and waning of performance across repeated testings.

Different clinicians have different standards for inferring abnormality. My own approach with older people is to give the benefit of the doubt when performance is not clearly poor enough to warrant a diagnosis. This approach may increase the rate of false-negative errors and cause frustration for the patient or family members who sense that something is wrong; in extreme cases, such errors may result in delay of service for a treatable disorder. However, false-positive diagnoses of brain impairment tend to be even more costly for older patients, leading to diminished expectations for improvement, exclusion from decisions about many basic life activities, and fewer referrals for useful services such as psychotherapy. Until both normal and abnormal aging are better understood and effective treatments are developed for degenerative brain diseases, the strategy of minimizing false-positive errors seems better than the alternative.

II

Common Neurological and Psychiatric Disorders

6

Delirium and Dementia

An Overview

Foremost among the mental disorders affecting older adults are the diffuse or multifocal brain syndromes known as *delirium* and *dementia*. In delirium, cognitive disturbance is transient or fluctuating; symptoms develop rapidly, generally as a result of a change in medical state. In dementia, cognitive loss is more persistent; in most cases, symptoms have a gradual onset and a stable or progressive course.

In many medical and community settings, the most common referral question for geriatric neuropsychologists is to evaluate the presence or extent of dementia. An opinion about the specific type of dementia (e.g., Alzheimer's disease or vascular dementia) may also be requested, and questions about an individual's competence and prognosis may be raised. However, before conclusions can be drawn about dementia, the possibility of delirium must be carefully considered, especially in patients with acute medical illness or multiple medications.

This chapter examines general diagnostic criteria for delirium and dementia and provides an overview of causes and treatments of these clinical syndromes. Several of the most common causes of dementia in the elderly—Alzheimer's disease, vascular disease, Parkinson's disease, and depression—are discussed in greater detail in Chapters 7 through 12.

DELIRIUM

Many older adults experience transient cognitive problems due to overmedication, worsening medical conditions, or changes in living arrangements (e.g., hospitalization or moving to a nursing home). These temporary cognitive disorders have been referred to as *confusional states*, *acute organic brain syndromes*, and currently, *delirium*. In hospitals and long-term care settings, delirium is at least as prevalent as dementia as a cause of cognitive problems, and accurate differentiation of the two conditions is needed to ensure proper medical and psychosocial intervention.

Diagnostic Criteria and Clinical Features

In the revised third edition of the *Diagnostic and Statistical Manual of the American Psychiatric Association* (DMS-III-R; American Psychiatric Association, 1987), the behavioral features necessary for a diagnosis of delirium include:

a. impaired attention;
b. disorganized thinking; and
c. two of more of the following problems:
   1. reduced level of consciousness;
   2. perceptual disturbances;
   3. altered psychomotor activity;
   4. disorientation;
   5. memory impairment.

Additional criteria are:

a. that the clinical features develop over a short period of time (hours or days) and tend to fluctuate; and
b. there must be evidence of a specific organic factor causing the mental disturbance or all reasonable nonorganic causes (e.g., mania) must have been ruled out (p. 103).

An important aspect of the DSM-III-R criteria is that they preclude the diagnosis of dementia in the presence of significant delirium, except in the case where there is a clear history of preexisting dementia. When in doubt as to the differentiation of dementia and delirium, the recommendation is to assign a provisional diagnosis of delirium, which "should lead to a more active therapeutic approach" (American Psychiatric Association, 1987, p. 103).

Symptoms of delirium vary considerably from patient to patient. The most consistent features are difficulties in maintaining or shifting attention and rambling, irrelevant, or incoherent speech which suggests disordered thinking (American Psychiatric Association, 1987; Liston, 1989). Disturbances of perception, including visual hallucinations and illusions, are also quite common.

Three clinical subtypes of delirium have been identified based on differing activity levels: a hyperactive type, characterized by excessive psychomotor activity; a hypoactive type, with reduced psychomotor activity and alertness; and a mixed type, with hyperactive and hypoactive features present at different times (Lipowski, 1980; Liston, 1989). Hyperactive and mixed types predominate in older patients (e.g., Koponen,

Hurri, Stenback, Mattila, Soininen, & Riekkinen, 1989a), although as Liston (1989) noted, hypoactive types may be more easily overlooked.

Prevalence and Risk Factors

Ten to fifteen percent of medical/surgical inpatients experience episodes of delirium, either at the time of hospitalization or during the course of treatment (Liston, 1989). Delirium can occur at any age, but children and the elderly have the highest risk of this disorder (Liston, 1989). Although specific prevalence estimates vary, delirious episodes have been reported for as many as 30% to 50% of older patients in medical or psychiatric settings (Lipowski, 1987; Liston, 1982).

Older patients with preexisting brain disease are at particularly high risk for delirium. For example, of the 69 elderly delirious patients studied by Koponen *et al.* (1989a), 54 (78%) also had dementia or Parkinson's disease.

Other predisposing factors for delirium noted by Liston (1989) are multiple medications, a history of drug or alcohol abuse, sensory loss, social isolation, unfamiliar environments, sleep deprivation, and weakened psychological defenses. These factors are particularly likely to trigger delirium in patients with dementia or other preexisting brain impairment.

Conditions That Can Cause Delirium

Delirium can result from any condition that disrupts cerebral metabolism or otherwise interferes with neuronal function (Lipowski, 1980). In their study of older psychiatric patients, Koponen *et al.* (1989a) found the predominant causes of delirium to be stroke (22% of cases), infection (13%), and adverse drug reactions (13%), followed by epileptic seizures (9%) and major life changes in patients with dementia (9%). Other common causes and precipitating factors are shown in Table 6.1.

Adverse Drug Reactions

The risk of adverse drug reactions is greatly increased among older adults (for thorough discussions, see Bressler, 1987; Divoll & Greenblatt, 1987; Ouslander, 1981; Simonson, 1984; Stewart, 1988). Age-related physiological changes (e.g., in gastrointestinal absorption, renal excretion, and protein binding) produce a general increase in sensitivity to medications (Divoll & Greenblatt, 1987; cf. Chapter 2); therefore, toxic effects may be observed even with standard or reduced drug doses. Elderly patients usually take multiple medications and, as a result, may experience drug–drug interactions; for example, in one study of nursing-home patients, each person was found to be taking four to nine prescription medications (Segal, Thompson, & Floyd, 1979). Older patients take many high-risk medications (e.g., psychotropics, anti-Parkinson drugs, antihypertensives, and analgesics) and may inadvertently increase adverse effects by taking these drugs incorrectly (Divoll & Greenblatt, 1987; Stewart, 1988).

TABLE 6.1. Conditions Commonly Associated with Delirium[a]

Central nervous system disorders	Cardiopulmonary disorders
Vascular disease	Myocardial infarction
Head trauma	Congestive heart failure
Seizures	Cardiac arrhythmias
Postictal states	Shock
Infection	Respiratory failure
Brain tumor	Miscellaneous conditions
Neurodegenerative disease (e.g., Alzheimer's)	Adverse medication reactions
Metabolic disorders	"Street drugs" (e.g., phencyclidine)
Uremia	Toxins or heavy metals
Liver failure	Severe physical or mental trauma
Anemia	Sepsis
Hypoglycemia	Sensory deprivation
Thiamine deficiency	Temperature dysregulation
Endocrinopathies	Postoperative states
Fluid or electrolyte imbalance	
Acid–base imbalance	

[a]From Liston (1989, p. 806). Copyright 1989 by the American Psychiatric Association. Adapted by permission.

Table 6.2 lists a few of the drugs that can adversely affect cognition in elderly patients. Psychoactive medications are listed first, since virtually any drug of this type can have adverse effects on cognitive function in susceptible individuals. Among the anticonvulsants, phenytoin tends to have the highest rate of adverse effects, followed by barbiturates such as phenobarbital; carbamazepine (Tegretol) tends to have fewer cognitive side effects (Trimble, 1987). Among antidepressants, risk of delirium is greatest for tricyclics with high anticholinergic activity (especially amitriptyline) and lower for certain other tricyclics (e.g., desipramine), monoamine oxidase inhibitors (e.g., phenelzine), and newer antidepressants such as trazodone (DeVane & Tingle, 1988). Anti-Parkinson drugs that block cholinergic activity (e.g., benztropine, trihexyphenidyl) produce delirium more often than those that enhance dopamine (e.g., levodopa, amantadine; cf. Chapter 9), and of the antipsychotics, thioridazine and chlorpromazine tend to affect cognition more than haloperidol (Haldol; cf. DeVane & Tingle, 1988). Long-acting benzodiazepines such as diazepam are more likely to produce adverse effects than shorter acting agents such as oxazepam (Serax) or lorazepam (Ativan). Psychotropic medications are frequently involved in drug–drug interactions with other medications noted in Table 6.2.

Brain Substrates

The brain mechanisms that give rise to delirium are poorly understood. Diffuse slowing of the EEG is commonly observed in delirium (e.g., Koponen, Partanen,

TABLE 6.2. Medications That Can Adversely Affect Cognition[a]

Medical condition	Type of medication	Common examples
Neurological and psychiatric	Anticonvulsants	Barbiturates, carbamazepine, psychiatric diazepam, phenytoin
	Anti-Parkinsonism agents	Amantadine, benztropine, levodopa, trihexyphenidyl
	Hypnotics and sedatives	Barbiturates, belladonna alkaloids, bromides, chloral hydrate, ethchlorvynol, glutethimide, methaqualone
	Psychotropics	Benzodiazepines, hydroxyzines, lithium salts, meprobamate, monoamine oxidase inhibitors, neuroleptics, tricyclic antidepressants
Cardiovascular	Antiarrhythmics	Procainamide, propranolol, quinidine
	Antihypertensives	Clonidine, methyldopa, reserpine
	Cardiac glycosides	Digitalis
	Coronary vasodilators	Nitrates
Gastrointestinal	Antidiarrheals	Atropine, belladonna, homatropine, hyoscyamine, scopolamine
	Antinauseants	Cyclizine, phenothiazines, homatropine–barbiturate preparations
	Antispasmodics	Methantheline, propantheline
Musculoskeletal	Anti-inflammatory agents	Corticosteroids, indomethacin, phenylbutazone, salicylates
	Muscle relaxants	Carisoprodol, diazepam
Respiratory-allergic	Antihistamines	Brompheniramine, chlorpheniramine, cyproheptadine, diphenhydramine, tripelennamine
	Antitussives	Opiates, synthetic narcotics
	Decongestants and expectorants	Phenylephrine, phenylpropanolamine, potassium preparations
Miscellaneous	Analgesics	Propoxyphene, opiates, phenacetin, salicylates, synthetic narcotics
	Anesthetics	Lidocaine, methohexital, methoxyflurane
	Antidiabetic agents	Insulin, oral hypoglycemics
	Antineoplastics	Corticosteroids, mitomycin, procarbazine
	Antituberculosis agents	Isoniazid, rifampin

[a]From Liston (1982, p. 57). Copyright 1982 by W. B. Saunders Co. Adapted by permission.

Paakkonen, Mattila, & Riekkinen, 1989b; Rabins & Folstein, 1982; Romano & Engel, 1944), and latencies of brain-stem and somatosensory evoked potentials (EPs) may also be increased (e.g., Trzepacz, Sclabassi, & Van Thiel, 1989). Delirium can result from vascular lesions in several anatomical regions, including prefrontal, temporal-occipital, and posterior parietal regions of the neocortex, the hippocampus, and the limbic areas (e.g., Koponen *et al.*, 1989a; Levine & Grek, 1984; Mesulam, 1979) and from tumors in several cortical and subcortical areas (Byrne, 1987). In general, older patients with pronounced cerebral atrophy on computerized tomography (CT) are more likely to become delirious than those with minimal atrophy (Koponen *et al.*, 1989a).

Assessment Procedures

Clinical Interview

Lipowski's recommended diagnostic procedure (1987) is an informal bedside evaluation designed to elicit key symptoms such as distractibility, disorganization, and inconsistencies among responses. He emphasized that "acute onset of cognitive and attentional deficits and abnormalities, whose severity fluctuates during the day and tends to worsen at night, is practically diagnostic" (p. 1791).

For an experienced clinician familiar with elderly patients, these procedures may well prove adequate. However, many medical professionals lack specialized experience with the aged and may work under time constraints that preclude the thorough clinical testing to which Lipowski (1987) referred. Under these circumstances, a brief objective screening measure would be of great assistance in ensuring that delirium is not overlooked.

A Delirium Rating Scale

Trzepacz, Baker, and Greenhouse (1988) devised a 10-item Delirium Rating Scale (DRS) that may help to objectify symptom severity when delirium is suspected (see Table 6.3). Items pertain not only to cognitive disturbance, but also to the time course and consistency of symptoms and to the presence and severity of associated clinical features (e.g., psychotic symptoms or mood, sleep, and motor disturbance). In the full version of the scale (see Trzepacz *et al.*, 1988), each item is introduced by a brief statement of the rationale for its selection and some rough guidelines for differentiating symptoms of delirium from those produced by other disorders (e.g., affective disorders or schizophrenia).

Preliminary findings on the DRS were reported for 20 medical/surgical patients with delirium and 9 control subjects in each of three groups (dementia, schizophrenia, and affective/personality disorder). Mean scores on this scale were markedly elevated for the delirium group compared to those of any of the comparison groups, with no overlap in distributions. For example, while delirious patients averaged 23.0 (± 4.8) points on the DRS, the mean score for dementia patients was only 4.6 (± 2.1). Scores correlated significantly with performance on a mental status exam and Trails B within the delirium group, and interrater reliability between two independent raters was very high (r = .97).

Although these results are encouraging, cross-validation studies are needed before the DRS can be recommended for diagnostic application; at present, however, it provides a useful checklist of clinical features to evaluate when delirium is suspected.

Neuropsychological Testing

Because attention and thinking are often severely impaired in delirium, extensive neuropsychological testing is generally inappropriate for patients with this disorder. Brief cognitive mental status exams such as the Mini-Mental State Examination

(MMSE) can be used to confirm the presence of cognitive deficits and to monitor changes in symptoms over time. Even on these brief exams, however, many delirious patients perform very poorly; for example, in a recent study of elderly delirious patients, 77% had MMSE scores of 20 or lower and 28% had scores of 10 or below (Koponen *et al.*, 1989a).

In patients for whom more extensive testing is possible, attention to qualitative features of performance may provide clues to differential diagnosis. Weicker (1987) found mental control items (e.g., counting backward from 20 or reciting the months or the alphabet) and clock-drawing tasks to be particularly useful in distinguishing dementia and delirium, delirious patients more often losing track or perseverating on these simple tasks.

Electrophysiological Measures

Because diffuse slowing on the electroencephalogram (EEG) is a common finding in delirium, the absence of such slowing may help to identify confusion due to severe psychiatric illness (e.g., psychotic depression) as opposed to delirium. EEGs can also be used to monitor resolution or worsening of delirium in patients who are unable to participate in cognitive testing.

Treatment

The importance of prompt treatment for delirium is underscored by the high mortality rates associated with this condition. Among elderly patients, 17% to 25% with delirium die within the first month of illness (Liston, 1982). Younger patients have a better chance of recovery from delirium than the elderly, and a more positive prognosis is observed if the episode is brief (Liston, 1982).

Treatment of delirium requires the identification and correction of underlying medical causes. Because of the wide range of conditions that can cause delirium (see Table 6.1), a very thorough diagnostic evaluation may be needed in some cases; however, the most common causes can usually be identified with relatively simple screening studies (e.g., urinalysis, blood chemistries, chest X ray, electrocardiogram, and EEG; see Liston, 1989).

Lipowski (1983, 1987) emphasized the frequency with which delirious states in the elderly are induced by medications and recommended that current medications be stopped (or dosages reduced) so that it can be determined if drugs are causing the mental disturbance. For some delirious patients, however, low doses of major tranquilizers such as haloperidol may be needed to control severe agitation (Lipowski, 1987).

Environmental and psychological factors can also affect recovery. Having a familiar person such as a relative stay with the patient, providing a modest and consistent amount of stimulation, and providing frequent reorientation have all been recommended as useful (Liston, 1982). Skilled nursing care or supervision by family caregivers is crucial for preventing falls and injuries that may result from disorganized and agitated behavior.

TABLE 6.3. Items Included in the Delirium Rating Scale[a]

Item 1. Temporal onset of symptoms
0. No significant change from long–standing behavior, essentially a chronic or chronic-recurrent disorder.
1. Gradual onset of symptoms, occurring within a six-month period.
2. Acute change in behavior or personality occurring over a month.
3. Abrupt change in behavior, usually occurring over a one- to three-day period.

Item 2. Perceptual disturbances
0. None evident by history or observation.
1. Feelings of depersonalization or derealization.
2. Visual illusions or misperceptions including macropsia or micropsia; e.g., may mistake bedclothes for something else.
3. Evidence that the patient is markedly confused about external reality; e.g., not discriminating between dreams and reality.

Item 3. Hallucination type
0. Hallucinations not present.
1. Auditory hallucinations only.
2. Visual hallucinations present by history or inferred by observation, with or without auditory hallucinations.
3. Tactile, olfactory, or gustatory hallucinations present with or without visual or auditory hallucinations.

Item 4. Delusions
0. Not present.
1. Delusions are systematized, i.e., well-organized and persistent.
2. Delusions are new and not part of a preexisting primary psychiatric disorder.
3. Delusions are not well circumscribed; are transient, poorly organized, and mostly in response to misperceived environmental cues.

Item 5. Psychomotor behavior
0. No significant retardation or agitation.
1. Mild restlessness, tremulousness, or anxiety evident by observation and a change from usual behavior.
2. Moderate agitation with pacing, removing IVs, etc.
3. Severe agitation, needs to be restrained, may be combative; or has significant withdrawal from the environment, but not due to major depression or schizophrenic catatonia.

Item 6. Cognitive status during formal testing
0. No cognitive deficits, or deficits that can be alternatively explained by lack of education or prior mental retardation.
1. Very mild cognitive deficits which may be attributed to inattention, pain, etc.
2. Cognitive deficit largely in one major area tested, e.g., memory.
3. Significant cognitive deficits that are diffuse; must include periods of disorientation, abnormal registration or recall, and reduced concentration.
4. Severe cognitive deficits, including motor or verbal perseverations, confabulations, disorientation to person, memory deficits, and inability to cooperate with formal testing.

Item 7. Physical disorder
0. None present or active.
1. Presence of any physical disorder that may affect mental state.
2. Specific drug, infection, metabolic, central nervous system lesion, or other medical problem that can be temporally implicated in causing the altered behavior or mental status.

Item 8. Sleep–wake cycle disturbance
0. Not present.
1. Occasional drowsiness during day and mild sleep continuity disturbance at night; may have nightmares but can distinguish them from reality.
2. Frequent napping and unable to sleep at night, constituting a significant disruption or a reversal of usual sleep–wake cycle.

TABLE 6.3. (*Continued*)

3. Drowsiness prominent, difficulty staying alert during interview, loss of self-control over alertness and somnolence.
4. Drifts into stuporous or comatose periods.

Item 9. Lability of mood

0. Not present.
1. Affect/mood somewhat altered and changes over the course of hours; patient states that mood changes are not under self-control.
2. Significant mood changes that are inappropriate to situation, including fear, anger, or tearfulness; rapid shifts of emotion.
3. Severe disinhibition of emotions, including temper outbursts, uncontrolled inappropriate laughter, or crying.

Item 10. Variability of symptoms

0. Symptoms stable and mostly present during daytime.
2. Symptoms worsen at night.
4. Fluctuating intensity of symptoms, so that they wax and wane during a 24-hour period.

[a]From Trzepacz, Baker, and Greenhouse (1988, pp. 95–97). Copyright 1988 by Elsevier Scientific Publishers Ireland Ltd. Adapted by permission.

It is also important to educate family members that symptoms of delirium may resolve slowly; the acute phase may be followed by a transitional phase in which attention appears to have returned to normal, but there are residual problems with cognition, affect, or behavior.

DEMENTIA

Dementia denotes a state of generalized and persistent cognitive decline that is severe enough to interfere with important everyday activities. Such cognitive incapacity was once called senility and was attributed to aging *per se* or to vague conditions such as "hardening of the arteries." Dementia is now recognized as a pathological brain syndrome that can result from a variety of causes.

Scope of the Problem

A recent review of epidemiological studies from several countries reported rates of mild dementia ranging from 0.5% to 16.3% and rates of moderate to severe dementia from 2.0% to 7.7% (Jorm, Korten, & Henderson, 1987; cf. Gurland & Cross, 1982; Mortimer, Schuman, & French, 1981). Prevalence is strongly age-dependent, with rates of dementia doubling for each five-year interval between 60 and 95 years (Jorm *et al.*, 1987). For example, less than 1% of 60- to 64-year-olds have moderate to severe dementia compared to nearly 40% of 90- to 95-year-olds.

Currently, 1.5 million Americans have such severe dementia that they are no longer able to function independently; another 1 to 5 million have mild or moderate dementia

(U.S. Congress, Office of Technology Assessment, 1987). By 2040, because of projected increases in the aged population, it has been estimated that more than 7 million Americans will be disabled because of dementia.

The total cost of caring for demented patients was estimated at $38 billion in 1983 (U.S. Congress, Office of Technology Assessment, 1987). Cost of institutional care alone is said to exceed $25 billion per year (Katzman, 1986). When these monetary debits are added to the loss of productivity and the emotional costs of the disease to the patient, family members, and friends, the enormity of problems associated with dementia readily becomes apparent.

Diagnostic Criteria

It is important to recognize that dementia is a *behavioral* syndrome; that is, when correctly applied, a label of *dementia* indicates that specific disturbances of cognition or personality are present.

In the DSM-III-R, the behavioral features required for a diagnosis of dementia are:

a. impairment in short- and long-term memory; and
b. at least one of the following:
   1. impairment of abstract thinking;
   2. impaired judgment;
   3. other disturbance of higher cortical functions, such as aphasia, apraxia, agnosia, and constructional difficulty; and
   4. personality change (p. 107).

These problems must be severe enough to interfere with work or interpersonal relationships and must reflect a decline from a more effective level of function. Exclusionary criteria must also be met before the label of dementia can be applied. Dementia cannot be diagnosed when cognitive disturbance occurs exclusively during the course of delirium (see above) or when symptoms of dementia can be accounted for by a nonorganic mental disorder (e.g., depression). If these causes have been excluded, an organic etiology can be assumed even if no specific organic cause has been identified.

The DSM-III-R criteria for dementia identify a general category of dysfunction that may result from many different illnesses (see below). They are useful, nonetheless, because they place restraints on the type and extent of deficits that warrant a diagnosis of dementia, and because they prompt the clinician to consider alternative diagnoses.

According to these criteria, dementia *cannot* be diagnosed on the basis of such medical diagnostic indicators as atrophy on the CT scan or white-matter lucencies on a magnetic resonance imaging (MRI) scan. If a person's behavior does not fit the positive diagnostic criteria, a diagnosis of dementia cannot be made. This is a crucial point, since there is considerable overlap in CT and MRI findings for neurologically healthy older people and those with dementing disorders. Second, the degree of decline must be severe enough to interfere with everyday life; psychometric decline alone would not be a basis for inferring dementia. This criterion is particularly useful in preventing overdiagnosis of dementia in normal older people. Third, an individual cannot be diagnosed as demented unless significant memory loss is apparent. Therefore, aphasia, apraxia, or reasoning deficits would not in themselves be sufficient for a diagnosis to be made. Finally, there must be some other form of deficit in addition to memory loss in order for this diagnosis to apply. This emphasis on diffuse or multifocal impairment helps to distinguish dementia from amnestic conditions that may have separate causes and treatments.

Conditions That Can Cause Dementia

There are many conditions that can produce a clinical syndrome of dementia, either routinely or occasionally (for additional information, see Cummings & Benson, 1983; National Institutes of Health, 1987; Strub & Black, 1988; U.S. Congress, Office of Technology Assessment, 1987).

Currently Irreversible Dementias

Table 6.4 provides a listing of illnesses that can produce persistent or progressive dementia. A few of these disorders invariably produce dementia (e.g., Alzheimer's, Pick's, or Creutzfeldt-Jakob's disease); for the remainder (e.g., Parkinson's, head trauma, metal exposure), dementia is observed only in some cases. Several of these conditions are preventable (e.g., toxic exposures, neurosyphilis), and for others (e.g., alcoholic dementia), partial recovery in cognitive function may be observed if the illness is controlled or arrested. However, in most cases, the deficits which result from these disorders are relatively permanent, and for neurodegenerative illnesses such as Alzheimer's disease, there is no means at present of preventing or reversing impairments.

"Reversible" Dementias

Medications, psychiatric illness, or nutritional and metabolic disorders can sometimes produce cognitive deficits that are difficult to distinguish from the dementias caused by structural brain damage. The latter conditions have been referred to either as *reversible dementias* (e.g., National Institute on Aging Task Force, 1980; National Institutes of Health, 1987) or as *conditions that simulate dementia* (U.S. Congress, Office of Technology Assessment, 1987).

Potentially reversible causes are listed in Table 6.5. Some of these conditions (e.g., medication reactions, metabolic disorders) are more likely to result in delirium than dementia; however, if the underlying problems go untreated for long periods of time, a dementia can sometimes develop. Sensory impairment, social isolation, and pain, while not usually considered causes of dementia, can greatly exacerbate mild organic brain changes or can lower cognitive performance to the point where dementia is suspected.

TABLE 6.4. Conditions That Can Cause Dementia[a]

Degenerative diseases	Infectious dementia
Alzheimer's disease	Acquired immune deficiency syndrome (AIDS)
Parkinson's disease	Creutzfeldt-Jakob's disease
Pick's disease	Progressive multifocal leukoencephalopathy
Huntington's disease	Postencephalitic dementia
Progressive supranuclear palsy	Behcet's syndrome
Cerebellar degenerations	Herpes encephalitis
Amyotrophic lateral sclerosis (ALS)	Fungal meningitis or encephalitis
Parkinson–ALS–dementia complex of Guam and other island areas	Bacterial meningitis or encephalitis
Rare genetic and metabolic diseases (e.g., Wilson's)	Parasitic encephalitis
Vascular dementia	Brain abscess
Multi-infarct dementia	Neurosyphilis
Cortical microinfarcts	Normal-pressure hydrocephalus
Lacunar dementia	Space-occupying lesions
Binswanger's disease	Chronic or acute subdural hematoma
Cerebral embolic disease	Primary brain tumor
Anoxic dementia	Metastatic tumors
Cardiac arrest	Multiple sclerosis
Cardiac failure (severe)	Autoimmune disorders
Carbon monoxide	Disseminated lupus erythematosus
Traumatic dementia	Vasculitis
Dementia pugilistica (boxer's dementia)	Toxic dementia
Head injuries	Alcholic dementia
	Metallic dementia (e.g., lead poisoning)
	Organic poisons (e.g., solvents, some insecticides)
	Other disorders
	Epilepsy
	Whipple's disease
	Heat stroke

[a]From U.S. Congress, Office of Technology Assessment (1987).

Prevalence of Different Dementias in Old Age

One of the best studies to date of the prevalence and reversibility of dementias in a clinical population is that of Larson, Reifler, Sumi, Canfield, and Chinn (1985). The sample for this study consisted of 200 consecutive referrals to a psychiatric outpatient program that specialized in diagnosis and treatment of cognitive impairment in elderly patients. Clinical diagnoses were assigned according to DSM-III criteria (American Psychiatric Association, 1980), supplemented by a thorough medical diagnostic workup. Several neuropsychological tests were also administered as part of the evaluation, including a mental status exam, a depression rating scale, and the Wechsler Adult Intelligence Scale (WAIS), Wechsler Memory Scale (WMS), and the Object Memory Evaluation. A multidisciplinary team reviewed all findings and identified a primary illness believed to be causing the dementia, as well as secondary psychiatric illnesses and medical conditions.

TABLE 6.5. Conditions That Can Simulate Dementia[a]

Psychiatric disorders	Metabolic disorders
Depression	Hyper- and hypothyroidism
Anxiety	Hypercalcemia (sodium)
Psychosis	Hyper- and hyponatremia (sodium)
Posttraumatic stress disorder	Hypoglycemia (glucose)
Adverse medication reactions	Hyperlipidemia
Sedatives	Hypercapnia (carbon dioxide)
Hypnotics	Kidney failure
Antianxiety agents	Liver failure
Antidepressants	Cushing's syndrome
Antiarrhythmics	Addison's disease
Antihypertensives	Hypopituitarism
Anticonvulsants	Remote effect of carcinoma
Antipsychotics	Other conditions
Digitalis and derivatives	Sensory deprivation (e.g., blindness or deafness)
Any drugs with anticholinergic side effects	Chronic or recurring pain
Nutritional disorders	Environmental change and isolation
Pellagra (vitamin B-6 deficiency)	Anesthesia or surgery
Thiamine deficiency	
Cobalamin (vitamin B-12) deficiency or pernicious anemia	
Folate deficiency	

[a]Adapted from Office of Technology Assessment, U.S. Congress (1987).

Alzheimer-type dementia was clearly the predominant clinical diagnosis in this sample, accounting for 69% of cases. However, 9% were judged to have no dementia or to have age-associated forgetfulness, and 17% were felt to have medical causes for their cognitive impairment. Foremost among the specific causes were drug effects, accounting for 5% of all cases; myxedema (hypothyroidism), accounting for 1.5%; and other metabolic diseases, affecting 2.5% of cases. Of the individuals judged to be without organic dementia, two-thirds (10 of 15, or 5% of the total sample) were diagnosed as having depression.

Many of these patients had more than one illness contributing to their cognitive problems. Depression was identified as a secondary cause in 24% of the patients, drug effects in 9.5%, and hypothyroidism in 3%. More than 60% of these patients had medical illnesses (e.g., hypertension, osteoarthritis, chronic obstructive pulmonary disease, congestive heart failure) that may also have contributed to cognitive problems.

Participants in this study were followed clinically over a one-year period. Of the 200 patients, 55 (27.5%) improved in cognitive function for a month or more; gains were generally attributed to removal of medications exacerbating dementia or to treatment of coexisting conditions. In about one-half of these patients, the improvement was sustained over the year, but for the remainder, gains were more transient. In only two cases—one with medication toxicity, the other with a history of alcohol abuse—was the initial dementia completely eliminated.

These data suggest that *curable* dementia is rare in older patients in comparison to conditions such as Alzheimer's disease or multi-infarct dementia. However, they also show that treatment of coexisting conditions (e.g., medical illness or depression) can result in noticeable clinical gains for many demented patients.

Larson *et al.*'s findings (1985) generally concur with other recent data on causes of dementia. For example, in a review of 32 prevalence studies, Clarfield (1988) found that Alzheimer-type dementia and multi-infarct dementia accounted for 56.8% and 13.3% of all reported cases, respectively. An additional 13.2% of cases were felt to be due to potentially reversible causes, most notably, medication reactions, depression, and metabolic disorders.

Assessment Procedures

The most important procedures in diagnosing dementia are a careful clinical evaluation of the patient, a mental status examination, and interviews with relatives or other informants that allow one to obtain a history of symptoms and to estimate how the patient is functioning in everyday settings (see Table 6.6; National Institutes of Health, 1987). If clinical assessment suggests a dementia, routine laboratory tests (see Table 6.6) are recommended to reveal reversible causes. If findings from these tests are negative, additional neurodiagnostic procedures (e.g., CT scans, EEGs, neuropsychological assessment) are commonly performed.

Mental Status Examination

A structured cognitive mental status examination is the standard procedure used in identifying patients whose cognitive problems are severe enough to raise a question of dementia. As noted in Chapter 4, there are many options to choose from in selecting a mental status exam. Very brief scales (e.g., the Mental Status Questionnaire; Kahn *et al.*, 1960) which tap only orientation and memory may be useful in certain settings (e.g., long-term care). However, for initial diagnostic assessments, somewhat longer scales, tapping a broader range of functions, are preferred. The Mini-Mental State Examination and the Neurobehavioral Cognitive Status Examination (see Chapter 4 for descriptions and critiques) are useful in this regard, as is the more extensive Dementia Rating Scale developed by Mattis (1976). The Mattis scale taps initiation and perseveration as well as language, visuospatial skills, and memory. However, it takes at least 45 minutes to administer to impaired older patients and is most appropriate in settings in which neuropsychological testing is not available to follow up on the deficits noted on brief mental status exams.

Functional Assessment

Careful evaluation of everyday functioning is very important when dementia is suspected. Functional assessment can help to validate impressions formed during

TABLE 6.6. Diagnostic Tests for Dementia[a]

Careful clinical history
Mental status examination
Physical examination
Routine laboratory tests
Complete blood count
Electrolyte panel
Screening metabolic panel
Thyroid function tests
Vitamin B-12 and folate levels
Tests for syphilis and, depending on history, for human immunodeficiency antibodies
Urinalysis
Electrocardiogram
Chest X ray
Other procedures that are commonly useful
Neuropsychological evaluation
Speech and language analysis
Formal psychiatric evaluation
CT scan of the head
Clinical EEG
Discontinuation of nonessential medications
Inpatient hospitalization
Tests that may be useful in specific cases
MRI scan of the head
Cerebral blood flow and brain metabolic studies (e.g., positron emission tomography)
Lumbar puncture
Specialized electrophysiological techniques (e.g., event-related potentials)
Brain biopsy

[a]Adapted from National Institutes of Health (1987, pp. 15–18).

clinical interviews and is crucial for making recommendations about treatment and levels of care.

Several structured rating scales have been devised to assess activities of daily living (ADLs; for detailed information, see Kane & Kane, 1981). These are usually completed by caregivers based on their observation of the patient at home. The Instrumental Activities of Daily Living (IADL) scale (Lawton & Brody, 1969), summarized in Table 6.7, covers several of the skills required for independent living (e.g., meal preparation, use of medications, financial management). Another popular questionnaire is the Blessed Dementia Rating Scale (Blessed *et al.*, 1968), which assesses practical functions (e.g., ability to find one's way in the neighborhood) as well as mood and personality changes). The IADL is easier to use than the Blessed, because it provides clear anchor points for rating different skills. However, the Blessed examines a broader range of problems and has been shown to correlate significantly with neuropathological findings in Alzheimer's disease (Blessed *et al.*, 1968).

Scores on these scales correlate significantly with findings from mental status

TABLE 6.7. Items from the Instrumental Activities of Daily Living (IADL) Scale[a]

A. Ability to use the telephone
Does not answer telephone at all (1); answers telephone but does not dial (2); dials a few well-known numbers (3); operates telephone on own initiative (4)

B. Shopping
Completely unable to shop (1); needs to be accompanied on any shopping trip (2); shops independently for small purchase (3); takes care of all shopping needs independently (4)

C. Food preparation
Needs to have meals prepared and served (1); heats and serves prepared meals, or prepares meals but does not maintain an adequate diet (2); prepares adequate meals if supplied with ingredients (3); plans, prepares, and serves adequate meals independently (4)

D. Housekeeping
Unable to participate in any housekeeping tasks (1); needs help with all home maintenance tasks (2); performs light daily tasks such as dishwashing (3); maintains house alone or with occasional assistance (4)

E. Laundry
All laundry must be done by others (1); launders a few small items (2); does most small items, depends on others for large items (3); does personal laundry completely (4)

F. Mode of transportation
Does not travel at all (1); travel limited to taxi or automobile with assistance of another (2); travels on public transportation when assisted or accompanied by another (3); travels independently on public transportation, taxi, or drives own car (4)

G. Responsibility for own medications
Is not capable of dispensing own medication (1); takes responsibility if medication is prepared in advance in separate dosages (2); takes independent responsibility but occasionally forgets a dosage (3); is responsible for taking medication in correct dosages at correct time (4)

H. Ability to handle finances
Incapable of handling money (1); manages day-to-day purchases but needs help with banking, major purchases, etc. (2); manages financial matters independently but, on occasion, has forgotten to pay a bill or has been overdrawn in bank account (3); manages financial matters independently, collects and keeps track of income (4)

I. Ability to perform household repairs or chores
Unable to do even simple household repairs or chores (1); can only do very simple tasks such as hanging a picture or mowing the lawn (2); with some help and direction can do moderately difficult household repairs such as fixing a leaky faucet (3); is able to independently perform most household chores or repairs (4)

J. Skill in driving an automobile
Is unable to drive an automobile (1); drives when someone is present to give directions, drives poorly, or drives very slowly and cautiously (2); drives alone but has some tendency to get lost or has occasional driving problems (3); drives alone, has good sense of direction, and good driving skills (4)

[a]Numerical ratings are in parentheses. From Lawton and Brody (1969, pp. 179–186). Copyright 1969 by The Gerontological Society of America. Adapted by permission.

examinations, but the strength of associations is quite low, particularly for patients with mild mental status impairments (Reed, Jagust, & Seab, 1989). Everyday functioning is presumably influenced by many factors other than cognitive impairment; in addition, functional ratings can sometimes be biased by the personal characteristics of the rater (La Rue, Watson, Plotkin, Larson, & Kukull, 1988).

Procedures have also been developed for objective evaluation of functional abilities. A recent example is the Direct Assessment of Functional Status scale developed by Loewenstein, Amigo, Duara, Guterman, Hurwitz, Berkowitz, Wilkie, Weinberg, Black, Gittelman, and Eisdorfer (1989a). Patients are observed in their attempts to tell time, use a telephone, make change, balance a checkbook, and other activities; an optional driving scale, assessing knowledge of actions required by different road signs, is also included. The total time required to complete this assessment is usually less than 30 minutes, and preliminary normative data are available for both English- and Spanish-speaking patients.

Direct evaluation of functional abilities eliminates the possible reporting biases of caregivers. However, results must still be interpreted cautiously, since real-life situations may impose more complex demands than those observed in clinical testing. For example, patients may be impaired in their ability to plan and organize everyday behavior (e.g., keeping track of when to pay their bills), even if they still retain relevant component skills (e.g., knowing how to write a check). For tasks which entail a high degree of risk (e.g., driving an automobile), direct observation by a professional examiner is needed to evaluate safety. In California, physicians are now required to report patients with dementing disorders to city or county health departments, which then inform the Department of Motor Vehicles of the need for follow-up testing.

Specialized Neurodiagnostic Procedures

Other more expensive and sophisticated neurodiagnostic procedures (e.g., CT or MRI scans, EEG, and neuropsychological assessment) are often included in dementia evaluations. A primary reason for conducting such tests is to rule out focal brain pathologies (e.g., tumor or stroke) that may be the cause of cognitive problems. The value of any particular test varies with the clinical history and presentation (National Institutes of Health, 1987). CT scans or MRI scans are particularly important when there has been an abrupt onset or relatively rapid rate of decline. EEG is especially helpful when there is fluctuation of symptoms, suggesting a possible delirium or seizure disorder. Neuropsychological testing is most applicable when patients have a mild level of impairment or an unusual combination of cognitive symptoms, or when establishing a baseline for monitoring cognitive changes over time. Chapters 7, 8, and 9 provide more detailed information about the utility and limits of these procedures in testing for certain forms of dementia.

Treatment

Experimental treatments are being actively investigated for many of the causes of dementia, including Alzheimer's disease, multi-infarct dementia, and Parkinson's disease (see Chapters 7, 8, and 9). However, since existing treatments usually cannot reverse the cognitive loss associated with these disorders, most clinical interventions for dementia patients focus on prevention and alleviation of "excess disabilities" (i.e., dysfunctions that result from coexisting illnesses or from limitations in the social or physical environment). Treatment of specific medical and mental disorders can produce clinical improvement in some cases and may help to slow the rate of decline in others (Group for the Advancement of Psychiatry, 1988; Jarvik & Winograd, 1988; cf. Larson *et al.*, 1985, discussed above).

The psychiatric symptoms that often accompany dementia (e.g., agitation, sleep disturbance, paranoia, or depression) can sometimes be treated through behavioral techniques or by changing a patient's environment. Problems with sleeping through the night may be helped by increasing physical activity during the day and limiting daytime naps. Agitation may be controlled in some cases by identifying and reducing provoking situations or by distracting the patient with other activities. One caregiver discovered that he could reduce his mother's anxiety and pacing in the late afternoon by giving her a book of blank checks and asking her to "pay the bills"; she had been responsible for handling the family finances in earlier years and was usually happy to work on this familiar (and distracting) task. Some caregivers are good at discovering these techniques on their own; many others can benefit from suggestions provided by more experienced caregivers (e.g., through support groups or telephone help lines) or by professionals familiar with behavioral management techniques.

Zarit, Orr, and Zarit (1985) provided an excellent guide to psychosocial interventions for families affected by dementia; their approach combines psychotherapeutic services to caregivers (e.g., support groups and individual psychotherapy) with training designed to improve the skills of caregivers in managing problem behaviors. They also stressed the importance of identifying day-care, respite, or residential programs that can reduce the physical and mental strains on caregivers. Self-help organizations such as the Alzheimer's Association sponsor support groups for dementia caregivers and provide a wealth of information about local community resources; books such as *The 36 Hour Day* (Mace & Rabins, 1981), *Dementia Care* (Mace, 1989), and *Parent Care* (Jarvik & Small, 1988) also provide helpful information.

Some patients with dementia require medications to control severe psychiatric and behavioral problems. However, because these patients are very sensitive to psychoactive medications, a conservative approach to drug treatment is strongly recommended (see guidelines and examples provided by the Group for Advancement of Psychiatry, 1988; Jarvik & Winograd, 1988; Spar & La Rue, 1990).

In contrast to individuals with focal brain impairments, patients with Alzheimer's disease or other progressive dementias generally cannot take advantage of cognitive remediation techniques such as visual imagery or verbal associations; tangible aids (e.g., reminder notes or calendars) may be helpful in some cases, but extensive attempts to retrain memory skills are not generally recommended (for some exceptions, see Camp & Stevens, 1990). Individual psychotherapy can be helpful for patients with mild dementia (Teri & Gallagher-Thompson, 1991), and in our experience, there may be benefits from groups where patients can discuss the social and personal adjustments created by memory problems.

SUMMARY AND CONCLUSIONS

An important first step in evaluating an older patient with cognitive problems is to determine if the individual's history and behavior meet diagnostic criteria for delirium. If this condition can be ruled out, a second step is to determine if conditions are met for a generic diagnosis of dementia. For many older patients, deficits will be too mild to warrant this diagnosis, and for others, alternate explanations of the cognitive deficits (e.g., depression) will be identified.

Health care professionals of all types need to be aware that some types of dementia can be reversed with appropriate treatment and that currently irreversible dementias are often compounded by adverse coexisting conditions. Those working in community settings may be in the position of advising the patient and family members about the need for additional diagnostic procedures to screen for treatable causes. Those in medical settings must be prepared to explain the purposes of various tests that may be included in dementia evaluations and to communicate findings in an effective way.

Attending to the total picture of a patient's problems can strengthen one's credibility and effectiveness in other aspects of therapeutic work with the patient and caregivers. Also, it is important to keep in mind how often patients and family members are sustained by the small positive changes that can result from effective treatment of coexisting conditions. Even a little improvement can make the difference between hope and despair in learning to cope with such difficult conditions.

7

Alzheimer's Disease

Alzheimer's disease (AD) first attracted attention as a rare debilitating illness affecting individuals in middle life. Early case summaries provide a poignant record of the onset of symptoms and of the devastating loss of functional ability that can result as the illness progresses. Alzheimer (1907/1987) described his initial case as follows:

> The first noticeable symptom of illness shown by this 51-year-old woman was suspiciousness of her husband. Soon, a rapidly increasing memory impairment became evident; she could no longer orient herself in her own dwelling, dragged objects here and there and hid them, and at times, believing that people were out to murder her, started to scream loudly. On observation at the institution, her entire demeanor bears the stamp of utter bewilderment. She is completely disoriented to time and place. (p. 7)

Another individual with autopsy-confirmed disease had the following symptoms:

> [The] patient [aged 61] was a quiet woman, always inclined to be apprehensive and to worry unduly. [Her] husband noticed a change in her behavior ten years previous to admission. At that time she showed a tendency to repeat things in her conversation, began to fail in her house duties and to do silly things. . . . Her memory began to fail and she was disoriented. She developed a "mania for dusting the house"; this she used to do twenty to thirty times a day. She used to rise in the small hours of the morning and to work frantically about the house. She collected photographs of her son and latterly used to embrace them and imagined she was feeding the baby. Lately she has been very restless and asked to go to mother (who is dead). (Stengel, 1943, p. 3)

In the decades since these examples were published, AD has been the topic of much basic and clinical research. It is now believed to be a common disorder with a strong predilection for old age. The cause of AD is still unknown and an autopsy is still required to confirm the diagnosis. However, much progress has been made in identifying clinical symptoms associated with the disease, permitting more accurate antemortem diagnosis, and in developing interventions that can minimize some of the more distressing symptoms for the patient and family.

This chapter begins by providing background information important for understanding Alzheimer's disease. Diagnostic terms are defined, overviews of neuropathology and epidemiology are provided, and some current perspectives on causes and treatments are briefly noted. The second section of the chapter examines clinical diagnostic criteria and discusses variations in presenting features and course. The final section reviews neuropsychological findings and provides guidelines for interpreting test results when AD is suspected.

BACKGROUND

Clarification of Terms

Several sets of diagnostic terms are used in discussing AD. Neuropathologically confirmed disease is referred to as *definite AD*, or sometimes, simply *AD*. When AD is merely suspected on the basis of clinical assessment, appropriate diagnostic terms include *dementia of Alzheimer type* (DAT) or *possible* or *probable AD*. The pathological diagnosis is based on the co-occurrence of neuritic plaques and neurofibrillary tangles in sufficient density and distribution throughout the brain (see "Neuropathology," below). The clinical diagnosis is made when there is a gradually progressive dementia without any other apparent cause (see "Clinical Features and Course," below).

Neuropathology

Neuroanatomical Findings

On autopsy, brains of AD patients often show signs of atrophy that exceed those observed in normal aging. Shrinkage is most readily apparent in the gyri of the association areas of the cerebral cortex and least obvious in primary motor and sensory areas of the cortex (Katzman, 1986).

Overall loss of brain cells in AD may not be much greater than that seen in normal aging (Katzman, 1986). However, 40% to 60% of large cortical neurons may be destroyed (Terry, Peck, DeTeresa, Schechter, & Horoupian, 1981), and there is additional neuronal loss in the hippocampus, entorhinal cortex, locus ceruleus, and nucleus basalis (Katzman, 1986). This pattern of cell death may serve to "disconnect" the hippocampus from other brain regions (Hyman, Van Hoesen, Damasio, & Barnes, 1984), helping to explain the prominent amnestic symptoms noted in this disorder (cf. Hyman, Van Hoesen, & Damasio, 1990).

The plaques and tangles that characterize AD are also selectively distributed. Concentrations tend to be highest in certain regions of the cortex (e.g., the temporal-parietal and frontal areas), the hippocampus, entorhinal cortex, and amygdala, and relatively low in the motor, primary sensory, and cerebellar regions (Katzman, 1986; Kemper, 1984). The selectivity of affected regions may help to explain the prominence of intellectual changes in the early and middle stages of AD, as opposed to motor or sensory impairments.

As discussed in Chapter 2, neither plaques nor tangles are unique to AD; however, their joint presence, in sufficient numbers, is characteristic of this disease (Khachaturian, 1985). Tangles are usually much more numerous and widespread throughout the brain than in age-matched controls, and in contrast to what is true of normal brains, plaques are likely to be noted in the frontal and temporal cortex (Zubenko, Moossy, Martinez, Rao, Kopp, & Hanin, 1989; cf. Chapter 2). In patients aged 75 years or older, tangles are sometimes lacking in cortical regions; however, a diagnosis of AD may still be made if the clinical criteria for dementia are clearly met and if the brain contains numerous plaques (Joachim, Morris, & Selkoe, 1988; Terry, Hansen, DeTeresa, Davies, Tobias, & Katzman, 1987).

Other common neuroanatomical findings in AD include deposition of amyloid in the lining of cerebral blood vessels, granulovacuolar degeneration, and excessive Hirano bodies and Lewy bodies relative to those found in normal elderly controls (see Chapter 2 for additional discussion of these changes).

Neurotransmitter Changes

Multiple neurotransmitter abnormalities have been documented in AD. The most striking changes occur in the cholinergic system. Choline acetyltransferase (CAT), the enzyme that synthesizes the neurotransmitter acetylcholine from its precursors (see Chapter 2), is decreased by as much as 90% in the cerebral cortices of AD patients (Bowen, Benton, Spillane, Smith, & Allen, 1982; Davies & Maloney, 1976; Perry *et al.*, 1978). This decline in central cholinergic activity has been attributed in part to the death or dysfunction of neurons in the nucleus basalis of Meynert in the basal forebrain. In severe cases of AD, more than 75% of the neurons in this region are depleted (Whitehouse, Price, Struble, Clark, Coyle, & DeLong, 1982).

Somatostatin, a peptide neurotransmitter that may be important for cortical connectivity, has been found to be reduced by 50% to 75% in the cerebral cortices of AD patients (Davies, Katzman, & Terry, 1980; Rossor, Emson, Mountjoy, Roth, & Iversen, 1980). Changes in a variety of other neurotransmitters have also been reported, but with less consistency than the cholinergic and somatostatin changes (Katzman, 1986). For example, although some AD patients have reduced levels of dopamine in the striatum, this reduction may be due to coexistent Parkinson's pathology, which has been noted in 15% or more of AD cases (Joachim *et al.*, 1988; Morris, McKeel, Fulling, Torack, & Berg, 1988; cf. Chapter 8).

Epidemiology

Autopsy investigations indicate that 50% to 60% of clinically demented individuals have brain changes consistent with AD, and that for another 10% to 20%, Alzheimer changes occur in combination with other neuropathology such as cerebral infarction or Parkinson changes (Katzman, 1986; Tomlinson, Blessed, & Roth, 1970).

Although DAT is not usually regarded as a primary cause of death, it has been estimated to be a contributing cause in more than 100,000 deaths per year in the United States (Terry, 1976). In the age range of 75 to 85 years, a person is more likely to develop DAT than to have a heart attack and is at about equal risk for AD and stroke (Katzman, 1986). DAT is much more common than some other notable neurodegenerative disorders, being 14 times as prevalent as multiple sclerosis and more than 100 times as prevalent as amyotrophic lateral sclerosis.

The primary risk factor for developing DAT is increasing age. Although estimates vary for different samples and diagnostic procedures, nearly all studies show a sharp increase in prevalence from middle age to advanced old age. A recent study that used the criteria of the National Institute of Neurological and Communicative Disorders and Stroke and the Alzheimer's Disease and Related Disorders Association (NINCDS-ADRDA) with a large community sample reported an increase in rates of probable AD from about 3.0% for 65- to 74- year-olds to 18.7% for 75- to 84-year-olds and 47.2% for those aged 85 years or older (Evans, Funkenstein, Albert, Scherr, Cook, Chown, Hebert, Hennekens, & Taylor, 1989). These percentages are as high as those reported in some previous studies for all forms of dementia combined (see Chapter 6), suggesting that DAT may be a more common disorder than previously assumed.

Close relatives of patients with DAT appear to be at greater risk of developing the disorder than the general population, but the magnitude of the risk to family members is still unclear (for recent reviews, see Chandra & Schoenberg, 1989; Kay, 1989). There are some families in which the occurrence of DAT follows an autosomal dominant mode of inheritance across several generations. Whether this is the typical mode of inheritance or is limited to only an occasional family is a matter of considerable debate. Several family history studies have provided data consistent with the autosomal dominant hypothesis, estimating a 50% risk of DAT in first-degree relatives who survive to old age (e.g., Huff, Auerbach, Chakravarti, & Boller, 1988; Mohs, Breitner, Silverman, & Davis, 1987). However, Heston, Mastri, Anderson, and White (1981), who conducted the only family history study based on autopsy-confirmed index cases, found that risks of this magnitude were restricted to certain families (i.e., those with more than one affected individual and where symptoms began before the age of 70 years). In about 60% of the families they studied, only a single individual (the index case) was afflicted with AD.

It is difficult to investigate a disease like AD with family-study methodology, since many individuals die for other reasons before they enter the prime risk period for the disease; evidence of dementia in earlier generations is usually vague and anecdotal, and autopsy confirmation is usually lacking for both index and secondary cases (cf. Heston, 1988). Therefore, a cautious approach is recommended in discussing the role of inheritance with family members who may be worried about their chances of developing AD. At present, most experts in the field draw a distinction between familial DAT (where there is a clear family history, often with an autosomal dominant pattern) and other cases where there is less evidence of an inherited pattern.

Women appear to be at slightly greater risk of developing DAT than men (Rocca, Amaducci, & Schoenberg, 1986); in addition, there are suggestions that people with a history of head injury may be apt to develop the disease (Heyman, Wilkinson, Stafford,

Helms, Sigmon, & Weinberg, 1984; Mortimer, French, Hutton, & Schuman, 1985). Other possible risk factors, including viral or toxic exposure, medical illness, or stressful experiences, have not been confirmed in case control studies (Rocca *et al.*, 1986).

Causal Hypotheses

Relatively little is known about the causes of AD, although research on this topic is expanding very rapidly (for reviews, see Scheibel & Wechsler, 1986; Terry, 1988; Wurtman, Corkin, Ritter-Walker, & Growdon, 1990). In addition, since the clinical syndrome of DAT is such a broad disease category, many researchers believe that there may be multiple underlying causes that combine in various ways in different individuals.

Genetic Factors

A causal role for genetic factors in AD is suggested by the family history studies noted above and by similarities in neuropathological findings in AD and older Down's syndrome patients (e.g., Burger & Vogel, 1973; Glenner & Wong, 1984).

Recombinant-DNA techniques are being applied in searches for a possible gene locus for AD. Gusella and colleagues (St. George-Hyslop, Tanzi, Polinsky, Haines, Nee, Watkins, Myers, Feldman, Pollen, Drachman, Growdon, Bruni, Foncin, Salmon, Frommelt, Amaducci, Sorbi, Piacentini, Steward, Hobbs, Conneally, & Gusella, 1987), who studied four large families in which AD seemed to follow an autosomal dominant inheritance pattern, reported localization of the genetic defect for familial AD to chromosome 21. However, several other studies have not been able to replicate this finding (e.g., Roses, Pericak-Vance, Dawson, Haynes, Kaplan, Gaskell, Heyman, Clark, & Earl, 1988; Schellenberg, Bird, Wijsman, Moore, Boehnke, Bryant, Lampe, Nochlin, Sumi, Deeb, Beyreuther, & Martin, 1988). Therefore, while progress is clearly being made, the full range of genetic defects in AD has yet to be identified.

Environmental Factors

Studies of monozygotic twins suggest that nongenetic factors are also involved in the development and expression of DAT. One such study (Nee, Eldridge, Sunderland, Thomas, Katz, Thompson, Weingartner, Weiss, Julian, & Cohen, 1987) found that the concordance rate for DAT in identical (monozygotic) twins was only about 40%. Others have indicated that the age of onset of DAT may differ by as much as 6 to 15 years in identical twins (e.g., Jarvik, Ruth, & Matsuyama, 1980; Kay, 1989).

To date, epidemiological studies have not identified any specific environmental factors associated with DAT. However, the range of factors that have been investigated is still quite small, and research on this topic is continuing.

There has been considerable interest in the possible causative role of environmental toxins in DAT, especially aluminum. Aluminum is a known neurotoxin which some studies have found to be present in high concentrations in neurofibrillary tangles in AD brains (Perl & Brody, 1980). However, in recent years, aluminum buildup in AD has generally been interpreted as secondary to some more fundamental process, perhaps involving a breakdown of the blood–brain barrier.

An infectious agent model has also been proposed because of the established role of viral infections in some other neurodegenerative conditions (e.g., Creutzfeldt-Jakob's disease). However, animal studies have failed to demonstrate transmission of Alzheimer-type neuropathological changes from affected tissue, and there is no indication that AD can be transmitted through routine personal contact with DAT patients or blood transfusions.

Pathogenic Mechanisms

Investigators have been searching for a central pathogenic mechanism in AD, that is, a single change or set of changes from which other neuropathological features appear to follow. Identification of such a factor may help to organize the many separate findings on brain changes in AD and may greatly stimulate development of theories about the cause of the disorder.

One example of this line of inquiry is provided by recent research on the role of beta-amyloid in AD. The beta-amyloid protein is found in neuritic plaques and cerebral blood vessels in patients with AD, in older Down's syndrome patients, and to a lesser extent, in normal older adults (Joachim & Selkoe, 1989); recently, deposits have also been observed in nonneural tissues (e.g., skin and intestines) of patients with DAT (Joachim, Mori, & Selkoe, 1989). According to one recent hypothesis (Joachim & Selkoe, 1989), beta-amyloid may form as a result of genetic transcription or translation errors involving a larger, precursor protein located on chromosome 21. Whether beta-amyloid causes other neurobiological abnormalities in AD (e.g., plaques and tangles) or is a consequence of a still more basic process is still unknown. Shifts in brain immunoreactivity, breakdown of the blood–brain barrier, impairments of the intracellular microtubular system, or other fundamental changes may precede beta-amyloid deposition (Matsuyama & Jarvik, 1989; Scheibel, 1992).

Experimental Therapies

Since the mid-1970s, most of the experimental treatments for DAT have been aimed at correcting cholinergic neurotransmitter deficits. Choline and lecithin supplements have been prescribed in an attempt to increase acetylcholine concentrations; however, this approach has met with very limited clinical success (see Bartus *et al.*, 1982, for a review). A second line of treatments has focused on cholinesterase inhibitors such as physostigmine or tetrahydroaminoacridine (THA). These drugs inhibit the breakdown of whatever acetylcholine is available within the synaptic cleft (see Chapter 2 for discussion of the cholinergic system). Mild improvements have sometimes been noted with physostigmine (cf. Bartus *et al.*, 1982), and some longer term benefits have been reported for THA in a few individuals. However, the findings with respect to THA (Summers, Majovski, Marsh, Tachiki, & Kling, 1986) are controversial, and a multisite study is under way to provide a clearer picture of THA effects. Another approach has been to treat with drugs such as philocarpine, arecholine, or bethanechol that stimulate postsynaptic cholinergic receptors. These receptors are less affected by AD than other elements of the cholinergic system, so they may provide a more suitable brain substrate for drug enhancement (Tariot, Cohen, Welkowitz, Sunderland, Newhouse, Murphy, & Weingartner, 1988). Findings from this approach are also very preliminary, although mild symptomatic improvements have sometimes been observed. In the case of bethanechol infusion (Harbaugh, Roberts, Coombs, Saunders, & Reeder, 1984), where the drug is injected directly into the ventricles of the brain through a small subcutaneous tube, possible positive results have often been offset by the side effects associated with neurosurgery and chronic tube implantation.

Medications influencing dopamine, serotonin, neuropeptides, and vasodilation have also been studied, all with negligible or modest effects (see Drachman & Swearer, 1992, for a review). However, at least 15 new drugs designed to improve cognitive function are currently being tested in the United States (Pharmaceutical Manufacturers Association, 1989). Human studies of nerve growth factor, which may prolong survival of damaged cholinergic neurons, are also being planned (Drachman & Swearer, 1990; Russell, 1988).

CLINICAL FEATURES AND COURSE

Generalizations about the clinical presentation of DAT are complicated by the insidious onset and progressive nature of the illness. Until recently, standards for rating the severity of DAT have been lacking, so that it has been difficult for investigators to compare their observations or to describe the natural history of the disease. Contemporary studies are providing a clearer picture of the cognitive and behavioral disturbances in different stages of DAT; however, they also provide evidence of heterogeneity in early symptoms and in the rate of decline over time.

The following sections review clinical and research criteria for diagnosing DAT, describe some severity rating scales, and take a closer look at individual differences in clinical presentation and course.

Dementia of the Alzheimer Type

In the revision of the third edition of the *Diagnostic and Statistical Manual* (DSM-III-R; American Psychiatric Association, 1987, p. 121), a diagnosis of Primary Degenerative Dementia of the Alzheimer Type (DAT) is made under the following conditions:

1. A dementia, as defined in Chapter 6, is present.
2. There was insidious onset with a generally progressive deteriorating course.
3. All specific causes of dementia have been excluded by history, physical examination, and laboratory tests (see Chapter 6).

Possible or Probable AD

In clinical research, DSM-III-R criteria are often supplemented with diagnostic standards provided by a panel of experts from the NINCDS-ADRDA (McKhann, Drachman, Folstein, Katzman, Price, & Stadlan, 1984). These criteria rank AD diagnoses on a continuum of certainty (see Table 7.1).

A diagnosis of probable AD is made in individuals with two or more areas of cognitive impairment, a history of gradual decline, and negative medical diagnostic findings for specific causes. Other clinical findings that either support the impression of probable AD or raise doubts about the diagnosis are noted in Table 7.1. Autopsy verification rates of 80% or higher have been reported for probable AD cases (e.g., Morris *et al.*, 1988; Tierney, Fisher, Lewis, Zorzitto, Snow, Reid, & Nieuwstraten, 1988).

A diagnosis of possible AD can be made when onset or course is atypical, coexisting illness is present, or only a single, progressive cognitive impairment has been identified. The possible AD category fits many of the patients referred for clinical diagnostic assessments, since a high percentage have medical or psychiatric illness that may be contributing to their impairments (see Chapter 6).

Neurodiagnostic Findings

Computer Tomography and Magnetic Resonance Imaging Scans

Standard computer tomography (CT) and magnetic resonance imaging (MRI) scans are not sufficiently sensitive to confirm a diagnosis of AD (Katzman, 1986; McKhann *et al.*, 1984). On the average, the degree of atrophy detected on these tests is greater for AD patients than for controls (Albert & Stafford, 1988; cf. Chapter 2); however, when findings are examined individually, a substantial proportion of AD patients show no more atrophy than expected for age alone. In dementia evaluations, therefore, CT and MRI scans are used primarily to screen for other types of brain lesions (e.g., tumors or strokes).

Cerebral Metabolic Studies

Positron emission tomography (PET) scan procedures are being increasingly used to study cerebral metabolic patterns in AD. Most research has focused on glucose metabolism using fluoro-D-glucose (FDG) techniques (see Chapter 2 for a description). The most common finding to date is regional hypometabolism, which is most apparent in the parietal or temporoparietal regions in the early stages of disease (for reviews, see Metter, 1988; Riege & Metter, 1988). As severity of illness increases, metabolic changes are often observed in frontal regions as well.

Studies suggest that parietal hypometabolism may be observed even in mild DAT, when memory loss is the sole neuropsychological deficit (e.g., Grady, Haxby, Horwitz, Sundaram, Berg, Schapiro, Friedland, & Rapoport, 1988; Kuhl, Small, Riege, Fuji-

TABLE 7.1. Criteria for Diagnosis of Probable and Possible AD[a]

Probable AD

Diagnostic criteria
1. Dementia established by clinical examination, mental status testing, and neuropsychological assessment.
2. Deficits in two or more areas of cognition.
3. Progressive worsening of memory and other cognitive functions.
4. No disturbance of consciousness.
5. Onset between the ages of 40 and 90 years, usually after age 65.
6. Absence of systemic disorders or other brain disease that could account for the decline in memory and cognitive function.

Additional findings that support the diagnosis
1. Progressive deterioration of cognitive functions such as language, motor skills, and perception.
2. Impaired activities of daily living and altered patterns of behavior.
3. Family history of similar disorders.
4. Any of the following laboatory findings:
   a. Normal lumbar puncture.
   b. Normal pattern or nonspecific changes in EEG, such as increased slow-wave activity.
   c. Evidence of cerebral atrophy on CT which is progressive on serial examinations.

Other findings consistent with the diagnosis
1. Plateaus in the progression of symptoms.
2. Associated symptoms of depression; insomnia; incontinence; delusions; illusions; hallucinations; catastrophic verbal, emotional, or physical outbursts; sexual disorders; and weight loss.
3. Neurological abnormalities, including motor signs such as increased muscle tone, myoclonus, or gait disorder, especially in more advanced disease.
4. Seizures in advanced disease.
5. CT normal for age.

Clinical features that make the diagnosis uncertain or unlikely
1. Sudden, apoplectic onset.
2. Focal neurological findings such as hemiparesis, sensory loss, visual field deficits, and incoordination early in the course of illness.
3. Seizures or gait disturbance at the onset or very early in the course of illness.

Possible AD

A diagnosis of possible AD may be made when
1. There is evidence of dementia with atypical presentation or course, in the absence of other neurological, psychiatric, or systemic disorders sufficient to cause dementia.
2. A second systemic or brain disorder is present that might produce dementia, but that is not considered the sole cause of cognitive impairment.
3. There is a single, severe cognitive deficit that is gradually progressive and does not have a specific identified cause.

[a]From McKhann, Drachman, Folstein, Katzman, Price, and Stadlan (1984, p. 940). Copyright 1984 by Edgell Communications, Inc. Adapted by permission.

kawa, Metter, Benson, Ashford, Mazziotta, Maltese, & Dorsey, 1987). As a result, there is considerable interest in monitoring PET changes in patients with questionable DAT and in individuals who are believed to be at increased genetic risk of developing AD.

The application of PET procedures in dementia is still considered experimental. Methodological techniques are being perfected (see Chapter 2), and as Riege and Metter (1988) noted, there is substantial overlap in current metabolic findings for DAT and normal aging. To date, therefore, PET has not been recommended as a routine diagnostic procedure in dementia evaluations (see Tables 6.6 and 7.1).

Electroencephalographic Findings

The most common electroencephalographic (EEG) finding for patients with DAT is generalized slowing of the background rhythm. On the average, the degree of slowing is greater in DAT than in normal aging; however, overlap between groups is substantial, particularly in mild dementia. Generalized slowing can also be caused by many brain impairments other than AD (see Chapter 6). Therefore, like atrophy on CT, diffuse slowing on clinical EEG cannot be used to confirm a diagnosis of AD.

More sensitive electrophysiological techniques, including evoked-response procedures and computerized spectral analysis (see Chapter 2 for descriptions) have also been used with DAT patients. Late components of the evoked response (especially the P300, a measure of central decision-making speed) are often slowed in patients with DAT, whereas early components (which reflect simple sensory processing) are normal for age (e.g., Ball, Marsh, Schubarth, Brown, & Strandburg, 1989; cf. Chapter 2). Brain mapping by computerized EEG also shows differences between patients with DAT and normal controls (Duffy & McAnulty, 1988; cf. Chapter 2) and may eventually prove useful in distinguishing DAT from vascular dementia (Leuchter, Spar, Walter, & Weiner, 1987). However, like PET scans, these techniques are not routinely recommended for dementia evaluations.

Severity Rating Scales

To achieve greater consensus in the use of terms such as *mild* versus *moderate* or *early* versus *advanced dementia*, several systems have been developed to define clinical stages of DAT. One of the most widely used is the Clinical Dementia Rating (CDR; Berg, 1988b; Hughes, Berg, Danziger, Coben, & Martin, 1982) summarized in Table 7.2.

CDR scores are assigned on the basis of a detailed clinical interview involving both the patient and a close informant; the interview is guided by a set of questions and instructions called the Initial Subject Protocol and takes about 90 minutes. The informant provides a history of the illness and rates the patient with respect to memory and problem solving; self-care abilities are rated on the Blessed Dementia Rating Scale (Blessed *et al.*, 1968). The patient is then given brief tests of memory, orientation, abstraction, calculation, judgment, and problem solving, with performance rated on a

TABLE 7.2. Clinical Dementia Rating (CDR)[a]

	Impairment				
	None 0	Questionable 0.5	Mild 1	Moderate 2	Severe 3
Memory	No memory loss or slight inconsistent forgetfulness.	Consistent slight forgetfulness; partial recall of events; "benign" forgetfulness.	Moderate memory loss; more marked for recent events; interferes with everyday activities.	Severe memory loss; only highly learned mateial retained; new mateial rapidly lost.	Severe memory loss; only fragments remain.
Orientation	Fully oriented.	Fully oriented except for slight difficulty with time relationships.	Moderate difficulty with time relationships; oriented for place at exam; may have geographic disorientation elsewhere.	Severe difficulty with time relationships; usually disoriented in time, often to place.	Oriented to person only.
Judgment and problem solving	Solves everyday problems well; judgment good in relation to past performance.	Slight impairment in solving problems, similarities, differences.	Moderate difficulty in handling problems, similarities, differences; social judgment usually maintained.	Severely impaired in handling problems, similarities, differences; social judgment usually impaired.	Unable to make judgments or solve problems.
Community affairs	Independent function at usual level in job, shopping, business and financial affairs, volunteer and social groups.	Slight impairment in these activities.	Unable to function independently at these activities though may still be engaged in some; appears normal to casual inspection.	No pretense of independent function outside home; appears well enough to be taken to functions outside a family home.	Appears too ill to be taken to functions outside a family home.
Home and hobbies	Life at home, hobbies, intellectual interests well maintained.	Life at home, hobbies, intellectual interests slightly impaired.	Mild but definite impairment of function at home; more difficult chores abandoned; more complicated hobbies, interests abandoned.	Only simple chores preserved; restricted interests, poorly sustained.	No significant function in home.
Personal care	Fully capable of self-care.	Fully capable of self-care.	Needs prompting.	Requires help in dressing, hygiene, keeping of personal effects.	Requires much help with personal care; frequent incontinence.

[a]From Berg (1988b, p. 89). Adapted by permission.

continuum; the Short Portable Mental Status Questionnaire (Pfeiffer, 1975), the Face-Hand Test (Zarit, Miller, & Kahn, 1978), and verbal tasks from the Boston Diagnostic Aphasia Examination (Goodglass & Kaplan, 1983) are also administered.

Based on interview and test results, ratings are assigned in six categories: memory, orientation, judgment and problem-solving, community affairs, home and hobbies, and personal care (see Table 7.2). Ratings are made only in relation to the subject's past performance, not in relation to general population norms. In determining an overall CDR score, memory is weighted most heavily, and guidelines are provided for assigning overall ratings when there are discrepant rankings across the six categories. Interrater reliabilities for CDR scores are quite high (kappa = .74) for examiners who have been trained in use of the scale (Burke, Miller, Rubin, Morris, Coben, Duchek, Wittels, & Berg, 1988).

Perhaps because it focuses on the early stages of decline and operationalizes the distinction between questionable and mild dementia, the CDR has been adopted in many recent studies as a means of grouping subjects and of summarizing changes in global functional levels observed over time. Also, as discussed below, subjects with CDR ratings of 0 and 1 generally perform quite distinctively on neuropsychological testing.

An alternative rating system is provided by the Global Deterioration Scale (GDS; Reisberg, Ferris, de Leon, & Crook, 1982a). GDS scores range from a low of 1 (corresponding to normal function) to a high of 7 (late dementia). In this system, the term *dementia* is not applied until GDS Stage 4; patients at this level are no longer capable of independent living, often have some disorientation, and are usually unable to recall some important aspects of personal history. The GDS also appears to have acceptable validity and reliability when used by experienced examiners (Reisberg *et al.*, 1982a; Reisberg, Ferris, de Leon, Sinaiko, Franssen, Kluger, Mir, Borenstein, George, Shulman, Steinberg, & Cohen, 1988).

Another instrument that can be used to measure severity of DAT is the Alzheimer's Disease Assessment Scale (ADAS; Rosen, Mohs, & Davis, 1984). The ADAS includes an 11-item cognitive subscale and a 9-item noncognitive subscale. Scores on the cognitive subscale are derived from brief tests of memory, orientation, language, design copying, and ideational praxis (preparing a letter for mailing), and from ratings of behavior during testing. The noncognitive subscale rates the severity of emotional and behavioral problems such as tearfulness, depression, distractibility, and delusions, based on behavioral observations during testing and information provided by a family member or caregiver. The ADAS does not define stages of illness; however, it provides a brief and reliable index for tracking treatment response or longitudinal changes (Kramer-Ginzberg, Mohs, Aryan, Lobel, Silverman, Davidson, & Davis, 1988).

Decline over Time

It is very difficult to pinpoint the beginnings of an illness such as DAT. The symptoms (e.g., forgetting of recent events, word-finding problems, occasionally getting lost) overlap with normal aging changes and with the everyday cognitive lapses that even healthy young people experience. With hindsight, family members often remember a particular incident (e.g., a year when the patient found himself unable to do income taxes) that signaled the beginning of serious problems, but the validity of these retrospective impressions has not been determined. Careful prospective studies would be needed to provide a clear picture of the earliest phases of DAT, but to date, no systematic data of this type are available.

The natural history of DAT is also hard to specify. A few years ago, it was thought that the illness had a course of approximately five years from the time of diagnosis to death, with death occurring from a variety of conditions to which demented, progressively debilitated individuals become increasing susceptible (e.g., pneumonia). Two factors have altered this picture. First, diagnoses of DAT are often made at an earlier point in the illness than was the case 10 or 20 years ago. This reflects the general public's increased awareness of DAT as a disease (in distinction to "old age" as a cause of decline) and the dissemination to the medical community of guidelines for diagnostic evaluation (see Chapter 6). Second, at least in the United States, the quality of basic medical care available to older adults has improved. Coexisting medical conditions are identified more often and treated more aggressively, with the result that individuals afflicted with DAT often live for many years.

The development of severity rating scales has enabled a reexamination of rates and patterns of decline. A number of prospective studies are under way, tracing patterns of longitudinal change for groups of DAT patients with various levels of dementing illness (e.g., Berg, 1988b; Botwinick, Storandt, & Berg, 1986; Kramer-Ginzburg *et al.*, 1988; Reisberg, 1985; Rubin, Morris, Grant, & Vendegna, 1989).

Preliminary findings have been reported for 16 patients initially rated as having questionable DAT (CDR = 0.5) who were followed for a seven-year period (Rubin *et al.*, 1989). For a majority (n = 11, or 69%), symptoms either worsened to the point where a clear dementia was present (2 had CDRs = 1; 8 had CDRs $\geqslant$ 2) or AD was confirmed by autopsy. However, for 3 patients (19%), symptoms did *not* worsen over time. For the remaining 2 individuals, outcomes were unclear because of complicating brain disorders (tumor, cerebral infarction).

Berg (1988b) described follow-up findings on 43 DAT patients with mild dementia (CDR = 1). After an interval of about five years, 30% of these patients had died, and 80% of the survivors were severely demented (CDR = 3). Longitudinal neuropsychological findings have also been described for some of these subjects (Botwinick *et al.*, 1986). Across a span of four years, mean scores declined significantly on many different tests (e.g., 79% decline on Wechsler Memory Scale [WMS] Logical Memory; 74% on Wechsler Adult Intelligence Scale—Revised [WAIS-R] Digit Symbol). However, a few patients (5 of 18, or 28%) showed negligible decline, even on very sensitive tests.

Results of these studies indicate that most individuals who meet research diagnostic criteria for dementia are likely to undergo further declines within a few years. However, for some patients with questionable or mild DAT (perhaps as many as 20% to 25%), symptoms may fail to progress or may do so very slowly.

Why some cases of dementia worsen more rapidly than others is not known. This makes it difficult to answer caregivers' questions about how quickly, and how far, their afflicted relative is likely to decline in the future. In general, the more severe the cognitive impairment at diagnostic evaluation, the more likely it is that additional declines will occur in the next one to two years. However, management of coexisting illness can affect the course (see Chapter 6), as can the quality of the social environment. It is also important to note that the prognosis for patients with clinical complications (e.g., with coexisting symptoms of depression, significant medical illness, or multiple medications) may be quite different from that of carefully screened research subjects. Therefore, while it is essential to communicate to caregivers that DAT is likely to worsen over time, more specific predictions usually cannot be justified.

Heterogeneity in Symptoms

The problems that patients with DAT experience in the early and middle stages of the disease can be quite variable. Memory loss is usually the first problem reported by family members and is the most consistent impairment observed on clinical examination. Certain language and visuospatial deficits are also very common (see "Neuropsychological Findings," below). Nonetheless, several studies have identified subgroups of patients with DAT in whom either language or visuospatial functioning appears to be spared early in the disease (e.g., Martin, Browers, Cox, Teleska, Fedio, Foster, & Chase, 1986; Naugle, Cullum, Bigler, & Massman, 1985).

Changes in personality, affect, and behavior are even more heterogeneous. No single form of personality change has been observed in DAT, despite clinical lore suggesting that apathy is typical. One study (Reisberg, Borenstein, Salob, Ferris, Franssen, & Georgotas, 1987) found that 58% of patients with moderate to severe DAT (GDS scores $\geq$ 4) had significant behavioral problems, most commonly involving delusions, agitation, and diurnal rhythm disturbances. Another (Rubin, Morris, Storandt, & Berg, 1987) found behavioral changes in 75% of patients with mild DAT (CDR = 1); passive symptoms were the most common (e.g., withdrawal, lack of interest), occurring in two-thirds of the subjects, but agitated and self-centered symptoms were also common, occurring in about one-third of the patients. Prevalence estimates for depression in DAT vary widely. A few investigations have found major depression to be absent in DAT (e.g., Cummings, Miller, Hill, & Neshkes, 1987); however, others have described depressive symptoms in 30% to 86% of cases (e.g., Merriam, Aronson, Gaston, Wey, & Katz, 1988; Reifler, Larson, Teri, & Poulsen, 1986).

Although there is much discussion in the current literature about diagnostic subgroups within DAT, findings are not consistent enough to warrant a search for subtypes in routine clinical assessments (see critical discussion by Jorm, 1985). Apparent preservations in cognitive performance can sometimes be explained on the basis of premorbid superiority in a particular skill (cf. Naugle *et al.*, 1985); in other cases, low performance in one cognitive area, or a prominent behavioral or psychiatric symptom, can be explained by coexisting conditions (e.g., stroke, psychosis, or depression). Therefore, while there is ample evidence for heterogeneity in clinical symptoms, and in neurobiological findings as well (see Friedland, 1988, for a review), more research is needed to determine the causes and clinical significance of these variations.

NEUROPSYCHOLOGICAL FINDINGS

There is an extensive neuropsychological literature pertaining to DAT, and new studies are being published at a rapidly increasing rate. Reviews of this literature have been provided by Kaszniak (1986), Moss and Albert (1988), Poon (1986), and Riege and Metter (1988), and abstracts of pertinent studies are now available from the Psychological Abstracts Information Service of the American Psychological Association (Costa, Whitfield, & Stewart, 1989).

The following pages describe some of the outcomes of this research that are relevant to clinical assessment. The first section gives an overview of the range and severity of deficits that can be expected in early stages of DAT. The next sections provide a closer examination of test findings in specific areas (e.g., attention, memory, and language). A summary of test outcomes that support a diagnosis of DAT is provided at the end of the chapter.

Scope of Impairment in Early DAT

The severity of cognitive deficits and the number of different neuropsychological areas that are affected in DAT vary with the stage of illness and, to a lesser extent, with other individual difference factors.

Table 7.3 compares performance of patients with questionable or mild DAT (CDR = 0.5 or 1) to healthy older individuals on some well-known clinical tests (for descriptions, see Chapter 4), based on findings from the Washington University studies of aging and dementia (Storandt & Hill, 1989). The three groups were similar in age (mean = 71.6 to 73.9 years) and did not differ in education (mean = 12.8 years). All participants were given a thorough clinical interview to determine severity of DAT (see procedures for CDR ratings described above) and were carefully screened so that individuals with depression, reversible dementias, and complicating medical conditions were excluded.

Two trends are suggested by a comparison of mean scores: (1) patients with mild DAT performed much worse than normal older adults on a wide range of cognitive tests, and (2) those with questionable DAT had difficulties on the same types of tests as those with mild DAT, although to a lesser degree. Some tests provided better statistical differentiation of groups than others (especially WMS Logical Memory, WAIS Digit Symbol, and the Boston Naming Test), a finding suggesting that certain cognitive

TABLE 7.3. Test Performance in Mild and Questionable DAT Compared to Normal Aging[a]

Measure	Mild dementia	Questionable dementia	No dementia	ω^2
	Diagnostic group			
WAIS (raw scores)				
Information	8.77 (5.47)	14.10 (5.54)	20.14 (4.55)	.49
Comprehension	11.91 (6.22)	18.29 (5.06)	22.24 (3.13)	.47
Digit Symbol	18.94 (12.63)	31.93 (10.40)	45.42 (10.33)	.52
Block Design	12.47 (11.12)	19.32 (10.05)	29.11 (7.47)	.38
WMS				
Mental Control	4.53 (2.57)	5.58 (2.30)	7.20 (1.92)	.21
Digit Span				
Forward	5.76 (1.23)	6.17 (1.34)	6.81 (1.41)	.12
Backward	3.15 (1.38)	4.10 (1.32)	5.15 (1.31)	.30
Logical Memory	1.73 (1.76)	4.68 (2.12)	9.01 (2.48)	.69
Associate Learning				
Easy pairs	10.76 (4.15)	13.46 (2.61)	16.39 (1.59)	.41
Hard pairs	0.27 (0.67)	1.46 (2.07)	4.83 (2.94)	.47
Associate Learning (recognition)				
Easy pairs	5.68 (0.66)	5.85 (0.42)	6.00 (0.00)	.08
Hard pairs	1.79 (1.28)	3.20 (0.95)	3.96 (0.24)	.54
Visual Retention Test				
Total correct	2.08 (1.76)	3.73 (1.67)	5.55 (1.68)	.44
Total errors	16.82 (5.21)	11.66 (4.13)	7.12 (3.35)	.50
Word Fluency				
Letter "S"	6.76 (4.83)	11.51 (5.80)	14.25 (5.49)	.27
Letter "P"	6.35 (4.24)	10.63 (5.08)	13.66 (0.24)	.30
Boston Naming Test	28.53 (15.92)	43.00 (12.76)	53.64 (5.13)	.47
Trail Making Test (Part A)	103.71 (50.40)	68.22 (32.89)	42.14 (12.52)	.41
Crossing-Off Task	123.68 (39.15)	144.63 (45.53)	170.94 (35.30)	.22

[a]Table values are mean scores with standard deviations in parentheses; ω^2 is percentage of variance accounted for by a given measure. From Storandt and Hill (1989, p. 384). Copyright 1989 by the American Medical Association. Adapted by permission.

functions (e.g., verbal recall, speeded psychomotor integration) may be particularly affected by early DAT. However, the primary message conveyed by these results is that even in early stages, DAT can undermine many different cognitive skills.

Another study (Huff, Becker, Belle, Nebes, Holland, & Boller, 1987) described neuropsychological test findings for patients diagnosed with possible or probable AD based on NINCDS-ADRDA criteria. This sample (n = 79; mean age = 67 years) was also carefully screened for the exclusion of other illnesses that could influence cognitive function. Ratings of dementia severity were not provided; however, the general level of impairment was noted to be mild (e.g., patients were capable of giving informed consent and of completing a lengthy test battery).

Neuropsychological tests were given to evaluate performance in five different areas (orientation, attention, memory, language, visuoconstruction, and visual perception); the battery included many well-known tests (e.g., the Boston Naming Test, the Rey-Osterrieth Complex Figure Test, story recall, letter cancellation), but administration and scoring procedures were modified for several measures. Composite scores were computed for each area, and individual performances were classified as intact or impaired relative to a matched control group. A relatively stringent criterion was used to infer impairment (i.e., ≤ the 5th percentile for normal controls).

Table 7.4 summarizes the patterns of cognitive deficits observed in this sample. Only a few patients (5%) who were felt to have AD on clinical grounds were free of impairments on testing. Another small group (12%) had only one area in which a deficit was clearly apparent. The great majority of patients (83%) were impaired in two or more areas. Memory and language deficits were most commonly observed, affecting 87% and 72% of patients, respectively; deficits in visual discrimination, attention, and visuoconstruction were noted for 44% to 49% of cases.

These studies demonstrate the general sensitivity of neuropsychological tests to early DAT and provide support for the use of these tests as a diagnostic tool. However, they also illustrate the importance of integrating test results with other types of clinical data (cf. Chapters 4 and 5), particularly in very early DAT.

TABLE 7.4. Patterns of Cognitive Deficit in DAT and Normal Aging[a]

	Number (percentage) with pattern	
Pattern	DAT patients (n = 79)	Normal elderly (n = 86)
No deficit	4 (5%)	68 (79%)
One deficit	9 (12%)	15 (17%)
Orientation only	1	2
Memory only	6	1
Language only	1	1
Construction only	0	4
Visual only	0	4
Attention	1	3
Two deficits	12 (15%)	2 (3%)
Memory and orientation	4	0
Memory and language	5	2
Memory and construction	1	0
Language and attention	1	0
Construction and attention	1	0
Three or more deficits	62 (68%)	1 (1%)

[a]From Huff, Becker, Belle, Nebes, Holland, and Boller (1987, p. 1122). Copyright 1987 by Edgell Communications, Inc. Adapted by permission.

Storandt and Hill (1989) found that only a small set of tests (WMS Logical Memory, WAIS Digit Symbol, and the Boston Naming Test) was required to distinguish patients with mild dementia (CDR = 1) from healthy controls. However, none of the tests that they studied, either alone or in combination, reliably differentiated patients with questionable dementia (CDR = 0.5) from the normal elderly group. Storandt and Hill concluded that absolute levels of performance on cognitive tests may not be helpful in identifying very mild dementia unless premorbid abilities of individual patients can be taken into account. Huff *et al.* (1987) also suggested that a history of intellectual deterioration may be a more sensitive diagnostic indicator than cognitive test scores obtained from a single evaluation.

These studies did not interpret performance qualitatively, and they did not compare declines to estimates of premorbid ability. Somewhat better diagnostic accuracy might have been achieved in questionable cases if these procedures had been applied, or if newer tests, potentially more sensitive to early symptoms, had been included (see discussion below). Nonetheless, it is clear that standard cognitive tests cannot always detect the beginning stages of DAT.

Attention

Most patients with mild DAT perform quite well on simple tests of concentration and vigilance, such as WAIS Digit Span, WMS Mental Control, and number cancellation (Reisberg *et al.*, 1988; Storandt, Botwinick, & Danziger, 1986; Vitaliano, Breen, Albert, Russo, & Prinz, 1984). On the average, scores are slightly below expectations for age (see Table 7.3); however, distributions overlap considerably for patients and controls. As severity of illness increases, performance declines quite sharply on these tasks. For example, when patients with mild DAT (CDR = 1) were retested 2.5 years after their initial evaluation, mean scores for forward and backward Digit Span were only 4.3 (± 2.3) and 1.7 (± 1.6), respectively (Storandt *et al.*, 1986).

Changes in complex attentional processes may be noted much earlier in the course of DAT. Grady *et al.* (1988) followed a small group of DAT patients whose impairments were initially confined to memory loss; the next area of deficit to emerge for most patients was on tasks requiring sustained attention to complex task demands and cognitive flexibility (e.g., Trail Making Test, Part B, or interference condition of the Stroop Color-Word Interference Test). This finding is consistent with those of other studies which show good differentiation of mild DAT and normal aging based on WAIS Digit Symbol scores (e.g., Storandt & Hill, 1989). Whether it is the attentional demands of these tasks that lead to diminished performance is somewhat unclear, since these measures require the combined application of several different cognitive skills (see Chapter 4).

Some patients with DAT have more severe attentional problems than others (see Table 7.4). The reasons for these individual differences are just beginning to be explored. Severity of attentional deficits may be related to norepinephrine levels, which, in turn, may reflect the extent of locus ceruleus degeneration (Freed, Corkin, Growdon, &

Nissen, 1988). Reduced innervation to the frontal cortex has also been proposed as a mechanism for attentional problems in DAT (Becker, 1988). Clinically, it is important to be aware that mild to moderate attentional problems are not inconsistent with DAT, although care must be exercised in ruling out alternative causes of these problems such as delirium or depression (see Chapters 6 and 11).

Learning and Memory

Primary Memory

DAT clearly affects primary memory, but the severity of deficits is usually mild in early stages (Kaszniak, Poon, & Riege, 1986; Riege & Metter, 1988). In learning word lists, for example, patients with DAT still exhibit recency in free recall, preferentially retrieving the last-presented items (Miller, 1975); however, the number of items in primary memory is usually reduced compared to that in age-matched controls (Wilson, Bacon, Fox, & Kaszniak, 1983). Mild deficits can also be expected on digit span, word span, and block span tasks (Kaszniak *et al.*, 1986).

Greater impairments are noted when primary memory is tested under divided-attention conditions; for example, patients may find it hard to recall a list of three words for even a minute's time if the interval is filled with a distraction task such as counting backward (Morris & Baddeley, 1988). Based on these and other findings, Baddeley (1986) and Becker (1988) have proposed a two-factor model of memory loss in DAT, involving deficits in both a central executive system and in secondary-memory functions. The central executive system controls primary memory and coordinates resources for various mental tasks; when this system is impaired, problems are observed on primary-memory tasks, on tests of divided attention or attentional switching, and tasks which require quick access to lexical/semantic memory (e.g., verbal fluency tasks). For a subset of patients with DAT, executive system deficits can be quite severe and may equal or exceed secondary-memory impairment (Becker, 1988).

Secondary Memory

Learning and Recall. As Table 7.3 illustrates, patients with mild DAT (CDR = 1) generally perform much worse than healthy older adults on clinical measures of secondary memory such as Logical Memory, Associate Learning, or the Visual Retention Test (see Chapter 4 for a description of these tests and the Appendix for additional age norms). On the average, patients with this level of dementia remembered fewer than two items on immediate Logical Memory (cf. Butters *et al.*, 1987), showed almost no evidence of learning hard word pairs (cf. La Rue *et al.*, 1986a), and correctly reproduced only 2 of 10 designs immediately after presentation (cf. Eslinger, Damasio, Benton, & Van Allen, 1985; La Rue *et al.*, 1986a). These scores were much lower than those of the healthy elderly group (see Table 7.3) and also fall into the impaired ranges of norms reported in other studies (see Tables A.1 and A.2 in the Appendix).

List-learning tasks such as the Object Memory Evaluation, Selective Reminding Test, and California Verbal Learning Test are also very sensitive to the memory disorder associated with DAT (see Table 4.3 for a description of these measures). La Rue *et al.*, (1986a) found that the Object Memory Evaluation distinguished patients with mild DAT from both normal older adults and depressed patients with greater accuracy than either paired-associate learning or the Visual Retention Test. On the Object Memory Evaluation, patients with DAT were impaired on measures of learning (Storage, Ineffective Reminders) as well as on measures of retrieval (Retrieval, Repeated Retrieval); they recalled an average of only 2 to 3 items (out of 10) per trial and, by the fifth learning trial, had a mean Storage score of only about 4 items. By contrast, normal and depressed subjects recalled an average of 9 and 7 items per trial, respectively, and stored 8 to 10 items by Trial 5. A similar pattern of results has been reported for the verbal Selective Reminding Test; that is, patients with DAT, compared to normal adults, tend to have difficulty with all aspects of the task (Hart *et al.*, 1987a; Masur *et al.*, 1989), whereas in depression, impairments are frequently restricted to retrieval problems (Hart *et al.*, 1987a; see Chapter 11 for additional discussion of memory loss in depression). In classification analyses, storage deficits have been found to have fairly low sensitivity but very high specificity for DAT compared to normal aging (Masur *et al.*, 1989).

Intrusion Errors. Butters *et al.* (1987) examined errors made by patients with mild DAT on paragraph recall tasks similar to Logical Memory. The procedure differed from the standard clinical task in that four stories were presented (instead of two), and there was a 30-second period of distraction prior to recall. Under these conditions, DAT patients remembered very few correct facts (an average of only about 4 units of information for the four stories, each with a total of 23 units); they also made multiple errors of intrusion, interjecting details from stories that had been presented earlier or adding unrelated details. Proportionately, about 35% of their responses conveyed correct information, 25% consisted of prior-story intrusions, and 40% were extrastory intrusions.

The results of this study provide further evidence of the very severe impairments that one is likely to observe in DAT patients on story recall; in addition, they suggest that recall attempts may be dominated by *incorrect* responses (i.e., intrusions). This finding contrasts with findings for normal older adults, who make fewer intrusion errors overall and rarely confuse details of different stories (Butters *et al.*, 1987; cf. Chapter 4).

Intrusions may constitute 20% or more of DAT patients' responses on paired-associate learning tests (La Rue *et al.*, 1986a; Whitehead, 1973) and up to 50% of their responses on certain list-learning tests, especially under delayed- or cued-recall conditions (Kramer, Delis, Blusewicz, Brandt, Ober, & Strauss, 1988). On these tasks, too, intrusions are very rare for healthy older adults (La Rue *et al.*, 1986a; Kramer *et al.*, 1988; cf. Chapter 4).

Intrusions are observed more often in DAT than in Huntington's disease (Butters *et al.*, 1987; Kramer *et al.*, 1988), multi-infarct dementia (Fuld, Katzman, Davies, & Terry, 1982; Reed, Jagust, & Seab, 1988; cf. Chapter 9), or major depression (La Rue *et al.*, 1986a; Whitehead, 1973; cf. Chapter 11). This finding suggests that monitoring of intrusions may help in differentiating DAT from other dementing disorders. However, frequent intrusions cannot be considered pathognomonic of DAT, since they are also noted in alcoholic Korsakoff's syndrome and certain other neurological disorders (Butters *et al.*, 1987; Shindler, Caplan, & Hier, 1984). In addition, some patients with DAT make very few intrusion errors, even during lengthy assessments (La Rue *et al.*, 1986a; Ober, Koss, Friedland, & Delis, 1985). Therefore, the absence of this type of error should not be used to rule out the possibility of DAT.

Recognition Memory. The pervasiveness of memory problems in DAT is also apparent on recognition tests. As shown in Table 7.3, when patients with mild DAT were tested for multiple-choice recognition of word pairs from WMS Associate Learning, they correctly identified only two of the four hard pairs immediately after learning. Deficits have also been documented in mild DAT on the recognition components of the California Verbal Learning Test (Kramer *et al.*, 1988) and the Selective Reminding Test (Hart *et al.*, 1987a), and on tasks assessing recognition of pictures (e.g., Miller & Lewis, 1977), faces, and spatial locations (Moss, Albert, Butters, & Payne, 1986; Salmon, Granholm, McCullough, Butters, & Grant, 1989).

Unlike normal older adults or most patients with depression, patients with DAT often make frequent false-positive errors on recognition memory tasks. For example, when tested for recognition of the word list used in the California Verbal Learning Test, patients with mild DAT had as many false-positive errors as correct recognitions; by contrast, in the normal elderly group, correct recognitions exceeded false-positive errors in a ratio of nearly 7 to 1 (Kramer *et al.*, 1988).

Patients with mild DAT sometimes perform above chance levels on simple recognition tests, a finding suggesting partial preservation of the capacity for new learning. On the Object Memory Evaluation, for example, patients with mild DAT recognized 74% of items that they had previously failed to recall (La Rue, 1989); this level exceeded the level that would be expected by chance (33% correct) but was below the perfect recognition performance expected in normal aging (Fuld, 1981). These findings underscore the importance of interpreting recognition scores relative to appropriate norms.

Delayed Recall and Recognition. On recall tasks such as Logical Memory, healthy older adults usually retain a high percentage of the information that they initially remembered following delays of 20 minutes to 30 minutes (see Chapter 4); good retention has also been reported for many patients with Parkinson's disease or major depression (see Chapters 8 and 11). Among DAT patients, however, there is often a sharp decline in memory performance between immediate and delayed evaluations.

Kopelman (1986) reported an average retention score of only 9.4% for DAT patients on Logical Memory after a 45-minute delay; healthy controls and depressed inpatients performed much better, with mean retention scores of 82% and 73%, respectively. Recall declined by 50% or more for all of the 16 DAT patients, whereas none of the normal or depressed subjects exhibited such pronounced decline. The mean delayed-recall score was only 0.3 in the DAT group, suggesting that many of these patients remembered nothing about the stories. Patients with Korsakoff's syndrome also had severe difficulties on delayed recall.

Since rapid forgetting is not an invariant finding in DAT (see Becker, Boller, Saxton, & McGonigle-Gibson, 1987), good retention scores should not be used as evidence against this diagnosis. However, when present, poor retention scores can strengthen an impression of DAT if alterative explanations (e.g., severe alcohol abuse) have been excluded.

Cuing and Encoding Enhancement. In normal aging, learning and recall can be enhanced quite easily by activities that increase depth of encoding during learning or by providing cues at the time of recall (see Chapter 3). Unfortunately, in DAT, these procedures usually produce much less improvement in performance (e.g., Davis & Mumford, 1984; Grober & Buschke, 1987; Weingartner, Kay, Smallberg, Ebert, Gillin, & Sitaram, 1981b).

Several clinical tests have been developed that evaluate benefits of cuing and encoding enhancement. For example, in the Delayed Word Recall Test (see Table 4.3 for a description), patients first make up sentences about each of 10 words and, after a short delay, are tested for recall of the words. The process of creating sentences presumably encourages semantic encoding of the to-be-remembered words. In a preliminary study of this measure, patients with mild DAT generally recalled two or fewer words after delay, compared to a mean score of six for healthy older adults, a finding suggesting that the patients were generally unable to capitalize on the encoding activity (Knopman & Ryberg, 1989). The Controlled Learning with Cued Recall procedure developed by Grober and Buschke (1987) provides semantic cues during learning and again at the time of recall (see Table 4.3). Normal older adults perform very well under these optimized conditions; by contrast, patients with mild DAT still experience deficits in recall. A validation study (Grober *et al.*, 1988) found that the cued learning and recall procedure distinguished patients with very mild DAT with greater accuracy than either standard free recall or recognition memory testing. The California Verbal Learning Test (Delis *et al.*, 1987; see Table 4.3) also includes procedures for testing cued recall and for examining spontaneous organization during learning.

In interpreting performance on cued recall, it is important to control for the possibility that correct responses will be produced by chance. That is, if strong associative cues are provided (e.g., presenting *night* as a cue for *day*), patients may sometimes produce a correct response by free-associating with the cue word (Granholm & Butters, 1988). As with recognition memory, therefore, it is important to evaluate cued-recall scores relative to established norms that control for guessing probabilities.

Link with Semantic Memory. Several investigations have linked DAT patients' problems with new learning to a breakdown in their ability to access semantic memory; that is, new information may be difficult to learn because it cannot be readily processed in terms of its semantic features or related to general knowledge (e.g., Flicker, Ferris, Crook,

& Bartus, 1987; Martin & Fedio, 1983; Weingartner *et al.*, 1981b). In mild DAT, performance on tests of verbal free recall is strongly correlated with scores on verbal fluency tests in which words must be rapidly retrieved from semantic memory stores (Weingartner *et al.*, 1981b). Also, patients with mild DAT generally have as much difficulty learning semantically organized word lists as learning those in which items are presented in a random order (Weingartner *et al.*, 1981b). And as noted above, patients with DAT obtain little benefit from encoding-enhancement activities or semantic retrieval cues.

There are many indications of erosion in semantic memory processes in DAT. Patients with this disorder have difficulty succinctly defining words (Houlihan, Abrahams, La Rue, & Jarvik, 1985) and matching abstract pictures to printed words (Martin & Fedio, 1983); verbal fluency and confrontation naming are also reduced in many cases (see "Language," below).

Is Procedural Memory Spared? In studies of amnesia, a distinction has been made between *declarative* (or *explicit*) *memory* and *procedural* (or *implicit*) *memory* (Cohen, 1984; Mishkin, Malamut, & Bachevalier, 1984; Squire, 1986). Declarative memory deals with specific facts or experiences of which the individual is generally consciously aware. By contrast, procedural learning usually takes places without conscious monitoring and is demonstrated only through action or performance. Different brain regions are believed to be involved in the these two types of learning, since amnestic patients who are unable to learn new facts may still show benefits of practice in performing motor skills.

Eslinger and Damasio (1986) reported good performance for DAT patients on a perceptual-motor learning task (pursuit rotor), and Moscovitch (1982) found that with practice, DAT patients improved their speed in reading mirror-reversed text at a rate that was comparable to that of age-matched controls. However, Grober (1985) found DAT patients to be impaired on a mirror-reading task. In addition, several studies show that word-priming effects are diminished in DAT (e.g., Brandt, Spencer, McSorley, & Folstein, 1988; Shimamura, Salmon, Squire, & Butters, 1987). These findings provide additional evidence that memory deficits in DAT are broader in scope than those observed in many other disorders, including some cases of amnesia.

Remote Memory

In early stages of DAT, autobiographical memory is usually well preserved (Kaszniak *et al.*, 1986; Riege & Metter, 1988). However, when tested for recall of public events or prominent people from past decades, patients with mild DAT exhibit retrograde amnesia, recalling significantly more items from distant decades (e.g., the 1940s and 1950s) than more recent years (1960s through 1980s). This pattern appears even when cues are provided to aid remote recall (Beatty, Salmon, Butters, Heindel, & Granholm, 1988). Remote recall deficits correlate with global dementia severity, and by intermediate stages of DAT, a decline in recall is apparent even for distant decades (Sagar, Cohen, Sullivan, Corkin, & Growdon, 1988).

Summary of Learning and Memory Changes

An amnestic picture is expected in DAT. In early stages, this is most clearly demonstrated on secondary-memory tasks, such as story recall, paired-associate learning, copying designs from memory, and various list-learning tests. Serious deficits are noted in encoding as well as retrieval; as a result, patients with DAT also score below normative levels on recognition and cued-recall tasks. Imposing a delay may further accentuate problems in recognition and recall.

Compared to normal older adults, patients with DAT make more numerous errors of intrusion on verbal recall tasks and more false-positive errors on recognition testing. Procedures that usually enhance memory performance in normal older adults (e.g., organizing information by semantic categories) are often ineffective.

As DAT becomes more severe, impairments are noted in primary memory and in personally relevant aspects of remote memory. Semantic memory undergoes a significant erosion in DAT, and in contrast to many cases of amnesia, there may be a loss of procedural learning as well.

Language

Expressive Language

In the beginning stages of DAT, expressive language changes are generally subtle and do not greatly influence everyday communication. The most characteristic early problem is difficulty in accessing the lexicon, which may be manifested in several ways, including frequent circumlocutions, semantic paraphasias, use of vague superordinate or generic words, and explanatory paraphrasing (Hier, Hagenlocker, & Shindler, 1985). Deficits are apparent when narrative discourse is carefully analyzed and on tests of verbal fluency and confrontation naming.

Discourse. Patients with mild DAT usually speak fluently, but they convey less information than normal older adults in both oral and written discourse (Bayles & Kaszniak, 1987). For example, when they are asked to describe a picture, patients with mild DAT exhibit greater anomia than healthy controls, make more frequent use of empty words, and show a marked decrease in the number of relevant observations (Hier *et al.*, 1985).

Moderately impaired DAT patients tend to be more verbose but even less informative than mildly impaired patients. In late stages of illness, speech becomes laconic, and characteristics of Broca's aphasia (e.g., reduced phrase length, problems in articulation) may be observed (Hier *et al.*, 1985). Patients who do not become mute are still able to produce substantive words, but speech becomes increasingly telegraphic.

Complexity of syntax may be slightly reduced in early DAT, but syntactical difficulties are much less severe than lexical access problems (Bayles & Kaszniak, 1987). On picture-description tasks, for example, responses of patients with mild DAT are only slightly abnormal with respect to the number of prepositional phrases and subordinate clauses (Hier *et al.*, 1985). As the illness progresses, syntax is simplified, and some violations of grammatical rules emerge, particularly involving misuses of prepositions and incomplete sentences. Nonlinguistic abnormalities also become more apparent as DAT progresses. These include perseveration, palilalia (repeating of words), mutism, logorrhea (excessive talking), echolalia, and aposiopesis (stopping in the middle of a phrase).

According to Bayles and Kaszniak (1987), verbal description tasks (e.g., describing the Cookie-Theft picture from the Boston Diagnostic Aphasia Examination) are among the most sensitive test procedures for detecting language impairments in early DAT. However, scoring and interpretation of such measures may be difficult for examiners who lack training in clinical linguistics.

Verbal Fluency. Verbal fluency tasks can also be used to measure lexical access problems in early DAT (Appell, Kertesz, & Fisman, 1982; Benson, 1979; Corkin, Growdon, Nissen, Huff, Freed, & Sagar, 1984; Huff, Corkin, & Growdon, 1986). Both qualitative and quantitative changes in fluency have been documented in DAT. For example, when asked to name objects in a supermarket, normal older adults proceed in a systematic fashion from one superordinate category to another (e.g., vegetables, dairy products). By contrast, patients with mild to moderate dementia generate fewer categories as well as fewer exemplars per category (Martin & Fedio, 1983; Ober, Dronkers, Koss, Delis, & Friedland, 1986). Patients with DAT make more frequent errors of perseveration (i.e., repeating the same item two or more times) than normal older adults (Butters *et al.*, 1987) and may lose track of the type of item that they are trying to name (e.g., switching to fruits when they have been asked to name vegetables).

Some studies report greater impairment in DAT on category-naming tasks than on tests that require the naming of words beginning with specified letters (e.g., Sunderland, Tariot, Murphy, Weingartner, Meuller, and Cohen, 1985; Weingartner *et al.*, 1981b). Others have found category naming to be superior to letter naming (Hart *et al.*, 1987a; Ober *et al.*, 1986; Rosen, 1980). The particular letters and categories chosen may explain these conflicting results, and in general, a decrease can be anticipated on both types of fluency tasks.

Table 7.3 provides an example of the level of verbal fluency that can be expected of patients with mild DAT. On the average, patients with this level of illness named only about 6 words per minute for each of two letters, compared to mean scores of 13 to 14 words per minute for normal controls. Standard deviations were quite large in both groups, however, a finding suggesting considerable variability in fluency in both normal and demented individuals.

To evaluate the extent of fluency loss for a given patient, it is important to refer to age- and education-adjusted norms (see Chapter 4). Frequent perseverative errors or loss of set should raise a question of impairment, even if the total fluency score is only in a borderline-impaired range.

Confrontation Naming. Impairment of naming ability is one of the most commonly reported language deficits in patients with DAT (Hart, 1988). Problems have been observed on name recognition tests that minimize demands on verbal production (e.g., Huff *et al.*, 1986) and on traditional confrontation naming tasks such as the Boston Naming Test.

Storandt and Hill (1989) found the Boston Naming Test to be one of the best clinical measures for distinguishing mild DAT and normal aging. On the average, patients with mild DAT correctly named only about 28 items on the 60-item version of this test, compared to nearly 54 items for normal controls (see Table 7.3). Patients with questionable DAT also tended to perform below controls, but there was substantial overlap in distributions.

Although visual-perceptual deficits may contribute to some of the naming errors in DAT (Bayles & Kaszniak, 1987; Kirschner, Webb, & Kelly, 1984), perceptual errors account for only a small percentage of mistakes made by DAT patients on the Boston Naming Test (Martin & Fedio, 1983). Semantic association errors are very common and may differ qualitatively from those observed in normal aging (e.g., remote associations, or general category labels, are more prevalent in DAT). In addition, many patients with DAT perseverate in their naming responses (Bayles & Kaszniak, 1987).

Verbal Intelligence Subtests. Expressive language deficits can also be observed in the eroded quality of responses on verbal subtests from the WAIS or WAIS-R, especially Vocabulary. In a study at UCLA, we compared patients with mild DAT, depressed patients, and healthy elderly adults on WAIS Vocabulary performance, matching for total score across the three different groups (Houlihan *et al.*, 1985). Despite the equivalence of performance based on standard scoring, we observed a lower rate of perfect synonyms and a higher rate of poor explanations in the DAT group than the depressed or healthy elderly individuals.

Repetition. The ability to repeat words or phrases remains relatively intact in the early stages of DAT; however, problems may be noted in repeating sentences composed of low-frequency words or with novel or ambiguous content (Bayles & Kaszniak, 1987; Hart, 1988).

Reading Aloud. Patients with DAT can read single words out loud with remarkable accuracy (Hart, 1988), and as a result, word reading has sometimes been used to estimate premorbid intellectual ability (Nelson & McKenna, 1975). Sentence and prose reading are usually more impaired than word reading, perhaps as a result of visual scanning deficits (Hart, 1988). As discussed below, comprehension of written material is much more impaired than the mechanics of oral reading (Bayles & Kaszniak, 1987).

Writing. The presence of agraphia has sometimes been used as basis for subtyping patients with DAT (e.g., Breitner & Folstein, 1984), but there has been little systematic study of different levels of writing ability. Hart (1988) noted that some patients who are able to give accurate personal information when questioned orally may be completely unable to write such information. Bayles and Kaszniak (1987) reported only mild problems with the orthography of writing in mild to moderate DAT. However, when patients were asked to write a description of a picture, an increase in perseverations and sentence fragments and a decrease in vocabulary diversity were observed even in early stages.

Receptive Language

Auditory Comprehension. Mild to moderate deficits have been reported in early DAT on simple auditory comprehension subtests from the Boston Diagnostic Aphasia Examination, including word discrimination and verbal commands (Bayles & Kaszniak, 1987); more severe impairment is observed on the Complex Ideational Material scale (Bayles & Kaszniak, 1987; Rosen, 1983).

On the Token Test, performance of DAT patients declines as they are required to decode progressively more information, or when correct execution involves several steps (cf. Hart, 1988). The latter problem may be due to inadequate short-term memory, perceptual disability, and/or deficient motor programming rather than auditory language comprehension *per se*, since Token Test performance is significantly correlated with scores on the WAIS and WMS (Hart, 1988) as well as the Mini-Mental State Examination (MMSE; Swihart, Panisset, Becker, Beyer, & Boller, 1989).

Reading Comprehension. DAT patients have been reported to be less accurate in executing commands presented in writing as opposed to orally, a finding suggesting that they do not make use of the continuing presence of the written material to extract information (Hart, 1988). In general, auditory comprehension appears to fare better than reading comprehension, and reading for meaning is more likely to be impaired than reading aloud.

Does DAT Produce Aphasia?

Different usages of the term *aphasia* have led to some confusion in discussing language problems in DAT (see Bayles & Kaszniak, 1987, for a thorough discussion). Investigators who use *aphasia* as a descriptive term (connoting language impairment) usually find it to be common in DAT (e.g., Cummings & Benson, 1983; Kertesz, 1985). Others reserve the term *aphasia* for circumscribed language problems resulting from focal brain injury; these investigators draw a distinction between aphasia and the linguistic-cognitive changes which arise from progressive dementias.

On a descriptive level, similarities have been observed between language deficits in DAT and several different aphasic syndromes, including anomic, transcortical sensory, Wernicke's, and global aphasia (Appell *et al.*, 1982). In early stages, language in DAT patients most often resembles that of patients with anomic or transcortical sensory aphasia, while in late DAT, there is greater resemblance to Wernicke's aphasia (e.g., Hier *et al.*, 1985). There is less overlap in symptoms with Broca's or transcortical motor aphasia, since motor aspects of language function are well preserved until very late stages of DAT.

There have been a few case examples in which language impairments appeared as the first sign of DAT, preceding serious memory impairment (e.g., Kirshner, Webb, Kelly, & Wells, 1984b). These examples are rare, however, and in most cases, language problems follow or co-occur with amnestic symptoms. Therefore, as Bayles and Kaszniak (1987) pointed out, DAT can usually be distinguished from simple aphasia on the basis of memory tests and by clinical history.

Visuospatial Impairments

WAIS or WAIS-R Performance Subtests

Lowered Performance IQ and large Verbal IQ–Performance IQ (VIQ-PIQ) discrepancies are consistent with DAT but are not specific to this disorder (McFie, 1975; Miller, 1980; Wells & Buchanan, 1977). Certain WAIS or WAIS-R Performance subtests (e.g., Digit Symbol and Block Design) are especially sensitive to the distinction between normal aging and mild DAT (Storandt *et al.*, 1984), but deficits on these tests are also observed in depression and dementing disorders other than DAT (e.g., Parkinson's disease; cf. Chapter 8).

Hart *et al.* (1987b) provided a detailed comparison of Digit Symbol performance in patients with mild DAT (CDR ratings of 0.5 or 1.0) or major depression and in healthy normal controls. Depressed and demented groups completed many fewer items within the 90-second time limit than controls (mean raw scores = 27.0, 25.1, and 43.7, for depressed, demented, and control groups, respectively). However, on a test of incidental memory for the digit–symbol pairs, much poorer performance was noted for the demented patients than for those with depression. Of 15 mild DAT patients, 8 failed to recall any of the nine pairs, and no DAT patient recalled more than two pairs; by contrast, only 3 of 15 depressed patients recalled two or fewer of the nine digit–symbol pairs.

Correlations between WAIS Performance subtests and regional glucose metabolic rates have been documented in small groups of DAT patients. Patients with pronounced impairments on Block Design often show reduced metabolic activity of the right posterior parietal lobe, with somewhat weaker associations noted in the left parietal area (Chase, Fedio, Foster, Brooks, Di Chiro, & Mansi, 1984; Martin *et al.*, 1986). By contrast, patients with minimal visuospatial problems usually have normal metabolic function in the parietal regions. Therefore, variability between patients in the severity of visuospatial problems may mirror individual differences in brain substrates for DAT.

Copying and Recognition Tasks

In the early stages of DAT, patients often perform within normal limits on simple design-copying tasks, including the interlocking pentagons from the MMSE (Galasko *et al.*, 1990; Teng, Chui, Schneider, & Metzger, 1987), designs from the Mattis Dementia Rating Scale (Moss & Albert, 1988), and even the direct-copy version of the Visual Retention Test (Storandt *et al.*, 1986). However, as the disease progresses, copying ability declines quite sharply (Rosen, 1983; Storandt *et al.*, 1986; Teng *et al.*, 1987), and gross errors may be observed. Patients may perseverate on copying tasks or may be drawn to the concrete content of stimuli or instructions (Moss & Albert, 1988).

Rosen (1983) compared normal elderly subjects and patients with mild DAT on copying and immediate recall of designs from WMS Visual Reproduction. Both groups did much better on direct copying than on recall; however, because of the poor performance of normal subjects on the memory version (e.g., six of nine had scores of only one or two correct; cf. Chapter 4), the copying task proved to be a better procedure for distinguishing the control and mild DAT groups. Moderately impaired DAT patients were essentially unable to perform the copying task and scored at chance level on a matching-to-sample task involving the four designs.

Eslinger and Benton (1983) compared a mixed dementia sample (including DAT, multi-infarct dementia, and other conditions) with normal elderly controls on Judgment of Line Orientation and the Facial Recognition Test. Defective scores (i.e., performance that was worse than that of 92% of normals) were observed on one or both tests for 87.5% of the dementia patients. Marked disparities in performance across the two tests were much more common among dementia patients than among controls. Eslinger and Benton suggested that either very poor performance on visuoperceptual tests or prominent discrepancies in performance across such measures may be sufficient to raise a question of dementia as opposed to normal aging.

Topographical Orientation

Difficulty in finding one's way around familiar and unfamiliar places is a prominent practical problem for patients with DAT, but there have been few studies directly examining topographical orientation. On a computerized road map test, where the patient's task was to indicate whether turns on a map are to the left or to the right, mildly impaired DAT patients had greater problems than normal older adults (Flicker, Ferris, Crook, Reisberg, & Bartus, 1988), a finding suggesting impaired right–left orientation. However, this may be only a small part of DAT patients' topographical difficulties.

In an early study examining ability to solve simple mazes, Williams (1956) suggested that the bases of spatial disorientation are quite complex. Dementia patients tended to forget instructions and showed minimal benefits of practice or training. In addition, many patients were overly "attracted to the goal"; that is, they tended to proceed directly from the starting point to a visible end point, ignoring instructions to avoid obstacles.

Recently, Henderson, Mack, and Williams (1989) related DAT patients' performance on neuropsychological measures to caregivers' reports of topographical disorientation. Thirty-nine percent of the patients had frequent problems with topographical orientation, including wandering, getting lost indoors, getting lost on familiar streets, or being unable to recognize familiar surroundings. Performance on house- and clock-drawing tests was significantly related to topographical problems, as was severity of impairment on a verbal memory test; by contrast, naming problems and global mental status scores did not correlate significantly with everyday topographical impairment. The researchers suggested that a combination of memory and visuoconstructive impairments noted on testing may be helpful in identifying patients at risk of wandering.

Problem Solving and Executive Functions

Logical Reasoning and Abstraction

Impairments on WAIS and WAIS-R subtests measuring abstraction and practical reasoning are commonly observed in patients with mild to moderate DAT (Storandt & Hill, 1989; Storandt *et al.*, 1984). As shown in Table 7.3, for example, Comprehension scores are considerably reduced in mild DAT compared to those of normal controls. However, these measures generally do not discriminate between DAT and normal aging as well as some other measures (e.g., secondary-memory tasks or WAIS Digit Symbol).

Nonverbal reasoning may be intact on simple screening tests early in the course of disease (Moss & Albert, 1988), but on measures such as Progressive Matrices (see Chapter 4), substantial deficits are likely, even in early stages (Knopman & Ryberg, 1989). Concept identification tasks (e.g., the Category Test; see Chapter 4) are often too difficult for patients with DAT to complete validly.

Tests of verbal and nonverbal abstraction are strongly affected by background factors such as level of education, so that it is difficult to determine whether acquired deficit has occurred in older people with limited formal education. Therefore, these tests may be less useful than measures of memory or language function in differential diagnostic applications. Also, in patients who obtain normal scores on reasoning tasks (e.g., Comprehension), everyday judgment may still be impaired because of memory problems.

Cognitive Flexibility

As noted in earlier sections, patients with mild DAT often have problems on tasks which require flexibility in thinking or action (e.g., Digit Symbol, Trails A and B, the Wisconsin Card Sort Test; see Chapter 4). The mean scores for Digit Symbol and Trail A shown in Table 7.3 provide an indication of the severity of the changes that may be expected on these measures. Qualitative analysis of behavior provides further evidence of impairment. On Digit Symbol, some patients with mild DAT are unable to comprehend instructions or to complete the sample items without continuing correction; others understand the task initially but quickly lose set and may begin to copy numbers instead of symbols. Trail A is often completed correctly, although slowly, but on Trail B, the complexity of alternating sequences exceeds the capacity of a high proportion of patients.

Personality and Affect

The personality changes that accompany DAT vary widely from patient to patient (see "Heterogeneity in Symptoms," above). In some cases, core features of an individual's personality are accentuated (e.g., a quiet and reserved person may withdraw completely from social contacts, or an aggressive and competitive person may become angry and violent). In others, new characteristics emerge (e.g., a complaining, critical individual may become more accepting and pleasant, or a mild-mannered person may suddenly become angry and explosive). In general, there is a loss of complexity and subtlety in personality, and the ability to control emotional and interpersonal behavior is gradually undermined.

Psychodiagnostic assessment may be helpful in ruling out psychiatric disorder if the diagnosis of DAT is uncertain and can help to confirm coexisting psychiatric problems in patients with mild DAT. Standard psychodiagnostic measures (e.g., the Minnesota Multiphasic Personality Inventory or the Thematic Apperception Test) can be used with good effect in very early stages of DAT; however, as severity of illness increases, problems with attention and comprehension usually render such tests invalid.

Observer-rated scales assessing psychiatric symptoms are useful in tracking the effects of psychiatric interventions for patients with DAT. Appropriate measures include the noncognitive subscale from the Alzheimer's Disease Assessment Scale (see "Severity Rating Scales," above), the Behavioral Pathology in Alzheimer's Disease Rating Scale (Reisberg *et al.*, 1987), the Relative's Assessment of Global Symptomatology–Elderly (Table 4.8), and the Brief Psychiatric Rating Scale (Overall & Gorham, 1962).

Several new scales have been developed for measuring depression in patients with DAT, including the Dementia Mood Assessment Scale (Sunderland, Alterman, Yount, Hill, Tariot, Newhouse, Mueller, Mellow, & Cohen, 1988) and the Cornell Scale of Depression in Dementia (Alexopoulos, Abrams, Young, & Shamoian, 1988). These scales emphasize the behavioral and vegetative aspects of depression and minimize reliance on subjective reports of anxiety, guilt, and mood state. As a result, they may be more sensitive to depression in patients with aphasia or severe dementia than traditional depression rating scales (see Table 4.8).

A WAIS Profile for DAT?

Both Verbal and Performance IQ are likely to be decreased in mild DAT (see mean scores for WAIS subtests in Table 7.3). In questionable DAT, deficits on intelligence testing are milder and more variable; patients whose premorbid intellectual ability was in the superior range may still score at average levels on IQ summary scores, and earlier areas of competence (e.g., arithmetic for a bookkeeper, vocabulary for a writer) may still be reflected in the pattern of subtest scores (cf. Naugle *et al.*, 1985). Qualitative analysis of performance is important, since subtle changes in verbal abilities, perceptual analysis, or mental flexibility may be apparent, even if total scores are within normal limits (see "Language" and "Visuospatial Impairments," above).

Fuld (1984) proposed that the following WAIS profile (based on age-corrected scores) may be useful in distinguishing DAT from other dementing disorders.

$$A > B > C \leqslant D, A > D$$

where A = (Information + Vocabulary)/2
B = (Similarities + Digit Span)/2
C = (Digit Symbol + Block Design)/2
D = Object Assembly.

This profile was developed from research with young adults who had experimentally induced cholinergic deficiency; since DAT also involves prominent cholinergic deficits, Fuld hypothesized that this profile may be common among patients with DAT. In an initial study examining this idea, she found the profile in 44% (15 of 33) DAT patients, compared to only 8% (1 of 13) of individuals with multi-infarct dementia.

Several later investigations have supported the specificity of this profile for DAT. Brinkman and Braun (1984) found the profile to be present in 13 of 23 DAT patients, compared to only 2 of 39 with multi-infarct dementia. Satz, Van Gorp, Soper, and Mitrushina (1987) found the profile in only 12% of healthy older adults, and Bornstein, Termeer, Longbrake, Heger, and North (1989) observed it in only about 16% of patients with major depression.

However, other studies have raised doubts about the clinical utility of this WAIS pattern. For example, Filley, Kobayashi, and Heaton (1987) found that only 9 of 41 DAT patients (22%) exhibited the profile, compared to 5 of 30 (17%) patients with other conditions (depression, alcohol-related cognitive deficits, and delirium). They concluded, as Fuld (1984) did initially, that the sensitivity of the profile is too low for a negative finding to be used to rule out DAT, and in addition, they estimated that the predictive gain expected from a positive profile would be quite low in most clinical settings. This pessimistic view was supported by another study (Logsdon, Teri, Williams, Vitiello, & Prinz, 1989), in which positive Fuld profiles occurred with an equivalent low frequency (7% of cases) among DAT patients, depressed patients, and normal older volunteers.

Fuld's profile may eventually prove quite useful in identifying a particular subgroup of DAT patients. However, in light of its low overall sensitivity and conflicting findings about specificity, it seems premature to place much confidence in this profile for clinical assessments. Overall, memory and language tests appear more useful in evaluating patients with suspected DAT than intelligence test results; however, in a patient who otherwise meets criteria for dementia, a positive profile may provide an additional indication for considering a diagnosis of DAT.

A Severe Impairment Battery

For DAT patients with moderate to severe disease (e.g., CRD Stages 2 or 3 or GDS ratings of 4 or more), standard neuropsychological procedures are usually too difficult or demanding to yield meaningful results. Especially within the context of treatment intervention research, there is a need for simpler measures that can quantify limited cognitive capacities and detect small improvements or declines in such skills. Saxton, McGonigle-Gibson, Swihart, Miller, and Boller (1990) compiled a Severe Impairment Battery consisting of simple tasks assessing attention, orientation, language memory, and visuospatial skills; in an initial study, nonzero scores were obtained on each subscale even for patients whose scores on the Mini-Mental State Examination were very low (0–4). This procedure shows some promise for identifying residual strengths among very impaired patients and for providing an index of changes in cognition in the middle to later stages of dementia.

Synopsis of Neuropsychological Findings

Patients who meet research diagnostic criteria for DAT usually perform much more poorly than healthy older adults on a wide range of neuropsychological measures. In everyday clinical settings, however, differentiation can be more difficult, since many patients have complicating medical illnesses or unclear histories.

Table 7.5 lists some of the neuropsychological findings that are most consistent with mild DAT. Problems in secondary memory, word finding, and complex, speeded psychomotor integration are among the most likely areas of impairment. These may be accompanied by other types of problems (e.g., attentional deficits, visuoconstructive impairments) in individual cases. Qualitative analysis of performance can be helpful in cases where quantitative deficit is mild or questionable (see Table 7.5). The qualitative features noted in the table tend to be more common in DAT than in normal aging or in several other neurological and psychiatric disorders (e.g., Parkinson's disease or depression); therefore, their presence can help to strengthen an impression of DAT.

Neuropsychological testing has not provided a solution to the problem of early identification of DAT. There is great overlap in performance for normal older adults and patients with questionable DAT on standard clinical tests; whether newer tests (e.g., Controlled Learning with Cued Recall) will prove more effective in this respect remains to be seen. At present, since there is no cure for DAT, the benefits of very early detection are limited; however, as more effective treatments are developed, this issue is likely to become much more important to patients and their families.

SUMMARY AND CONCLUSIONS

DAT is the most common form of cognitive impairment in older adults. The primary risk factors for developing DAT are increasing age and a family history of dementia. A host of neurobiological changes are observed in this disease, but little is known about why these changes occur, or which are most crucial in producing cognitive and behavioral problems.

TABLE 7.5. Summary of Neuropsychological Test Findings in DAT[a]

I. *Typical presentation*
Disproportionate loss of memory, accompanied by
A. Deficits in cognitive flexibility and speeded perceptual-motor integration;
B. Deficits in language production and comprehension; and/or
C. Visuospatial impairments.

II. *Variations in presentation* (present in some cases)
Moderate deficits in attention and short-term memory.
Depression, psychosis, anxiety, or agitation.
Differential severity of language vs. visuospatial impairments.

III. *Most informative tests*
A. Secondary memory measures.
1. Quantitative deficit relative to age/education norms on all such tests.
2. Qualitative features present in many cases;
Logical Memory—Intrusions, confabulation; ≥50% decline on delayed recall.
Associate Learning—Intrusions; additional decline on delayed recall.
Object Memory Evaluation—Impairment in storage as well as retrieval; impaired recognition relative to norms.
Visual Reproduction Test—Omission of complete figure; gross distortions; perseveration from one design to the next.
B. Semantic memory/language processes
1. Quantitative deficit relative to age/education norms.
2. Qualitative features present in many cases:
Boston Naming Test—Marked circumlocution; remote semantic associations; perseverations.
Controlled Oral Word Association Test—Perseveration; loss of set.
Picture description—Fluent, but many vague terms; word-finding problems.

IV. *Findings that raise a question about the diagnosis*
Any of the following in early stages of illness:
A. Focal neurological signs and symptoms.
B. Motor impairments (e.g., gait disturbance, tremor).
C. Speech problems.
D. Severe attention deficits.

V. *Cautions*
Very early DAT cannot be reliably distinguished from normal aging by cognitive tests.
Autopsy is required to confirm AD pathology.

[a]From La Rue *et al.* (1992b, p. 650). Adapted by permission.

Neuropsychological assessment is one of the standard diagnostic procedures recommended for evaluation of suspected DAT. Tests of memory, language, and psychomotor integration are particularly sensitive to mild DAT and are generally more useful in detecting early illness than CT or clinical EEG. However, cognitive test findings must be combined with other measures to rule out alternative conditions.

Neuropsychological evaluation can be helpful in making recommendations for levels of supervision and care and, in some cases, can form the basis for more specific behavioral management plans. Family members sometimes fail to understand the extent of a patient's memory or reasoning problems, and in these cases, test results can be very useful in providing education about the disease and in identifying ways to work around some of the more troublesome impairments. Cognitive testing also provides an objective means of tracking the effectiveness of interventions. To date, no clearly effective drugs have been identified for alleviating symptoms of DAT, but five years from now, the therapeutic picture may be much more hopeful; in the interim, use of services such as caregiver support groups, adult day care, and in-home respite can often help to lighten the burden of dementia care.

8

Parkinson's Disease

A second important neurodegenerative disorder with a predilection for later life is Parkinson's disease (PD). PD is principally a movement disorder; however, cognitive and emotional problems are common in this disease, and a substantial percentage of PD patients develop a clear dementia.

In evaluating the mental status of patients with PD, examiners must learn to look beyond the slowness of speech and motor actions to form a valid picture of strengths and impairments. Neuropsychological testing can provide more accurate information about cognitive status than brief mental status exams and may help to determine if impairments fit a picture expected with PD, or whether additional pathology (e.g., delirium, depression, or dementia of Alzheimer type) may be present.

In the first section of this chapter, clinical features and diagnostic criteria are described, and neuropathology, epidemiology, and treatments are briefly reviewed. A discussion of dementia in PD is then presented, followed by a review of neuropsychological findings.

BACKGROUND

Clarification of Terms

As in dementia and Alzheimer's disease (AD), it is important to distinguish between the clinical symptom complex of Parkinsonism and Parkinson's disease (PD, also called *idiopathic PD*). *Parkinsonism* is a generic term which refers to a cluster of motor impairments. Principal features include:

1. Hypokinesia (i.e., difficulty in initiating movement).

2. Bradykinesia (i.e., slowness of movement).
3. Tremor, typically, a 4- to 8-cps resting tremor present in the limbs, face, or tongue.
4. Rigidity, consisting of resistance to passive manipulation of limbs or trunk.
5. Postural changes, including stooped posture and impaired righting reflexes, resulting in poor balance.
6. Gait disturbance (e.g., a shuffling, unsteady gait, or many rapid, small steps, called *festination*).
7. Ocular disturbance, including decreased volitional upgaze, impaired convergence, lack of smooth volitional and pursuit eye movements, and reduced accommodation to light.
8. Autonomic disorders (e.g., postural hypotension, a loss of muscle tone in the large bowel, and esophageal spasm).

Parkinsonism can result from a variety of specific illnesses (e.g., encephalitis lethargica) and toxic exposures (manganese poisoning) and is commonly observed as a side effect of neuroleptic medication (cf. Cummings & Benson, 1983; Koller, 1987). In PD, no specific cause can be identified, and symptoms have a gradual onset and progressive course. PD is by far the most common cause of Parkinsonism, particularly in older adults. Therefore, in the remainder of this chapter, the discussion pertains only to PD, and not to the broader category of illnesses resulting in Parkinsonism.

Diagnostic Procedures

A diagnosis of PD is established on the basis of clinical neurological examination, combined with medical history and laboratory tests which are negative for specific causes (cf. Cummings & Benson, 1983; Koller, 1987). Routine blood, urine, and cerebrospinal fluid tests are normal in PD. Slowing may be noted on electrophysiological measures such as electroencephalography (EEG) or event-related potentials (ERP), and cortical atrophy may be observed on computerized tomography (CT); however, these findings are not specific to PD (see Chapters 2 and 7). Specialized positron emission tomography (PET) procedures have been used to confirm the neurotransmitter deficiencies of PD (e.g., Brooks & Frackowiak, 1989; Martin & Palmer, 1989; Nahmias, Garnett, Firnau, & Lang, 1985), but these techniques are not routinely available for clinical diagnostic evaluation.

Clinical Features and Course

Tremor is the most common presenting symptom in PD, although a variety of other motor symptoms may be the initial sign, and in a small percentage of cases, depression or other psychiatric problems antedate motor problems (Cummings & Benson, 1983; Hoehn & Yahr, 1967; Mayeux, 1987). Different symptoms often worsen at independent rates.

A Severity Rating Scale

To provide a standard for classifying degree of disability due to PD, Hoehn and Yahr (1967) proposed a continuum of five arbitrary stages defined as follows:

I. Unilateral motor symptoms, usually with minimal functional impairment.
II. Bilateral or midline motor symptoms, without impairment of balance.
III. First sign of impaired righting reflexes (e.g., trouble with maintaining steadiness during turns); there is some restriction of everyday activities, but the patient is still physically capable of living independently.
IV. Fully developed, severely disabling disease; the patient is still able to walk and stand without assistance but is markedly incapacitated in other activities.
V. Patient is confined to a bed or wheelchair unless assisted. (p. 433)

Decline over Time

Wide variation has been reported in rates of progression of PD symptoms. A majority of patients experience significant disability within 10 to 15 years of diagnosis, and about one in four has rapidly progressive disease, becoming severely disabled within five years. In some patients, PD has a more benign course, with disability limited to Stage I or II for 10 or more years (Hoehn & Yahr, 1967).

Before anti-Parkinson drugs became available, the average length of survival following diagnosis of PD was 9 or 10 years; now, average life expectancy has increased to 13 or 14 years (Marttila, 1987). Some patients survive for 30 or more years with this condition.

Neuropathology

The most consistent neuropathological features of PD are neuron loss in the substantia nigra and other pigmented brain-stem nuclei and the presence of Lewy bodies in many of the neurons that remain in these regions (Gibb, 1989).

Lewy bodies are distinctive intracellular structures composed of packed filaments with a granular core. They increase in prevalence in normal aging (Chapter 2) and are associated with cell death in brain regions where they occur (Langston & Forno, 1978). Lewy bodies occur in the greatest concentrations in the substantia nigra and locus ceruleus but are also found in the nucleus basalis, dorsal vagal nucleus, autonomic ganglia, and hypothalamus; about a third of patients with PD have Lewy bodies in cortical regions (Gibb, 1989).

The substantia nigra is a principal site of dopaminergic neurons. Cell death in this region produces dopamine deficiency in associated brain regions, including the striatum and frontal cortex (see Figure 8.1). Several other neurotransmitters are also disrupted in PD, although not to the extent of dopamine (Cummings & Benson, 1983).

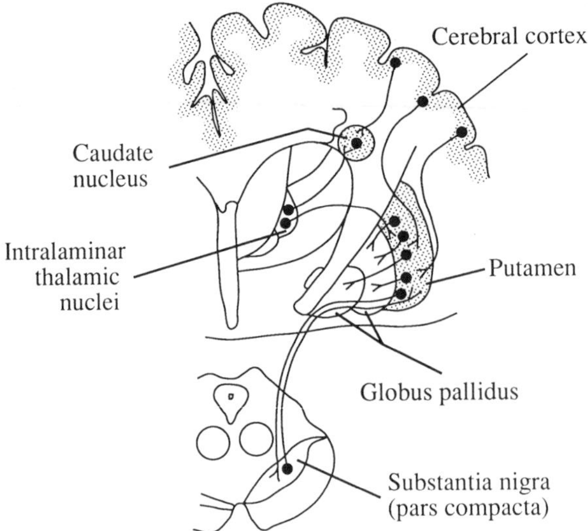

FIGURE 8.1. Afferent and efferent connections between the substantia nigra and other brain structures. The putamen, caudate nucleus, and globus pallidus are referred to collectively as the *corpus striatum*. (From Barr and Kiernan, 1988, p. 212. Copyright 1988 by J. B. Lippincott Company. Reprinted by permission.)

Dopamine depletion is considered the primary cause of the motor disturbances observed in PD (Cummings & Benson, 1983). The cognitive and emotional changes that accompany this disease may have a similar, or more complex, pathophysiological basis (see "Dementia in PD," below).

The presence of mild degrees of PD pathology in normal older adults suggests that a threshold of brain changes (estimated at 60% nigral neuronal loss and 80% striatal dopamine loss by Gibb, 1989) must be crossed before symptoms are observed. There may be a lengthy preclinical period prior to symptom expression, so that most people grow old and die without symptomatic PD, although many have some of the brain changes associated with this disease.

Some patients with PD have cortical plaques and tangles consistent with AD (see Chapter 7). This coexisting AD pathology may account for some of the more severe cases of cognitive decline that are sometimes observed in PD (see "Dementia in PD," below).

Epidemiology

PD is primarily a disease of late middle age and beyond. The average age at onset ranges between 59 and 62 years in different epidemiological studies. Incidence is very low before the age of 40 years and then increases sharply to the age of 70 to 79 years, when 1 or 2 persons out of every 1,000 develop the disease (Marttila, 1987). In later old age, the incidence of PD may decline (Marttila, 1987), although the reliability of this trend has been questioned on methodological grounds (e.g., Wolters & Calne, 1989).

Clinical surveys have suggested that PD is more common in men than in women, but epidemiological studies indicate that the risk is similar for the two sexes (Marttila, 1987; Rajput, Offord, Beard, & Kurland, 1984). PD may be more common in Caucasian populations than in other racial groups, and in Europe and the United States than in Southeast Asia; however, no geographic region or racial group has been found to be entirely free of the disease. Differing case identification procedures may be responsible for some of the apparent racial and geographic trends.

Few clear risk factors for PD have been identified other than advancing age. PD patients are less likely to have a history of tobacco smoking than the general population (e.g., Kessler & Diamond, 1971), and certain personality traits (e.g., introversion, emotional inflexibility, depressive features) may be overrepresented among PD patients compared to unaffected family members (Ward, Duvoisin, Ince, Nutt, Eldridge, & Calne, 1984). Interpretations of these associations vary, but the possibility that they reflect subclinical PD cannot be discounted (Marttila, 1987).

Causal Hypotheses

Accelerated Aging

The increased susceptibility of older adults to PD, combined with evidence of normal aging changes in the dopaminergic nigrostriatal system, suggests "an unavoidable mingling" of aging and PD-related decline (Langston, 1989). There is a steady loss of dopaminergic neurons and striatal dopamine throughout life, which may accelerate after age 65 (see Chapter 2), and effects of these changes may be compounded by reduced neuronal plasticity of the aged brain (Wolters & Calne, 1989).

The nigrostriatal dopaminergic system may be particularly vulnerable to lifelong wear and tear resulting from accumulation of free radicals, neuromelanin, or other products of dopamine oxidation. However, it is not clear yet whether normal aging changes in the nigrostriatal system are the same as those found in PD (see Calne, Crippa, Comi, Horowski, & Trabucchi, 1989, for detailed discussions). Wear and tear occurs in all aging people, but only a small percentage develop PD. Therefore, some "trigger factor" capable of causing an acceleration of the normal aging process must be involved (Langston, 1989), or an alternate explanation, less directly related to aging, may apply.

Aging Combined with Environmental Insult

Calne and Langston (1983) proposed that an environmental insult to the substantia nigra may occur at some point early in life, causing partial loss of dopaminergic neurons, which is later compounded by normal aging nigrostriatal changes. The two factors may eventually result in symptomatic PD, when a threshold of dopamine depletion (80% or greater) is crossed.

More recent evidence (McGeer, Itagaki, Akiyama, & McGeer, 1988) indicates that dopaminergic cell death occurs at a much faster rate in PD patients than in age-matched controls. This finding suggests that PD is an active process, rather than a "burned out" disease unmasked by normal aging (Langston, 1989). However, early environmental insults may cause surviving nigral neurons to be especially vulnerable to normal oxidative stress, thereby explaining a subsequent increase in rate of neuronal depletion (Langston, 1989).

Toxins

Barbeau (1984) proposed that factors such as stress or toxins may play a role in determining why some individuals develop PD and others do not. The prevalence of PD was found to vary in Quebec Province, with the highest rates noted in regions with intense agricultural activity and heavy use of pesticides (Barbeau, Roy, Cloutier, Plasse, & Paris, 1986). Furthermore, a higher percentage of PD patients than controls were found to have a gene associated with a defect in liver detoxification, which may have rendered them susceptible to the pesticide effects.

Interest in environmental toxins in PD has also been stimulated by the discovery of Parkinsonism caused by 1-methyl-4-phenyl-1,2,3,6-tetrahydropyridine (MPTP). Originally tested as a possible anti-Parkinson agent, MPTP was later sold on the illicit drug market as synthetic heroin. Several individuals who injected MPTP suddenly developed most of the features of PD (Langston, Ballard, Tetrud, & Irwin, 1983). Additional studies have shown the condition to be permanent, although responsive to standard anti-Parkinson therapies and have demonstrated that the primary lesion is a degeneration of the substantia nigra. Animal research suggests a link between MPTP effects and aging; that is, injection of MPTP produces extensive nigral cell degeneration in older mice but minimal change in young, mature mice (Ricaurte, Langston, Irwin, DeLanney, & Forno, 1985). Therefore, there may be an age-related sensitivity to environmental toxins such as MPTP.

Genetic Factors

Specific roles of hereditary factors in PD have been proposed (e.g., possible familial subtypes, or genetic susceptibility to toxins as discussed above), but in general, research suggests that heredity is less directly involved in PD than in some other neurodegenerative disorders (e.g., Huntington's disease, or even AD). In a widely cited twin study (Duvoisin, Eldridge, Williams, Nutt, & Calne, 1981; Ward, Duvoisin, Ince, Nutt, Eldridge, & Calne, 1983), the concordance rate for PD in monozygotic twins was found to be very low, and no difference in concordance was observed for monozygotic and dizygotic pairs. In addition, family studies report that prevalence of PD in parents and siblings of patients is only marginally increased relative to general population expectations (see Lang, 1987, for a review).

Approaches to Treatment

Symptomatic Therapies

Two classes of drugs are commonly used to alleviate symptoms of PD: those that increase dopaminergic activity (to compensate for dopamine depletion caused by nigrostriatal cell loss), and those that decrease cholinergic activity (to adjust neurotransmitter equilibrium disrupted by dopamine depletion).

The most widely used dopaminergic drug is levodopa, a dopamine precursor which is usually given in combination with a second drug, carbidopa (as in Sinemet), which helps to reduce peripheral side effects. Since its introduction in the early 1960s (Barbeau, Sourkes, & Murphy, 1962; Birkmayer & Hornykiewicz, 1961), levodopa has been recognized as a clearly effective symptomatic treatment (see Sacks, 1990, for dramatic examples of clinical benefit). It may take several weeks of treatment with levodopa for optimal response to be observed, but a majority of patients eventually experience some relief of motor symptoms (Cummings & Benson, 1983; Quinn, 1987).

Unfortunately, levodopa has many negative side effects. Psychiatric side effects are common and include nightmares, disturbed sleep patterns, perceptual illusions and hallucinations, hypersexuality, hypomania or mania, and delirium (Cummings & Benson, 1983; Mayeux, 1987). Long-term treatment with levodopa/carbidopa results in other complications (Lesser, Fahn, Snider, Cote, Isgreen, & Barrett, 1979). Treatment response begins to fluctuate, and in the extreme, "on-off" phenomena may be observed, with frequent, marked fluctuations in symptoms that often have no clear relationship to dose scheduling. Many patients also develop dyskinesias, including bizarre and dramatic involuntary movements (e.g., orofacial dyskinesia, chorea, or dystonic limbs). Currently, treatment with levodopa is often delayed as long as possible (i.e., until symptoms interfere with work or other essential activities), to prevent development of severe treatment complications in early stages of disease.

Other dopaminergic drugs (e.g., amantadine, Symmetrel, or bromocriptine, Parlodel) or anticholinergics (e.g., trihexyphenidyl, Artane) are sometimes substituted for levodopa in patients with mild disease or may be combined with levodopa to help to augment symptomatic relief. However, these drugs are generally less effective in controlling motor symptoms, and they also have negative side effects (Le Witt, 1987; Obeso & Martinez-Lage, 1987). A recent randomized comparison in newly treated PD patients found that bromocriptine helped only about 7% of patients after two years, compared to 59% treated with low-dose levodopa/carbidopa (Hely, Morris, Rail, Reid, O'Sullivan, Williamson, Genge, & Broe, 1989); bromocriptine also produced more confusion, postural hypotension, and nausea than levodopa/carbidopa.

Anticholinergic drugs such as trihexyphenidyl produce peripheral side effects such as dry mouth, constipation, and urinary retention; they frequently cause delirium and may exacerbate memory and language problems in patients without delirium (Koller, 1984; Obeso & Martinez-Lage, 1987; Sadeh, Braham, & Modan, 1982). Cognitive side effects are particularly likely in elderly patients or those with preexisting cognitive impairment, since acetylcholine levels are already reduced in aging and dementia (Chapters 2 and 7).

Experimental Therapies

The medications noted so far may postpone the emergence of disabling symptoms for several years but do not reverse underlying brain changes. Other treatments are now being tested that may have a more direct impact on pathology. For example, following the hypothesis that PD may be caused by a toxic substance such as MPTP (see "Causal Hypotheses," above), monoamine oxidase inhibitors such as deprenyl (which block conversion of MPTP to an active neurotoxin, MPP+) have been examined in several clinical trials. In the first prospective study to be reported, Tetrud and Langston (1989) observed beneficial effects of deprenyl compared to placebo in a three-year study of patients with early PD. The deprenyl-treated group was able to continue without levodopa therapy for a significantly longer period of time than controls (an average of 548 days compared to 312 days), and the rate of progression of motor symptoms was slowed by 40% to 83% on various assessment scales. Group differences did not appear to be due to antidepressant effects of deprenyl, since depressive symptoms did not differ for the drug and placebo groups. While these results are promising, they are based on a relatively small number of subjects (44 completing the study), and some researchers (e.g., Lees, 1987) are skeptical about the magnitude of effects that are likely to result from deprenyl. A large, multi-institutional study (DATATOP; Shoulson, 1989) will provide more definitive information on the effectiveness of this approach.

More radical approaches to treatment include attempts at grafting new tissue into the basal ganglia or other subcortical structures, using tissue transplanted from the patient's own adrenal gland or from aborted human fetuses (see Lindvall, 1989, for a review). Researchers agree that this approach is in a very early, experimental stage, and that major therapeutic benefits remain to be demonstrated. Older, cognitively impaired PD patients may suffer persistent mental status changes as a result of such surgery, leading to the recommendation that these patients be excluded from experimental surgical trials (Allen, Burns, Tulipan, & Parker, 1989).

DEMENTIA IN PD

The possibility that PD may result in dementia has been the subject of much research and even more debate. Both historically and at present, some experts consider dementia to be a routine part of the disease, whereas others find cognitive disturbance in a minority of PD patients. Different definitions of dementia and methods of ascertainment contribute to the debate; overlapping neuropathology between PD and DAT also complicates the picture.

Prevalence

Clinical surveys of hospitalized patients have estimated a 30% to 40% rate of dementia in PD patients (see Brown & Marsden, 1984, for a review). However, diagnostic criteria have been poorly specified in many of these studies, and as a result, estimates may be inflated by the inclusion of patients with delirium, aging changes, or cognitive impairment unrelated to PD. Adjusting for diagnostic limitations, Brown and Marsden (1984) suggested that the true prevalence of dementia in PD was closer to 20%. Even this reduced estimate has been challenged in more recent studies. For example, when Mayeux, Stern, Rosenstein, Marder, Hauser, Cote, and Fahn (1988) applied the criteria for dementia from the third edition of the *Diagnostic and Statistical Manual* (DSM-III; American Psychiatric Association, 1980) in their chart-review study of 339 idiopathic PD patients, the overall rate of dementia was only 10.9%. Although clear dementia appears to develop in only a minority of PD patients, rates exceed those expected for age alone. Mayeux *et al.* (1988) found that dementia was 3.75 times more likely in PD patients than in a normal aging comparison sample. More conservative estimates, based on multiple studies, suggest that dementia is twice as common among PD patients as in the general population (Gibb, 1989).

Coexistence of Alzheimer's and Parkinson's Changes

Several autopsy studies of demented PD patients have shown AD neuropathology (e.g., cortical plaques and tangles) coexisting with PD brain changes, leading to the suggestion that dementia in PD is actually dementia of Alzheimer type (DAT) (e.g., Boller, Mizutani, Roessmann, & Gambetti, 1980; Hakim & Mathieson, 1979). Demonstrations of cell loss in the nucleus basalis (e.g., Whitehouse, Hedreen, White, & Price, 1983) and reduced cortical choline acetyltransferase (CAT) levels (e.g., Perry, Tomlinson, Candy, Blessed, Foster, Bloxham, & Perry, 1983) in demented PD patients also tended to support this idea.

However, a later study (Perry, Curtis, Dick, Candy, Atack, Bloxham, Blessed, Fairbairn, Tomlinson, & Perry, 1985) found dementia in PD patients who did not have an excess of plaques and tangles. These patients had reduced cortical CAT, which correlated with mental impairment, but not with plaques or tangles. This finding suggests that reduced CAT, and associated mental decline, may result from the primary pathology of PD (Lewy bodies and nucleus basalis cell death) rather than coexisting Alzheimer changes.

Based on a review of the literature, Gibb (1989) suggested that a combination of cortical and subcortical pathology may be required for true dementia to emerge, and that several different neuropathological subgroups may combine to account for the 10% to 20% prevalence of dementia in PD. Pertinent subgroups may include PD patients with true, coexistent AD (a 5% to 7% rate would be expected on the basis of age); patients with preclinical AD plus extensive PD neuropathology; and PD patients with extensive cortical Lewy body pathology.

Subcortical Dementia

Some investigators (e.g., Cummings & Benson, 1983, 1984, 1988) have maintained that dementia is much more common in PD than the previous discussion suggests. However, this dementia is described as mild in severity and lacking in many of the clinical features that characterize DAT (e.g., aphasia or severe amnesia). The dementia of PD is said to be of a "subcortical" type, because impairments resemble those of other conditions where brain lesions occur primarily in subcortical structures (e.g., progressive supranuclear palsy or Huntington's disease).

In subcortical dementias, cognitive deficits are attributed to disruption of a complex "frontal system" composed of interconnections between the substantia nigra, neostriatum, thalamus, midbrain tegmentum, and frontal cortex (Cummings & Benson, 1983, 1988; see Figure 8.1). Table 8.1 contrasts the clinical features of subcortical dementia with those observed in disorders with extensive cortical brain pathology (e.g., DAT).

The concept of subcortical dementia is controversial, and its proponents acknowledge that more research is needed to clarify the role of subcortical structures in human cognitive function (cf. Chui, 1989; Whitehouse, 1986). Neuropsychological studies provide only partial support for the subcortical versus cortical distinction (see "Neuropsychological Findings," below). There are some notable similarities between PD patients' performance and that of patients with damage to the frontal lobes. However, for many patients with PD, deficits are so mild and circumscribed that a diagnosis of dementia may not be warranted. The specificity of some of the distinguishing clinical features also appears to be quite low. For example, although Table 8.1 lists affective

TABLE 8.1. Clinical Features That Distinguish Cortical and Subcortical Dementias[a]

Characteristic	Subcortical	Cortical
Mental status		
Language	No aphasia	Aphasia
Memory	Forgetful (retrieval deficits)	Amnesia (learning is impaired)
Cognition	Impaired (poor problem-solving produced by slowness, forgetfulness, and impaired strategy and planning)	Severely disturbed (agnosia, aphasia, acalculia, amnesia)
	Slow processing time	Response time relatively normal
Personality	Apathetic	Unconcerned or euphoric
Mood	Affective disorder common (depression or mania)	Normal
Motor system		
Speech	Dysarthric	Normal[b]
Posture	Abnormal	Normal[b]
Gait	Abnormal	Normal[b]
Motor speed	Slow	Normal[b]
Movement disorder	Common (chorea, tremor, rigidity, ataxia)	Absent

[a]From Cummings and Benson (1984, p. 875). Copyright 1984 by the American Medical Association. Adapted by permission.
[b]May be abnormal in later stages of Alzheimer's or Pick's disease.

disorder as specific to subcortical dementia, many studies report substantial depression in DAT as well (see Chapter 7); DAT patients may also exhibit slowing on motor and reaction time tasks (e.g., Ferris, Crook, Sathananthan, & Gerson, 1976; Miller, 1974; Pirozzolo & Hansch, 1981) and usually suffer impairment in planning and formulating strategies (see Chapter 7). On neuropsychological testing, therefore, there is often greater similarity in performance between DAT patients and PD patients with cognitive impairments than Table 8.1 would suggest.

NEUROPSYCHOLOGICAL FINDINGS

The following pages take a closer look at cognitive and emotional functioning in PD. The first section describes neuropsychological performance of patients who have recently been diagnosed with PD and who have not begun treatment with anti-Parkinson medications. Research with these patients provides the clearest picture of the impact of PD pathology on cognition and behavior. The second section reviews a larger set of studies assessing patients with more severe PD who are being treated with various anti-Parkinson medications. These patients are commonly referred for neuropsychological testing to assess the severity of cognitive problems and to evaluate mood disturbance or other psychiatric symptoms. A third section discusses neuropsychological findings on demented PD patients and compares their performance to that of patients with DAT. The final section presents a summary of test findings in specific cognitive areas.

Cognitive Deficits in Early, Untreated PD

To determine how patients in the early stages of PD perform on neuropsychological tests, Lees and Smith (1983) selected 30 individuals newly diagnosed with PD and compared them with an equal number of age-matched, hospitalized controls. The PD patients were all relatively young (65 years or less), had normal brain CT scans, and had no evidence of depression or cerebrovascular lesions. The mean duration of disease from the first reported symptom was 2.4 years, and motor disability was generally quite mild (83% were at either Stage I or Stage II on the Hoehn and Yahr scale). None of these patients had been treated with anti-Parkinson medications. Control subjects were primarily orthopedic surgery patients, and all were without brain disease.

On the Wechsler Adult Intelligence Scale (WAIS), no differences were observed in either Verbal or Performance IQ between the early PD patients and controls, and for both groups, mean scores were in the normal range (varying from 103 to 111). PD patients also performed as well as controls on a word-reading test, a result suggesting similar premorbid intelligence (Nelson & McKenna, 1975), and on recognition memory for faces and words. On a modified version of the Wisconsin Card Sort Test, there were no differences in total errors; however, PD patients made more perseverative errors and tended to identify fewer categories than controls. Similar trends were observed on verbal fluency testing. Mean fluency scores did not differ for patients and controls; however, a subset of subjects with PD had difficulty shifting from one letter category to the next and perseverated in naming specific words. Several patients appeared to be incapable of terminating a pattern of response that they knew to be incorrect, or of translating their correct grasp of concepts into task-relevant behaviors.

Hietanen and Teravainen (1986) also studied early PD patients (mean duration of illness = 2.3 years) who had never received anti-Parkinson medication. This sample was similar in average age to that of Lees and Smith (1983); however, a wider range of ages was included (32 to 81 years), and motor symptoms tended to be more severe (43% were at Hoehn and Yahr Stages I and II). An extensive test battery was used, consisting of several WAIS and Wechsler Memory Scale (WMS) subtests, a variety of psychomotor measures (Purdue Pegboard, finger tapping, writing speed, simple and choice reaction time), and the Trail Making and Stroop Color-Word Interference tests, which require cognitive flexibility in addition to motor speed (see Chapter 4).

The largest differences between patients and controls were noted on psychomotor tasks. Reaction times were about 30% longer in PD, Purdue Pegboard scores were reduced by about 20%, and on the Trail Making and Stroop tests, performance times were slowed by 30% to 36% compared to those of controls. Mild impairments were noted on secondary-memory measures from the WMS (immediate Logical Memory, Associate Learning, and Visual Reproduction), but not on Digit Span. Purdue Pegboard scores correctly classified 91% of PD patients and 82% of controls, in contrast to WMS Logical Memory, which identified only 60% of patients and 61% of controls.

Weingartner, Burns, Diebel, and LeWitt (1984) provided additional data on memory loss in early PD. They compared a small group of untreated PD patients (mean age = 65 years) with healthy, matched controls on an information-processing battery examining different types of memory. These patients were well educated (mean = 14 years) and scored above average on the WAIS (mean Full IQ = 129) and the WMS (mean Memory Quotient = 126); motor disability was also mild (5 of 6 were at Hoehn and Yahr Stages I or II). Patients with "significant depression" on psychiatric screening were excluded.

No problems were noted for PD patients in semantic memory processes (verbal fluency, recognizing degraded pictures) or automatic memory processes (frequency monitoring or recall of input modality). However, on effortful memory tasks (e.g., free recall of words or pictures and serial list learning), performance was consistently lower for PD patients than for controls. Problems were most apparent on early learning trials; as items were presented more often, PD patients were generally able to match the performance of controls.

These studies indicate that neuropsychological deficits in early PD are likely to be confined to three areas: (1) psychomotor slowing; (2) loss of cognitive flexibility; and (3) mildly reduced learning and recall. Intelligence and language are usually unimpaired, and in most cases, motor problems are more striking clinically than cognitive impairments.

Changes in cognitive flexibility and memory are reminiscent of problems which result from focal damage to the frontal lobes (Caltagirone, Carlesimo, Nocentini, &

Vicari, 1989; Cools, Van Den Bercken, Horstink, Van Spaendonck, & Berger, 1984; Flowers & Robertson, 1985; Lees & Smith, 1983; Pillon, Dubois, Lhermitte, & Agid, 1986; Taylor, Saint-Cyr, & Lang, 1986). Specific similarities on testing include perseveration and problems in achieving or switching categories on sorting and verbal fluency tasks, difficulties in recall of temporally ordered stimuli (as in serial recall), and disconnection between behavior and a verbalized plan or solution (for excellent summaries of frontal lobe deficits, see Schachter, 1987; Stuss & Benson, 1984). Everyday behavior of PD patients may also include subtle signs of frontal impairment (e.g., loss of spontaneity, lack of initiative, and a tendency toward repetition; see Lees & Smith, 1983). This finding lends some support to the notion that cognitive loss in PD is mediated by changes in subcortical systems that influence the frontal lobes (e.g., Cummings & Benson, 1983, 1988).

Nonetheless, most patients with early PD would not qualify for a clinical diagnosis of dementia. They usually score in the normal range on cognitive mental status examinations and generally do not have sufficient cognitive impairment to interfere with work or social interactions (Lees & Smith, 1983). Although specialized tests may unmask a memory impairment, clinical measures such as the WMS do not reliably separate these patients from controls. Even on discriminating tasks such as the Wisconsin Card Sort Test, differences may be confined to qualitative indicators such as a tendency to perseverate.

Moderate to Severe PD

Patients who have been under treatment for PD for several years often have more substantial neuropsychological impairments. This section provides an overview of deficits observed on testing and then examines clinical factors that may influence the severity of cognitive losses.

Scope of Impairment

The mean scores shown in Table 8.2 illustrate the range and severity of neuropsychological deficit that can be expected in later stages of PD. These data were provided by Pirozzolo, Hansch, Mortimer, Webster, and Kuskowski (1982), based on a comparison of 60 PD patients (mean age = 63 years; mean education = 11 years) with an equal number of matched controls. Patients had been ill for an average of nine years, and all were receiving anti-Parkinson medications, primarily levodopa/carbidopa. Subjects with a history of stroke, alcohol abuse, or other neurological conditions were excluded.

Group differences were negligible on verbal intelligence subscales (WAIS Vocabulary, Information) and on brief tests of apraxia (Christensen, 1975) and confrontation naming (Goodglass & Kaplan, 1972). Digit Span scores were slightly lower for PD patients than for controls but were well within normal limits for age. On all other tests, including measures of psychomotor speed, visuospatial ability, and learning and recall, PD patients performed substantially below controls.

Tests that combined motor speed requirements with cognitive flexibility and/or visuospatial processing demands provided the clearest distinction between groups. For example, in discriminant analysis, Digit Symbol scores correctly identified 72% of PD patients and 87% of controls. Nonetheless, tests that did *not* require speed or manual dexterity (e.g., visual discrimination and paired-associate recall) also provided fair discrimination, identifying 68% of patients and 85% of controls.

Pirozzolo *et al.* (1982) noted several similarities between cognitive decline in PD

TABLE 8.2. Test Performance in Moderate to Severe PD Compared to Normal Aging[a]

Measure	PD patients	Healthy controls
WAIS (age-scaled scores)		
Vocabulary	11.17 (2.79)	11.78 (2.04)
Information	11.58 (2.49)	12.33 (2.03)
Digit Span	11.35 (2.64)	12.92 (2.80)
Digit Symbol*	8.23 (3.05)	13.08 (2.45)
Block Design*	9.48 (3.35)	13.67 (3.05)
WMS		
Logical Memory (immediate)		
Paragraph I*	6.87 (4.26)	10.77 (3.80)
Paragraph II*	5.21 (3.31)	8.45 (3.11)
Logical Memory (delayed)		
Paragraph I*	4.65 (4.28)	8.30 (4.04)
Paragraph II*	3.00 (3.23)	6.45 (3.64)
Associate Learning (immediate)		
Easy pairs*	5.43 (0.91)	5.98 (0.13)
Hard pairs*	1.33 (1.32)	2.83 (1.17)
Associate Learning (delayed)		
Easy pairs*	5.29 (1.09)	5.91 (0.33)
Hard pairs*	0.98 (1.21)	2.23 (1.32)
Bender Gestalt (recall)*	3.36 (1.97)	5.12 (1.36)
Spatial Orientation*	10.80 (3.81)	14.82 (2.79)
Visual Discrimination*	16.48 (2.89)	19.25 (1.16)
Finger tapping		
Right*	30.27 (13.76)	50.07 (8.75)
Left*	30.13 (11.64)	46.73 (8.43)
Digit Cancellation (seconds)*	80.25 (42.03)	51.50 (15.59)
Trail Making Test		
Part A*	118.31 (81.72)	56.27 (1969)
Part B*	291.43 (175.54)	121.85 (92.69)
Object Naming	17.95 (0.22)	18.00 (0.00)
Apraxia Test	4.98 (0.16)	5.00 (0.00)
Depression (self-rated)*	51.45 (10.30)	38.86 (7.43)

[a]Table values are mean scores with standard deviations in parentheses. From Pirozzolo, Hansch, Mortimer, Webster, and Kuskowski (1982, p. 75). Copyright 1982 by Academic Press, Inc. Adapted by permission.

*$p < .001$.

and an accelerated aging process. Crystallized verbal intelligence remains an area of strength, while a variety of fluid intellectual processes appear to be undermined. And as is true of normal aging, neuropsychological deficits in PD are not restricted to tasks requiring speed or motor dexterity.

Whether patients with this level of performance should be described as demented is an open question. Some experts in the area (e.g., Cummings & Benson, 1988; Huber, Freidenberg, Shuttleworth, Paulson, & Christy, 1989) have maintained that this label is appropriate, since multiple areas of deficit are apparent in comparisons with age-matched controls. Others (e.g., Hietanen & Teravainen, 1988) believe that deficits are too mild to suggest a clear dementia. In Table 8.2, for example, mean age-scaled scores on WAIS subtests are not greatly below expectations for subjects with an average of 11 years of schooling, and on untimed memory tests (e.g., Logical Memory and Associate Learning), the level of deficit is best described as low-average or mildly impaired compared to age and education norms (see Tables A.1 and A.2 in the Appendix). In addition, Huber *et al.* (1989) found that even after an average of 10 years of illness, PD patients still obtained a mean Mini-Mental State Examination score of 24.6 (± 3.6).

In general, as discussed in Chapter 6, a diagnosis of dementia is warranted only in those cases where there is clear evidence of decline over time, and where there are impairments in work or social activities that can be attributed to cognitive loss.

Clinical Correlates of Cognitive Loss

Because the extent of cognitive decline varies so widely among PD patients, researchers have been attempting to identify factors that may be linked to cognitive change. These factors may shed some light on the neurobiology of cognitive problems in this disease and may be useful in identifying subgroups of patients who are at risk of cognitive loss.

Age at Onset. Clinical studies have sometimes reported a higher frequency of dementia in patients with late- as opposed to early-onset PD (e.g., Mayeux *et al.*, 1988). However, these findings have been based on clinical impression or brief mental status examinations, which do not take effects of aging into account.

To take a closer look at age effects, Hietanen and Teravainen (1988) studied 108 PD patients, excluding those who had been ill for more than 10 years or who had coexisting diseases that could affect intellectual performance. Patients were separated into an early-onset group (PD beginning before age 60) and a late-onset group. The average duration of illness for early- and late-onset patients was 3.7 and 3.4 years, respectively, and in both groups, a majority of patients received Hoehn and Yahr severity ratings of either II or III. Cognitive tests consisted of several WAIS and WMS subtests, reaction time testing, the Purdue Pegboard, Stroop's Color-Word Interference Test, and the Trail Making Test.

Early-onset PD patients scored significantly below age-matched controls on WAIS Block Design and Picture Completion, secondary-memory measures from the WMS, the cognitive flexibility measures (Stroop, Trail Making), and all of the psychomotor speed measures. Older PD patients were slower than controls on the psychomotor speed tests and had lower scores on Block Design, two of the WMS subtests, Stroop color naming (but not interference), and Trail B.

These findings indicate that early-onset patients also have cognitive impairments relative to age-matched controls, and that the same types of cognitive problems (psychomotor slowing, memory deficit on effort-demanding tasks, cognitive flexibility changes) affect both early- and late-onset patients. However, in older patients, deficits due to PD can combine with aging changes to give a global impression of dementia. In this study, for example, 25% of the older patients met DSM-III criteria for dementia, compared to only 2% of the early-onset group.

Coexisting Depression. Many of the studies discussed so far screened out potential subjects with serious depression. However, in clinical settings, cognitive problems often reflect the combined influence of PD and depression, since 40% to 60% of PD patients experience depression at some point in their illness (Cummings & Benson, 1983).

The potential confounding effects of depression were illustrated in a study by Starkstein, Bolduc, Preziosi, and Robinson (1989a). There were 94 PD patients who were classified into subgroups based on global severity of PD and presence or absence of depression as determined by standard observer-rated scales. The percentage of patients with depression ranged from 25% in the mildly impaired PD group (Hoehn and Yahr Stages I or II) to 60% among severely impaired PD patients (Hoehn and Yahr Stages IV or V). Cognitive impairment generally increased with severity of PD, but the subgroup with depression and severe PD tended to perform worse than all other groups, obtaining significantly lower scores on measures of frontal functions.

Severity of Motor Symptoms. Although there appears to be a rough parallel between progression of motor symptoms and worsening cognition in PD (cf. Huber *et al.*, 1989; Starkstein *et al.*, 1989a; and discussion above), correlations with specific motor symptoms (e.g., psychomotor slowing, tremor, or rigidity) are not so clear.

In one of the few investigations to use quantitative, instrument-assisted measures of motor symptoms, Mortimer, Pirozzolo, Hansch, and Webster (1982) found significant correlations between bradykinesia (slowness of movement) and performance on visuospatial tasks (r's = $-.34$ to $-.45$), but not on tests of memory or verbal intelligence. Rigidity and tremor were not related to cognitive scores.

Other studies have relied on clinical ratings of motor symptoms and have produced conflicting results. Riklan, Reynold, and Stellar (1989) and Taylor *et al.* (1986) found a correlation between memory loss and bradykinesia, but Hietanen and Teravainen (1986) did not. Another study (Pillon, Dubois, Cusimano, Bonnet, Lhermitte, & Agid, 1989) found that gait disturbance and dysarthria were more closely linked to cognitive performance than motor slowing *per se*.

Additional findings that question the strength of the connection between motor and cognitive problems come from studies which have tested patients in "on" and "off" phases of motor symptom severity. In general, there appears to be little change in cognitive performance through the course of these fluctuations (Brown, Marsden, Quinn, & Wyke, 1984; Delis, Direnfeld, Alexander, & Kaplan, 1982; Starkstein, Esteguy, Berthier, Garcia, & Leiguarda, 1989b; Taylor, Saint-Cyr, & Lang, 1987).

Mortimer *et al.* (1982) emphasized that the magnitude of correlations between cognitive and motor symptoms is modest at best. They suggested that motor slowing and visuospatial problems may share a common pathophysiological base (e.g., nigrostriatal degeneration), but that other brain pathology may be involved in producing memory loss or other cognitive impairments (for additional discussion, see Gibb, 1989; Mortimer, Jun, Kuskowski, & Webster, 1987; Pillon *et al.*, 1989).

Treatment Responsiveness. The effects of treatment on cognitive performance are also quite complicated. Some studies show mild benefits of levodopa on cognitive functions, particularly on psychomotor speeded tasks (cf. Cummings & Benson, 1983); however, this benefit has been attributed to a nonspecific "awakening" effect of medication and does not appear to prevent later worsening of cognitive performance (cf. Gibb, 1989).

Taylor *et al.* (1987) approached the question of treatment effects and cognitive function from a different perspective. They compared neuropsychological performance of healthy controls and subgroups of PD patients who differed in their response to treatment with dopamine enhancement medications (primarily levodopa/carbidopa). There were nine patients in each of four groups: early, untreated patients; those who had shown persistent good response to therapy; patients who had benefited from treatment but also suffered from medication-related fluctuations and dyskinesias; and a poor-response group who had initially responded to treatment but later showed generalized worsening of motor symptoms. Age, education, and estimated premorbid IQ were matched across all groups. An extensive neuropsychological battery was given, including psychomotor tests (e.g., Purdue Pegboard, Symbol Digit Modalities), memory tests (several WMS subtests and the Rey Auditory Verbal Learning Test), visuospatial measures (e.g., embedded figures, topographical orientation), and tests of executive function (e.g., Wisconsin Card Sort Test, Trail Making Test).

Results indicated that untreated patients, and those with either good response or fluctuating benefits, differed from controls on only a few measures (Wisconsin Card Sort Test, Rey Auditory Verbal Learning Test, a test of competing motor responses, and a delayed-recognition test for spatial location). Poor responders had more severe deficits on these tests and also had significant impairments on several other measures, including the Trail Making Test and verbal fluency.

The ability to respond to dopamine therapy was found to be a better predictor of cognitive impairment than duration of disease, length of treatment, or severity of motor impairment. For example, although patients in the fluctuating-response group had had a longer duration of illness than those in the poor-response group (mean = 13. 8 vs. 8.0 years), their cognitive performance, both in their best and worst motor phases, was no worse than that of an early, untreated group.

Taylor *et al.* (1987) speculated that individuals who lose their response to dopaminergic treatment may have different pathophysiological changes (e.g., cholinergic as well as dopaminergic loss or greater decline in neuronal plasticity) than those who continue to benefit from this therapy. These additional problems may be more directly involved in cognitive loss than the dopaminergic deficits *per se*.

Demented PD Patients

At least 10% to 20% of PD patients have such severe cognitive problems that they clearly meet diagnostic criteria for dementia. These patients probably represent a heterogeneous group in terms of neuropathology (see "Dementia in PD," above). Nonetheless, several investigations suggest that PD patients with dementia may have a somewhat different pattern of cognitive problems than DAT patients with comparable global intellectual impairment.

Helkala, Laulumaa, Soininen, and Riekkinen (1988) matched PD and DAT patients on Verbal and Performance IQs and on several basic visual, motor, and speech comprehension functions. PD patients had severe motor symptoms (most were at Hoehn and Yahr Stage IV) and were rated as having questionable to severe dementia on the Clinical Dementia Rating (CDR; see Chapter 7); their mean Verbal and Performance IQs were 84.2 and 65.7, respectively. DAT patients had comparable CDRs and similar IQ scores. Memory tests included recall of two stories (immediate, with interference, and after a 30-minute delay) and a list-learning task adapted from the Selective Reminding Test (see Chapter 4). No differences were noted between the groups on immediate recall of stories, total list learning, or estimates of short-term or long-term retrieval calculated from the learning phase. However, PD patients performed better on story recall following interference (where cues were used to prompt retrieval), on delayed recall of stories, and on recognition memory for list items.

Pillon *et al.* (1986) compared small groups of DAT and PD patients matched on age, education, and an index of deterioration based on a combination of cognitive tests. Although PD patients were impaired on secondary memory measures (WMS Logical Memory, Visual Reproduction, and Associate Learning), they were less impaired than DAT patients, particularly on Logical Memory. They showed relatively greater deficits than DAT patients on frontal lobe tests, including motor sequences and imitation, as well as on the Wisconsin Card Sort Test and verbal fluency (cf. Freedman & Oscar-Berman, 1986; Huber, Shuttleworth, Paulson, Bellchambers, & Clapp, 1986), and were described by relatives as having more inertia, indifference, and stereotypy in their everyday behavior.

Cummings, Darkins, Mendez, Hill, and Benson (1988) compared PD and DAT patients on a clinical speech and language battery. PD patients had notable problems with mechanical aspects of speech and writing, including reduced phrase length and grammatical complexity; altered speech rate, melody, pitch, and loudness; and impaired narrative writing and writing to dictation. Demented PD patients (i.e., those with Mini-Mental Status Examination scores ≤ 23) were more abnormal than nondemented PD patients in these respects and also had deficits in comprehension, naming, and word list generation. Closer examination indicated that 6 of 16 (38%) demented PD patients made naming errors and 4 (25%) had comprehension problems. DAT patients had less abnormality of motor aspects of language but had greater impairment on language measures (e.g., information content of spontaneous speech, word list generation, confrontation naming).

These studies suggest that neuropsychological testing has some potential for distinguishing dementia in PD from DAT even when the overall level of cognitive deficit is quite severe. However, since there is considerable overlap in distributions for the two disorders, even on discriminating measures, more work is needed to establish the clinical diagnostic utility of group trends. For example, one study (El-Awar, Becker, Hammond, Nebes, and Boller, 1987) reported a bimodal distribution of memory test scores among demented PD patients, with some doing as well as normal adults and others as poorly as patients with DAT. Others have also stressed that there is no single dementia syndrome characteristic of PD (Pirozzolo, Swihart, Rey, Jankovic, & Mortimer, 1988).

Toward a Neuropsychological Profile of PD

Table 8.3 summarizes the cognitive deficits that are most likely to be observed in PD.

Simple attention, as measured by forward digit span or registration of short lists of words, is well preserved, even in patients with severe motor symptoms (Huber, Shuttleworth, Paulson, Bellchambers, & Clapp, 1986; Huber *et al.*, 1989; Pillon *et al.*, 1986; Pirozzolo *et al.*, 1982). When attention is severely impaired, the possibility of medication toxicity or delirium should be carefully considered.

Mild problems on secondary-memory tasks can be expected in PD, even in early, untreated disease (Hietanen & Teravainen, 1986; Weingartner *et al.*, 1984). For patients in severe stages of PD, moderate to severe difficulties may be observed on effort-demanding tasks such as free recall of narrative, lists, or word pairs (Huber *et al.*, 1989; Pillon *et al.*, 1986). Rate of acquisition of new information is slowed, but with several repetitions of items, performance in PD can be expected to approximate normal levels (Weingartner *et al.*, 1984). PD patients usually perform well on recognition memory tasks (e.g., Lees & Smith, 1983) and usually do not show abnormal forgetting on delayed recall (Taylor *et al.*, 1986). Profound inability to learn new material, or failure to benefit from cuing or recognition prompts should raise a question of amnestic disorder or DAT. On remote-memory tasks, nondemented PD patients have been reported to have relatively good recall of the content of public and personal events, but noticeable problems in identifying the date at which these events occurred (Sagar *et al.*, 1988).

PD patients generally have slowing of speech and articulation problems, but their comprehension and use of language is not greatly impaired (Cummings *et al.*, 1988; Huber *et al.*, 1986, 1989). In early stages of PD, verbal fluency may be slightly reduced, and errors of perseveration or loss of set may be observed. In later stages of PD, fluency problems may increase in severity, and there may be some reduction in confrontation naming and verbally mediated intellectual processing (Huber *et al.*, 1989); however,

TABLE 8.3. Summary of Neuropsychological Test Findings in PD[a]

I. Typical presentation
   Disproportionate change in cognitive flexibility, accompanied by
   A. Mild memory deficit.
   B. Speech problems.
   C. Visuospatial impairment.
II. Most informative tests
   A. Cognitive flexibility/attentional switching
      1. Reduced speed of performance relative to age/education norms.
      2. Qualitative features present in many cases:
         Wisconsin Card Sort Test—Perseveration; difficulty in inferring or switching categories.
         Trails B—Difficulty comprehending task; loss of set.
   B. List-learning tests
      1. Storage, recognition, and rate of forgetting within normal limits.
      2. Impaired consistency of retrieval.
      3. Impaired recall of serial position.
      4. Low rate of intrusion errors.
III. Findings that raise a question about the diagnosis
   Any of the following in early stages of illness:
   A. Severe memory impairment.
   B. Severe attentional deficit.
   C. Deficits in language comprehension.
   D. Loss of verbal intellectual ability.
IV. Cautions
   Only a rough parallel should be expected between the severity of motor symptoms and the exent of cognitive loss.
   Depression is commonly observed and may exacerbate cognitive problems.
   10%–20% of patients have diffuse cognitive problems that are hard to distinguish from DAT.

[a]From La Rue *et al.* (1992b, p. 657). Adapted by permission.

these deficits are usually milder than those observed in DAT (Bayles & Tomoeda, 1983; Cummings *et al.*, 1988).

The literature is less consistent with respect to visuospatial impairments in PD (for critical commentary, see Brown & Marsden, 1986; Gibb, 1989). Minimal visuospatial impairment has been reported in early stages of disease, provided that tests do not require motor speed or dexterity (Huber *et al.*, 1989; Taylor *et al.*, 1986). In more severe PD, however, visuospatial problems may be quite prominent (Huber *et al.*, 1989; Pirozzolo *et al.*, 1982) and are not restricted to speeded tasks (Boller, Passafiume, Keefe, Rogers, Morrow, & Kim, 1984; Pirozzolo *et al.*, 1982).

Diminished cognitive flexibility is the most likely of all neuropsychological impairments in PD. Problems are subtle in early, untreated patients (Lees & Smith, 1983) and more obvious in later stages (Huber *et al.*, 1986, 1989; Pillon *et al.*, 1986). Perseveration and problems with inferring or switching categories may be expected. Deficits in flexibility, spontaneity, initiative, and judgment may also be apparent in everyday behavior (Lees & Smith, 1983; Pillon *et al.*, 1986).

PD versus Normal Aging

Significant overlap can be expected between the neuropsychological deficits observed in mild PD and normal aging. For both of these groups, the low points of the neuropsychological profile involve tests of complex, speeded psychomotor function, cognitive flexibility, and effortful learning and memory. Even in moderate to severe PD, cognitive differences are not as pronounced as those observed between mild DAT and normal aging. On brief mental status exams that do not have age-adjusted norms, elderly PD patients score in the impaired range more often than younger patients with this disease, a result contributing to an impression of increased dementia in older PD patients. However, on more detailed testing, the impact of PD on cognitive functions appears to be similar in young and old patients.

PD versus DAT

When cognitive test findings in PD are compared to those of patients with mild DAT (see Chapter 7), the clearest differences are observed in the areas of verbal intelligence (impaired in DAT; unimpaired in PD) and verbal memory (more profound impairment in DAT). Additional differences have been noted on speech and language tests and in the patterns of errors observed during learning and recall. In PD, articulation difficulties are relatively pronounced compared to language comprehension problems, whereas the reverse is true in DAT. PD patients are less likely to intrude irrelevant information during learning and recall and also show greater benefit from semantic cuing. PD and DAT both produce impairment on complex, speeded psychomotor tasks (e.g., Digit Symbol and Trail Making) and on demanding tests of cognitive flexibility (e.g., Wisconsin Card Sort). However, in PD, these problems are commonly the sole or most striking deficit on testing, while in DAT, memory loss is the most obvious clinical finding.

SUMMARY AND CONCLUSIONS

PD is a common disorder in older adults. Its cause is unknown, and there are no treatments yet that can reverse the neuropathological changes associated with this disease. However, symptomatic treatments are available that substantially reduce the impact of PD on everyday functioning.

Neuropathological hallmarks of PD include degenerative changes in the substantia nigra and other subcortical brain structures and disruption of dopaminergic neurotransmitter activity. Motor dysfunction is the most obvious clinical feature of PD; speech and motor actions are slowed, and tremor and gait disturbance are common.

Severe cognitive decline is the exception, rather than the rule, in PD. However, certain aspects of cognition are routinely disrupted by this disease, and more diffuse change is likely to be observed under some conditions. Whether cognitive deficits arise from the same brain pathology as motor impairments is currently unclear. Dopaminergic depletion may be responsible for the subtle changes noted in early PD, but other brain mechanisms may be involved when cognitive loss is severe.

The motor and speech difficulties that accompany PD can make it difficult to determine how well a patient is functioning emotionally and intellectually. Neuropsychological testing can provide some useful data on these questions. Since a patient with severe motor symptoms may have little or no cognitive impairment, testing often uncovers strengths that have been overlooked. Conversely, a person with PD who does well on intelligence and memory tests may still have loss of judgment or spontaneity that can detract from relationships at work or at home. Helping the patient and family members to understand these incongruities can give a firmer basis for deciding on the best and most necessary forms of care.

9

Vascular Dementia

Cerebrovascular disease is considered to be the second most common cause of dementia in older adults (see Chapter 6). Several cerebrovascular conditions can produce a dementia syndrome, and clinical features can vary considerably for different causes; however, by tradition, these disorders are often combined into a general category of *vascular dementia*.

Vascular dementia has not been as thoroughly researched as dementia of Alzheimer type (DAT) or Parkinson's disease (PD). There is disagreement among experts about the severity and pattern of cerebrovascular changes that are needed to produce dementia. Also, since an autopsy is required to rule out other brain pathologies such as Alzheimer's disease (AD), one can never be certain of a causal association between dementia and cerebrovascular changes observed on clinical examination (Brust, 1988). Nonetheless, with the development of neurodiagnostic techniques such as magnetic resonance imaging (MRI), positron emission tomography (PET), and single-photon emission tomography (SPECT), there has been renewed interest in exploring associations between cerebrovascular pathology and cognitive changes.

Neuropsychologists are frequently asked to try to distinguish between dementia due to vascular illness and DAT. As later sections of this chapter illustrate, test findings alone can contribute very little to answering this question. However, neuropsychological evaluation can be helpful for other reasons, e.g., to determine if problems are severe enough to warrant a diagnosis of dementia and to distinguish dementia from the focal brain impairments associated with stroke.

This chapter provides a brief review of neuropathology, epidemiology, and experimental therapies for vascular dementia. Diagnostic criteria and clinical features are reviewed in the second section, and neuropsychological findings are considered in a final section.

BACKGROUND

Neuropathology

Dementia can result from several types of cerebrovascular pathology (for detailed discussions, see Loeb, 1988a; Marshall, 1988; Meyer, Judd, Tawaklna, Rogers, & Mortel, 1986; Mirsen & Hachinski, 1988). Multiple bilateral hemispheric infarcts are considered the most common cause. However, a number of other conditions (e.g., subcortical arteriosclerotic leukoencephalopathy, or Binswanger's disease) are receiving increasing attention.

Cerebral Infarction

An infarct is an area where brain tissue has been destroyed because of insufficient oxygen supply (ischemia), generally as a result of blockage of a cerebral blood vessel. Large infarcts usually produce stroke, that is, focal neurological or neuropsychological deficits reflecting dysfunction of affected brain regions (Funkenstein, 1988). The site and extent of the lesion, history of prior brain injury, and coexisting medical conditions can all affect the deficits observed in stroke (for descriptions of stroke syndromes, see Baxter, 1987; Caplan & Stein, 1986; Funkenstein, 1988). Small infarcts can occur without any noticeable change in behavior ("silent stroke").

The likelihood of developing dementia from infarction varies with the number and distribution of cerebrovascular lesions. A single, strategically located infarct (e.g., in the thalamic, subthalamic, or mesencephalic brain regions) can sometimes produce dementia (Katz, Alexander, & Mandell, 1987); however, single infarcts probably account for only a small percentage of cases.

Tomlinson *et al.* (1970) found that most patients with vascular dementia had extensive, grossly visible infarction on autopsy. Usually, there were multiple infarcts in the cerebral gray matter, especially in regions supplied by the middle or posterior cerebral arteries. The aggregate volume of infarcted tissue generally exceeded 50 ml, and in severe cases of dementia, more than 100 ml of tissue was damaged or destroyed. These findings suggest that dementia is most likely to occur in patients with extensive cerebrovascular brain damage, and that generally, a history of one or more completed strokes can be expected.

Hachinski, Lassen, and Marshall (1974) and others (Cummings & Benson, 1983; Meyer *et al.*, 1986) have focused attention on the role of multiple, small cerebral infarcts (so-called lacunar infarcts) in dementia. Lacunar infarcts are minute (generally < 1 cm) cerebrovascular lesions concentrated in subcortical brain regions. Because of their small size and subcortical distribution, lacunar infarcts may not produce any of the obvious neurological symptoms usually associated with stroke. However, as they accumulate, they may begin to interfere with cognitive, sensory, and motor functions and may eventually produce a dementia (Hachinski *et al.*, 1974).

While it is generally agreed that lacunar infarcts can produce dementia, there is some question about the regularity with which this occurs (Brust, 1988; Liston & La Rue, 1983b). Patients who meet clinical criteria for vascular dementia frequently have evidence of lacunar infarcts on computerized tomography (CT) or MRI (see "Neurodiagnostic Tests," below). However, pathological studies suggest that a majority of lacunar infarcts are clinically silent, and that dementia is a relatively rare occurrence in patients with this infarction pattern (e.g., Fisher, 1982; Tuszynski, Petito, & Levy, 1989). Therefore, neuroradiological evidence of lacunar infarcts must be integrated with clinical data when a diagnosis of vascular dementia is considered (see "Neurodiagnostic Tests," below).

White Matter Disease

Binswanger's disease, or subcortical arteriosclerotic encephalopathy (Olszewski, 1962), has also been recognized as a cause of vascular dementia. The principal pathology in this disease is diffuse white matter degeneration in the area of the cerebral ventricles, with prominent loss of myelin and microvascular changes. These changes can result from arteriosclerotic disease of the small penetrating arterioles, causing decreased perfusion of the periventricular region, or from other, nonvascular causes. In many cases, white matter changes co-occur with lacunar infarcts and enlargement of the ventricles (Babikian & Ropper, 1987).

Binswanger's disease has generally been considered to be a rare condition. However, on CT or MRI scans, small areas of lucency or hyperintensity in the cerebral white matter are a very common finding, particularly in elderly patients. The clinical significance of these findings and their relationship to Binswanger's disease are still being investigated (see "Neurodiagnostic Tests," below).

Additional Causes

Occlusion of the carotid and vertebral arteries can sometimes produce dementia due to chronic low cerebral perfusion (Marshall, 1988; Meyer *et al.*, 1986), although stroke is a more common clinical outcome in these cases. Cerebral amyloidosis, sickle-cell anemia, and a number of other rare hereditary conditions can also produce dementia (Mirsen & Hachinski, 1988).

Prevalence and Risk Factors

Autopsy studies usually attribute 15% to 20% of dementia cases to cerebrovascular changes, and another 10% to 20% to mixed vascular/AD pathology (Mirsen & Hachinski, 1988; O'Brien, 1988). Comparable figures have been reported in epidemiological studies using clinical diagnostic procedures (Jorm *et al.*, 1987; Schoenberg, 1988). However, because vascular dementia is difficult to diagnose on either pathological or clinical grounds, prevalence estimates continue to be a topic of debate (for contrasting opinions, see Brust, 1988; O'Brien, 1988).

Advancing age is the primary risk factor for vascular dementia (Jorm *et al.*, 1987; Schoenberg, 1988). Men develop this condition more often than women, especially before the age of 70 years and in Oriental populations compared to Caucasians (Jorm *et al.*, 1987; Schoenberg, 1988).

Risk factors for stroke (e.g., hypertension, heart disease, hyperlipidemia, diabetes, cigarette smoking) have also been linked to the development of vascular dementia. For example, in a recent study of 175 patients with vascular dementia (Meyer, McClintic, Rogers, Sims, & Mortel, 1988a), 66% were found to be hypertensive, 47% had heart disease, and 37% were cigarette smokers; diabetes was noted in 20% and hyperlipidemia in 21% (cf. Liston & La Rue, 1983a,b; Loeb, 1980).

In the United States and some Western European countries, incidence rates for vascular dementia have declined substantially in recent years (Schoenberg, 1988), paralleling the decline in stroke in these same populations. For both of these conditions, therefore, improved control of risk factors appears to be having an impact on disease prevention.

Experimental Therapies

Once vascular pathology has progressed to the point where dementia is clinically evident, symptoms are very difficult to treat, and usually, there is continued decline in functioning (see "Clinical Course," below). However, several therapeutic approaches are being explored, and in vascular dementia, outcomes are slightly more positive than has been observed in DAT (for a review, see Meyer, McClintic, Sims, Rogers, & Mortel, 1988b).

One approach has been to treat some of the antecedent conditions associated with stroke. In one investigation (Meyer *et al.*, 1986), 52 patients who met strict diagnostic criteria for vascular dementia were followed for a two-year period, with reexaminations occurring at three-month intervals. Among hypertensive patients (35 of the total group of 52), cognitive performance improved or stabilized in those whose systolic blood pressure was controlled within a high-normal range (135 to 150 mm Hg). Among normotensive patients, individuals who stopped smoking tended to have a more favorable longitudinal course. No significant difference was observed for patients treated with aspirin compared to those who were not, although the trend was toward a more positive course in the aspirin-treated patients.

A larger study of the effects of aspirin was recently reported by the same research group (Meyer, Rogers, McClintic, Mortel, & Lotfi, 1989). One group of patients (n = 37) took 325 mg of aspirin daily for a period of up to three years; another group did not take aspirin but received similar clinical care. Aspirin-treated patients demonstrated slight improvements in cerebral perfusion and cognitive performance at follow-up assessments, whereas control subjects showed very little clinical change. There was also a nonsignificant trend toward fewer strokes in the aspirin-treated group.

It is important to note that patients in these studies were only mildly impaired at the initial evaluation and that a relatively lax criterion was used for judging cognitive improvement (a gain of 2 or more points on a mental status examination similar to the Mini-Mental State Examination; cf. Jacobs, Bernhard, Delgado, & Strain, 1977). Nonetheless, the findings offer some hope that symptoms of vascular dementia can be stabilized if detected in early stages.

Many other medications (vasodialators, calcium channel blockers, nootropic agents, etc.) have been investigated as possible treatments for vascular dementia. Most studies have found negligible effect of these drugs compared to placebo (for recent examples, see Dysken, Katz, Stallone, & Kuskowski, 1989; Nadeau, Malloy, & Andrew, 1988); a few have reported fairly consistent improvements in cognitive test scores, but not to a point that would be expected to influence everyday function (e.g., Jansen, Bruckner, & Jansen, 1985; Passeri & Cucinotta, 1989).

For patients whose dementia is related to arterial occlusion, surgical procedures (e.g., carotid endarterectomy, arterial grafting) are sometimes used in an attempt to alleviate symptoms or to prevent the occurrence of future strokes. There is now a large literature on carotid endarterectomy, where plaque is surgically removed from the carotid arteries. Improvement in cognitive test scores has sometimes been reported with these procedures, but well-controlled studies often show no clear benefit beyond that observed with spontaneous recovery (e.g., Casey, Ferguson, Kimura, & Hachinski, 1989; see Loeb, 1988b, for a review).

DIAGNOSTIC CRITERIA AND CLINICAL FEATURES

Multi-Infarct Dementia

Only one type of vascular dementia—multi-infarct dementia (MID)—is specifically recognized in the revised third edition of the *Diagnostic and Statistical Manual* (DSM-III-R; American Psychiatric Association, 1987). Diagnostic criteria for this disorder are as follows:

1. A dementia, as defined in Chapter 6, is present.
2. There has been a stepwise deteriorating course with "patchy" distribution of deficits early in the course.
3. Focal neurological signs and symptoms are present.
4. There is evidence from history, physical examination, or laboratory tests of significant cerebrovascular disease that is judged to be the cause of the dementia (p. 123).

These criteria, and their precursors in the third edition of the *Manual* (DSM-III; American Psychiatric Association, 1980) have been the subject of much criticism (Brust, 1988; Funkenstein, 1988; Liston & La Rue, 1983a,b; O'Brien, 1988). In effect, they identify patients with a history of stroke who have several areas of cognitive impairment, and who appear to be getting worse in an erratic fashion. Since an autopsy would be required to rule out AD pathology, a clinician can only assume that cerebrovascular disease is causing dementia in these cases. Patients with Binswanger's disease are likely to be overlooked, since they may not exhibit the focal neurological signs and symptoms expected with infarction. The vagueness of terms such as *stepwise deterioration* or *patchiness* of deficits creates additional problems, since examiners may interpret these criteria in many different ways.

Research Diagnostic Criteria

In clinical research, DSM-III-R criteria for MID are often supplemented with symptom rating scales and a variety of laboratory findings. The Hachinski Ischemic Score (see below) is commonly used to support the clinical diagnosis. Neurodiagnostic evidence of cerebrovascular disease (e.g., patchy cerebral blood flow reductions, signs of infarction on CT, or extensive white matter disease) may also be required for inclusion in research samples.

The Hachinski Ischemic Score

The Hachinski Ischemic Score (IS; Hachinski, Iliff, Zilhka, Du Boulay, McAllister, Marshall, Russell, & Symon, 1975) was developed as a clinical tool for identifying dementia that might be due to multiple infarction as opposed to DAT. The IS is usually completed on the basis of neurological examination and a review of medical history. Items (see Table 9.1) were derived from earlier clinical observations of patients with "arteriosclerotic dementia" (Roth, 1955; Slater & Roth, 1969; cf. Liston & La Rue, 1983a).

The IS was initially applied in a study of 24 relatively young (mean age = 64 years) demented subjects. A bimodal distribution of scores was observed, with 10 subjects scoring 7 or above and 14 scoring 4 or lower. Those with high scores were assumed to have MID and those with low scores to have DAT. Cerebral blood flow (CBF) assessment indicated reduced mean hemisphere flow in the MID group, but not the DAT group, relative to controls. There was a significant correlation between CBF and scores on a mental status examination in the MID group, which was interpreted as showing "a close relationship between decrease in CBF and mental deterioration when cerebrovascular disease is the cause" (p. 636). Autopsy findings to verify the clinical diagnoses were not presented.

In a subsequent validation study based on pathologically verified cases, Rosen, Terry, Fuld, Katzman, and Peck (1980) found that many of the IS items did not discriminate between MID, AD, and mixed MID/AD groups. Atherosclerosis was present in all cases, regardless of diagnosis, while preservation of personality was uniformly absent. Stepwise deterioration was absent for AD patients but was also lacking for 5 of 9 patients with MID or mixed MID/AD. Depression was noted in 3 of the 5 AD cases, compared to 4 of 9 MID and mixed cases. On the basis of these findings, Rosen *et al.* suggested that the IS be reduced to eight items (see footnote to Table 9.1). On this abbreviated IS, scores ranged from 0 to 2 for DAT patients, and from 4 to 10 for patients with MID or mixed MID/DAT.

TABLE 9.1. The Hachinski Ischemic Score[a]

Clinical feature	Score
Abrupt onset[b,c]	2
Stepwise deterioration[b]	1
Fluctuating course	2
Nocturnal confusion	1
Relative preservation of personality	1
Depression	1
Somatic complaints[b]	1
Emotional incontinence[b]	1
History of hypertension[b]	1
History of strokes[b,c]	2
Evidence of associated atherosclerosis	1
Focal neurological symptoms[b,c]	2
Focal neurological signs[b,c]	2

[a]From Hachinski, Iliff, Zilhka, Du Boulay, McAllister, Marshall, Russell, and Symon (1975, pp. 632–637). Adapted by permission.
[b]Revised Ischemic Score (Rosen *et al.*, 1980; see text).
[c]Modified Ischemic Score (Loeb, 1988a; see text).

Loeb (e.g., Loeb, 1980, 1988a; Loeb & Gandolfo, 1983) has proposed a different modification of the IS based on his own extensive work with vascular dementia patients. This system combines the four IS items that he has found to be most discriminating (abrupt onset, history of stroke, focal neurological symptoms, and focal neurological signs) with a CT finding of single or multiple low-density areas, with 2 points assigned for each positive item. Scores of 0 to 2 are considered consistent with DAT, and 5 to 10 with MID; scores of 3 or 4 are said to suggest a mixed disease state or other diagnosis.

Based on a review of the MID literature, Liston and La Rue (1983a) concluded that the IS may be most useful in *ruling out* MID. That is, individuals with very low scores would be unlikely to have suffered sufficient cerebrovascular impairment to produce a clear dementia. However, high scores are less specific and could result from a stroke unrelated to dementia or a mixed MID/AD condition, as well as from MID. Modified versions of the IS are preferable to the original form, since the original version includes several items with questionable diagnostic utility.

Neurodiagnostic Tests

CT and MRI Scans

CT scan findings of single or multiple low-density areas, consistent with infarction, are frequently used in support of a diagnosis of vascular dementia (Loeb, 1988a). However, these findings may be lacking in as many as 50% of the patients who meet clinical diagnostic criteria for vascular dementia (Ladurner, Iliff, & Lechner, 1982;

Loeb, 1980; Sluss, Gruenberg, Rabins, & Kramer, 1982), and they may be present in many individuals who do not have dementia.

MRI scans are more sensitive than CT to small infarcts of the lacunar type. With combined use of CT and MRI, Meyer *et al.* (1988a) reported that 65% of vascular dementia cases had evidence of multiple lacunar infarctions, either alone (43.4%) or in combination with other types of stroke lesions (21.1%).

CT and MRI scans can also detect small lesions in the cerebral white matter (leukoaraiosis, also called *periventricular lucencies*). These findings are sometimes interpreted as early signs of Binswanger's disease. A high percentage of patients diagnosed with vascular dementia have evidence of white matter lesions on MRI (Mirsen & Hachinski, 1988); however, these findings are also observed in 30% or more of DAT patients and 15% to 20% of neurologically normal older adults (George, de Leon, Gentes, Miller, London, Budzilovich, Ferris, & Chase, 1986; Mirsen & Hachinski, 1988; Rezek, Morris, Fulling, & Gado, 1987).

Research relating white matter changes to cognitive performance has produced equivocal results. Differences have sometimes been reported for patients with and without leukoaraiosis on mental status exams and neuropsychological tests (e.g., Gupta, Naheedy, Young, Ghobrial, Rubino, & Hindo, 1988); however, other studies find no association between white matter changes and cognitive test scores (e.g., Aharon-Peretz, Cummings, & Hill, 1988; Rao, Mittenberg, Bernardin, Haughton, & Leo, 1989).

In a careful study of white matter changes in patients with lacunar infarcts (Tanaka, Tanaka, Mizuno, & Yoshida, 1989), 15 of 33 were classified as nondemented by clinical and neuropsychological criteria (Mini-Mental State Examination and Wisconsin Card Sort Test scores), and 18 were judged to be either borderline impaired or definitely demented. Demented patients had much more extensive white matter lesions and greater brain atrophy than the nondemented patients. In these cases, therefore, dementia was observed only when there was a combination of pathological findings, that is, lacunar infarcts, extensive white matter changes, and pronounced cerebral atrophy.

Electroencephalographic Findings

An increased frequency of focal slow waves on electroencephalography (EEG) has been reported for patients with vascular dementia compared to those with DAT (Loeb, 1980, 1988a; Torres, 1988). However, these focal abnormalities are noted in only about 50% of vascular dementia cases (Harrison, Thomas, Du Boulay, & Marshall, 1979; Loeb, 1980). On computerized spectral analysis, MID patients present a more variable pattern of slowing than those with DAT (e.g., Leuchter *et al.*, 1987).

Cerebral Metabolic and Blood Flow Studies

Cerebral blood flow measured by PET, SPECT, or traditional xenon-inhalation techniques (Hachinski *et al.*, 1975; Perez, Mathew, Stump, & Meyer, 1977) has also been used in clinical research on MID (Cohen, Graham, Lake, Metter, Fitten, Kulkarni, Sevrin, Yamada, Chang, Woodruff, & Kling, 1986; Gemmel, Sharp, Evans, Besson, Lyall, & Smith, 1984). In DAT, blood flow reductions usually involve large areas, particularly the temporoparietal region (see Chapters 2 and 7); in MID, findings are less consistent and typically involve focal, asymmetric reductions. In addition, the time course of reductions may vary for the two diseases, with blood flow decline preceding clinical dementia in MID, but following the onset of symptoms in DAT (Rogers, Meyer, Mortel, Mahurin, & Judd, 1986).

In MID, blood flow reductions tend to be most severe in certain subcortical regions (e.g., the thalamus and portions of the striatum) but are also noted in moderate severity in the temporal and frontal cortex (see Figure 9.1). Changes in blood flow may be observed in regions where there is no visible infarction on CT or MRI, and in general, there appears to be a stronger association between behavioral deficits and blood flow than there is in infarction patterns (e.g., Kitagawa, Meyer, Tachibana, Mortel, & Rogers, 1984).

PET studies of cerebral glucose metabolism (fluoro-D-glucose technique) report outcomes similar to the blood flow findings. That is, hypometabolic regions are more discrete and regionally dispersed in MID than in DAT (e.g., Benson, Kuhl, Hawkins,

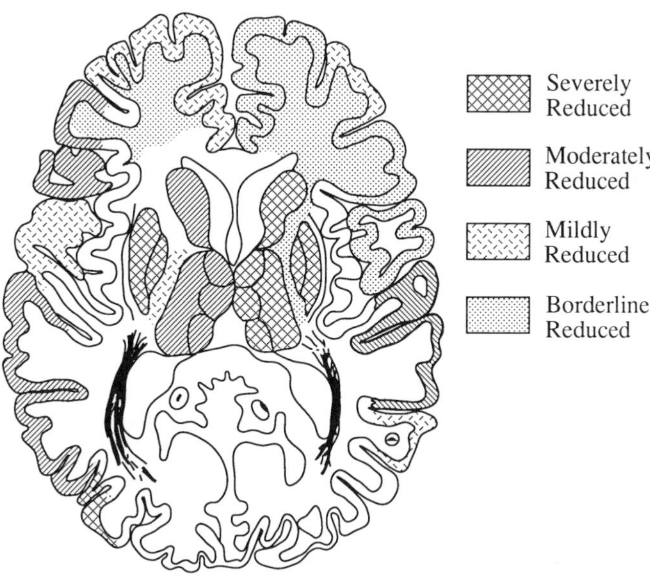

FIGURE 9.1. Local cerebral blood flow patterns in right-handed patients with multi-infarct dementia. (From Kitagawa, Meyer, Tachibana, Mortel, and Rogers, 1984, p. 1005. Copyright 1984 by the American Heart Association, Inc. Adapted by permission.)

Phelps, Cummings, & Tsai, 1983; Kuhl, Metter, Riege, Hawkins, Mazziotta, Phelps, & Kling, 1983; see also, Metter, 1988; Riege & Metter, 1988), and metabolic rates are often reduced in brain regions where there are no visible infarcts on CT or MRI (Kuhl, Metter, & Riege, 1985; Loewenstein, Barker, Chang, Apicella, Yoshii, Kothari, Levin, & Duara, 1989b).

Because there is no *specific* pattern of blood flow or metabolic findings associated with MID, tests such as PET or SPECT may be more useful in ruling out DAT than in confirming MID (Weinstein, Hijdra, van Royen, & Derix, 1989). However, in individual cases where MID is suspected, the regional dispersion of blood flow or metabolic changes may be useful in understanding specific behavioral and cognitive problems (see "Neuropsychological Findings," below).

Clinical Course

The course of illness appears shorter on the average in vascular dementia than in DAT, and more variable from person to person. In a recent follow-up study of 199 patients with DAT, 60 with MID, and 43 with mixed MID/DAT conditions, with roughly comparable degrees of initial impairment, Barclay, Zemcov, Blass, and Sansone (1985) found that 50% of the MID patients had died within 2.6 years after diagnosis, compared with 3.4 years for DAT patients. When measured from estimated onset of illness, 50% survival rates were observed at 6.7 years in MID versus 8.1 years in DAT. Survival curves diverged shortly after the point of diagnosis, but variability was greater in the MID group, particularly within the first two to three years. Behavioral deterioration was described as "relentless and progressive" in all groups.

Meyer *et al.* (1988a) followed vascular dementia patients diagnosed in very early stages of disease. Their findings present a more hopeful picture concerning clinical course. A mortality rate of 5.1% was reported in a sample of 175 patients followed for 31 months, and in the surviving patients, mild improvements in cerebral blood flow and cognitive performance were sometimes observed (see "Experimental Therapies," above).

NEUROPSYCHOLOGICAL FINDINGS

In contrast to the large literature on cognition in DAT, there have been relatively few studies of neuropsychological performance in vascular dementia. No criteria have been developed for rating the stage or severity of MID, and "patchiness" of deficits, as required by DSM-III-R, has not been operationalized. Sample sizes have typically been small, and in many studies, all patients with cerebrovascular pathology have been combined into a single group, regardless of the location or severity of lesions. These methodological limitations have made it difficult to identify the specific clinical-pathological associations necessary for differential diagnosis.

Performance on the Wechsler Adult Intelligence Scale

Severity of Impairment

An early investigation by Perez and colleagues (Perez, Rivera, Meyer, Gay, Taylor, & Mathew, 1975b) compared the Wechsler Adult Intelligence Scale (WAIS) performance of 42 subjects diagnosed with DAT, MID, or vertebrobasilar arterial insufficiency (VBI). Patients with MID were described as having focal neurological findings (e.g., hemiplegia, hemiparesis, dysphasia, or cortical sensory loss) and arteriographic evidence of atherosclerotic plaques and/or occluded cerebral vessels.

No significant differences were observed between the MID and VBI groups on IQ summary scales or any of the six subtests administered; mean Full Scale IQs were 87.7 and 97.2 for MID and VBI, respectively. The DAT group had significantly lower mean scores on all measures except Picture Completion; the estimated average Full Scale IQ in this group was only 64.6. Discriminant analyses correctly classified 90% of the Alzheimer's patients, 81% of the VBI patients, but only 56% of those with MID. The investigators concluded that intellectual deficits were similar for the three disorders, but that on the average, impairments were more severe in DAT. However, since the groups were not equated for overall degree of dementia or for duration of symptoms, there is a good possibility that DAT patients were simply at a more severe stage of illness.

Heterogeneity of Deficits

Perez *et al.* (1975b) also commented on the heterogeneity of deficits observed in the MID group. They concluded that "the MID group is less homogeneous than the other two groups, as might be predicted from the patchy nature of the disease process. The degree and pattern of cognitive deficit varies with each MID patient depending on the sites, location, extent, and number of cerebral infarctions" (p. 537).

The latter findings suggest that subtest scatter could be useful in identifying MID or in distinguishing this form of dementia from DAT. However, no criteria have been developed to indicate the extent or types of scatter that should be expected in MID. Since nearly one-half of normal adults have differences of 7 or more points between scaled scores on subtests of the WAIS-R (see Chapter 5), the mere presence of subtest scatter cannot be considered a strong indication of MID.

Subtest Profiles

As discussed in Chapter 7, Fuld (1984) and others have found that a certain WAIS profile is very rare in MID patients. However, since this profile is also lacking in as many as 50% of DAT patients, its absence cannot be used to differentiate between these conditions. To date, no specific WAIS or WAIS-R profiles have been proposed for vascular dementia.

Memory

Severity of Impairment

Perez, Gay, Taylor, and Rivera (1975a) compared 16 MID and 10 DAT patients on the Wechsler Memory Scale (WMS). DAT patients were significantly more impaired in overall memory quotient and all subtests except Information and Logical Memory. However, as in their earlier WAIS study, no evidence was provided to indicate that the two groups were comparable in overall dementia severity.

When severity of dementia is controlled, there appear to be few differences between MID and DAT patients on memory or other neuropsychological tests. This was illustrated in a recent study by Loewenstein, D'Elia, Guterman, Eisdorfer, Wilkie, La Rue, Mintzer, and Duara (1991) that compared 15 carefully diagnosed MID patients with an equal number of DAT patients. The MID patients all had multiple focal lesions on MRI which were outside of the immediate periventricular area; they also had significant cardiovascular risk factors and/or focal neurological symptoms.

Table 9.2 summarizes cognitive test scores for the MID and DAT groups. For these mildly impaired patients, the only differences to emerge were on the Retrieval index of the Object Memory Evaluation, where DAT patients had greater deficits, and on the prevalence of intrusion errors (see below).

TABLE 9.2. Neuropsychological Test Performance in Mild MID and DAT[a]

Cognitive measure	MID	DAT
Mini-Mental State Examination	23.5 (2.4)	22.9 (1.9)
WAIS-R (age-scaled scores)		
Similarities	7.4 (2.6)	9.2 (2.8)
Block Design	7.3 (2.9)	6.9 (2.5)
Object Assembly	6.1 (2.6)	7.2 (3.1)
WMS (raw scores)		
Logical Memory	4.8 (4.5)	3.9 (3.5)
Visual Reproduction	3.6 (2.4)	2.7 (1.8)
Object Memory Evaluation		
Retrieval*	30.2 (8.4)	18.5 (8.5)
Total Retention	9.7 (0.8)	8.7 (1.6)
Unrelated Intrusions**	0.3	1.9
Controlled Oral Word Association Test	22.6 (8.1)	24.8 (12.4)
Boston Naming Test (60 items)	38.1 (12.5)	38.5 (15.2)

[a]Table values are mean scores with standard deviations in parentheses. From Loewenstein, D'Elia, Guterman, Eisdorfer, Wilkie, La Rue, Mintzer, and Duara (1991, p. 111). Adapted by permission.
*$p < .01$
**$p < .05$.

Heterogeneity in Performance

La Rue (1989) reported that 3 of 9 inpatients with MID scored within normal limits on the Object Memory Evaluation, 2 had selective deficits (with retrieval more impaired than storage, or vice versa), and 4 were impaired in both storage and retrieval. Variability was related to the overall severity of dementia and to the presence or absence of depression. The patients with the greatest memory impairment had a mean Mini-Mental State Examination (MMSE) score of 17 compared to an average of 22 for those with normal memory scores; 3 of 4 patients with a secondary diagnosis of depression were impaired on all memory measures compared to only 1 of 5 nondepressed patients.

Intrusion Errors

In the study by Loewenstein *et al.* (1991), 73% of DAT patients made unrelated intrusions on the Object Memory Evaluation, compared to only 20% of MID patients. In additional groups of more severely impaired patients (with mean MMSE scores of 13 to 14), intrusions were observed for 86% of DAT patients and 64% of those with MID.

The investigators suggested that in DAT, intrusion errors are an integral part of the mnestic failure that accompanies the disorder, whereas in MID, deficits in recent memory may not be as severe or invariant early in the disease. Several other studies also provide some support for this conclusion (e.g., Fuld *et al.*, 1982; Loewenstein, Wilkie, Eisdorfer, Guterman, & Berkowitz, 1989c; Reed *et al.*, 1988; see Chapter 7).

Language

Hier *et al.* (1985) compared 26 patients with DAT and 13 with MID (excluding those with focal lesions in Wernicke's or Broca's areas) on a picture description task and several other language measures. MID patients were described as more laconic than DAT patients since they produced fewer words and shorter clauses during picture description. Increasing severity of MID was associated with a further decrease in word production and a greater number of incomplete sentences. However, moderately impaired MID patients retained the ability to make relevant observations and had less anomia than patients with DAT.

Powell, Cummings, Hill, and Benson (1988) compared 18 patients with MID and 14 with DAT on language tests adapted from the Boston Diagnostic Aphasia Examination, a dysarthria scale, and measures of reiterative speech disturbance (e.g., stuttering and echolalia). Both groups had moderately severe dementia, but the DAT group was slightly more impaired as judged by MMSE (means = 15.7 and 18.8 in the DAT and MID groups, respectively). The MID patients had IS scores of seven or higher, and all but one had CT scan evidence of focal cerebral infarctions. Mechanical aspects of speech (e.g., pitch, melody, articulation, and rate) were found to be more impaired in MID than in DAT (78% of MID patients had these problems, compared to 26% of DAT patients). By contrast, DAT patients had a greater reduction in confrontation naming and in the information content of spontaneous speech. Powell et al. suggested that "the diagnosis of DAT should be regarded skeptically in a demented patient with a melodic or articulatory abnormality" (p. 718), and that the presence of these abnormalities could be used in supporting a diagnosis of MID.

When DAT and MID groups have been equated for overall level of dementia (estimated by MMSE scores), at least two studies have found no differences on tests of verbal fluency and confrontation naming (Fischer, Gatterer, Marterer, & Danielczyk, 1988; Loewenstein *et al.*, 1991; see Table 9.2). Therefore, these tests appear to be less useful than analysis of narrative discourse in distinguishing vascular dementia and DAT.

Personality and Affect

Depression and emotional lability have been reported quite often in patients with vascular dementia (e.g., Roth, 1955; Rothschild, 1942; Slater & Roth, 1969), and as a result, both were included on the original version of the Hachinski IS (see Table 9.1). However, these features do not appear to distinguish between MID and DAT as well as the primary features of stroke (e.g., focal neurological signs and symptoms). Neither Rosen *et al.* (1980) nor Loeb and Gandolfo (1983) found a difference in rates of depression in DAT and MID groups, and "emotional incontinence" was noted in only one of nine patients with MID or mixed MID/AD (Rosen *et al.*, 1980). Cummings *et al.* (1987) reported higher scores on the Hamilton Depression Scale for patients with MID than for patients with DAT (means = 12.7 and 6.8, respectively), but scores were quite variable in both groups (range = 3 to 31 for MID patients), and only 4 of the 15 MID patients met criteria for major depression (see Chapter 11).

Is MID a Subcortical Dementia?

Since the lacunar infarcts and white matter changes commonly associated with MID are concentrated in subcortical structures, MID may be expected to share clinical features with subcortical brain disorders such as Parkinson's or Huntington's disease. As discussed in Chapter 8, subcortical disorders have been hypothesized to produce some unique neuropsychological findings, including motor slowing, forgetfulness, and impaired executive functions. Cummings and Benson (1983) suggested that in patients with a history of cerebrovascular disease, observation of this pattern on testing may be taken as support for a diagnosis of MID. By contrast, more pervasive deficits, including cortical as well as subcortical features, raise a question of DAT or a mixed MID/DAT condition.

Only a few studies have attempted to determine how closely the cognitive impairments of MID fit a subcortical pattern. Derix, Hijdra, and Verbeeten (1987) described six patients with clinical diagnoses of Binswanger's disease whose neuropsychological performance was felt to be consistent with subcortical dementia. All patients also had CT evidence of multiple infarcts which were predominantly lacunar. Deficits were reported in attention and concentration, memory, word finding, and visuoperceptual and visuoconstructive performance, but specific neuropsychological test scores were not provided. Two patients were also noted to have aphasia, which would usually be interpreted as a sign of cortical impairment.

Another study (Gupta *et al.*, 1988) compared neuropsychological performance of 27 elderly patients who had CT evidence of periventricular lucencies (leukoariaosis) with 17 age-matched controls with normal CT scans. All had been hospitalized for "various medical or neuropsychological problems." No differences were noted in WAIS Information or temporal orientation. However, patients with leukoaraiosis obtained significantly lower scores on WAIS Digit Symbol, WMS Logical Memory and Visual Reproduction, serial list learning, the Rey-Osterreith Complex Figure Test, verbal fluency, and serial 7's. These findings were interpreted as suggesting frontal system impairment of the type expected with subcortical dementia. However, this interpretation is open to question, since DAT patients also show impairment on these tests (see Chapter 7 and Table 7.3).

Searching for More Specific Brain–Behavior Patterns

Kitagawa *et al.* (1984) selected 15 well-defined cases of MID and examined relationships between infarction, cerebral blood flow patterns, and performance on a mental status examination. The patients in this sample all had a history of hypertension and had experienced small or transient strokes; they had focal neurological signs on examination, multiple cerebral infarcts on CT, and Hachinski IS scores of 7 or greater. Patients with recent strokes or severe strokes were excluded, as were patients with suspected Binswanger's disease. Regional cerebral blood flow was evaluated by means of a xenon inhalation procedure (see Chapter 2 for a description) monitored by computerized CT. Moderately or severely reduced flow was seen in the thalamus, the basal ganglia, and the temporal and frontal cortices (see Figure 9.1). Reductions in flow were described as bilateral but "patchy" in distribution.

Significant correlations (*r*'s ranged from .52 to .74) were noted between mental status scores (on a modified MMSE; cf. Jacobs *et al.*, 1977) and average blood flow readings in several regions. Reduced flow in the frontal regions correlated most strongly with deficits in orientation and impaired attention, whereas reductions in the temporal region correlated most strongly with memory and calculation deficits. Blood flow deficits in the thalamus tended to produce an "overall cognitive blunting" (i.e., poor performance on many aspects of the cognitive exam).

These findings illustrate the multifocal nature of brain impairment in MID and suggest that cortical brain regions are frequently involved in producing dementia symptoms. In some patients, there are obvious areas of infarction in the cortex (e.g., Tomlinson *et al.*, 1970); in others, these regions may be functionally impaired by disruption of projections from the thalamus, basal ganglia, or other subcortical structures. Therefore, while a subcortical dementia pattern can sometimes be observed in MID, a combination of cortical and subcortical features is not inconsistent with this diagnosis.

Synopsis of Neuropsychological Findings

The neuropsychological literature on vascular dementia is too limited and inconsistent to permit a listing of characteristic test outcomes. On the average, it appears that patients with MID do not differ greatly from those with DAT on standard clinical tests when the overall level of dementia is equated (cf. Erkinjuntti, 1987).

There are a few findings that can be considered *consistent with* a diagnosis of MID. Pronounced intertest variability would be expected for patients who have multiple, large cerebral infarctions in different cortical regions. By contrast, for patients with lacunar infarcts alone, or Binswanger's disease, intertest differences may not exceed those observed in normal test profiles or in patients with DAT. The presence of motor speech impairments is more common in MID than in DAT, as is the *absence* of intrusion errors. However, neither of these findings has been studied thoroughly enough to give firm estimates of diagnostic sensitivity and specificity. Patients with Binswanger's disease or infarcts limited to subcortical regions sometimes, but not invariably, have impairments that fit a pattern of subcortical dementia. For those with cortical infarcts, deficits consistent with established stroke syndromes (e.g., aphasia, apraxia, or agnosia) may be expected, in addition to memory impairment (see Table 9.3).

SUMMARY AND CONCLUSIONS

Age-related changes in the heart and vascular system predispose older patients to stroke and vascular dementia. Dementia occurs when there are multiple strokes that affect several different brain regions or when there is extensive degeneration in the deep cerebral white matter. Because the extent and distribution of brain lesions differs from patient to patient, clinical symptoms are also quite variable, so that it is difficult to generate uniform diagnostic criteria for vascular dementia.

TABLE 9.3. Summary of Neuropsychological Test Findings in Vascular Dementia

I. Common presentations
   A. Multiple large infarcts
      Expect deficits commensurate with location and extent of infarction.
   B. Lacunar infarcts/Binswanger's disease.
      Expect deficits resembling those of PD more than DAT.
II. Findings that raise a question about the diagnosis
   Absence of hypertension, heart disease, or other risk factors for stroke.
   Absence of focal neurological signs and symptoms.
III. Cautions
   Deep white matter changes and lacunar infarction are common in older adults and, in many cases, do not produce dementia.
   "Patchiness" of deficits has not been operationalized; intertest scatter *per se* is not specific to MID.
   AD and MID often coexist; an autopsy would be needed to rule out AD pathology.

A history of stroke or abrupt onset of cognitive problems, combined with focal neurological signs and symptoms, is the strongest clinical indication that dementia may be due to cerebrovascular changes as opposed to DAT. The presence of multiple infarcts or extensive white matter changes on CT or MRI, or patchy cerebral blood flow changes, provides additional support for this diagnosis when other criteria for dementia are met. However, any or all of these findings may be lacking in certain cases of MID, or they may be present in older individuals who do not have dementia.

Neuropsychological testing can help to determine if cognitive losses are severe enough to warrant a diagnosis of dementia and can distinguish between dementia and the focal impairments associated with stroke. However, testing is of limited use in distinguishing vascular dementia from DAT, partly because of methodological problems with existing studies. Most studies have combined patients with many different cerebrovascular lesions into a single group; mean scores obtained under this procedure often obscure brain–behavior patterns that may be present in individual cases. More restrictive sampling procedures may help to identify neuropsychological patterns specific to lacunar infarction or Binswanger's disease.

Distinguishing between vascular dementia and DAT has important, and relatively immediate, clinical implications. Patients with vascular dementia may benefit from a health regime that controls risk factors for stroke or from medications such as aspirin. Therefore, when vascular dementia is suspected, a strong effort should be made to enlist family support in making these changes. In addition, in patients with mild MID, some spontaneous recovery may occur, as is often the case with stroke. Therefore, it may be appropriate to encourage these patients to exercise existing skills and to make use of cognitive retraining procedures as their abilities permit.

10

Dementia

Case Examples

This chapter presents neuropsychological findings for four individuals with significant cognitive impairment. While each of these cases met clinical criteria for dementia, the pattern of impairments varied considerably from person to person. Suspected causes and contributing factors were also quite diverse. In two cases, there was significant depression, and in another, psychotic symptoms had been the first sign of neurological disease. The detracting effects of personal loss, relocation, and poor social supports are apparent in three of the cases but are particularly striking in the second example.

POSSIBLE EARLY DEMENTIA

The first example considers the possibility of early dementia in an individual whose history is complicated by depression and a recent episode of delirium. The patient was a 74-year-old woman whose baseline level of function was very high (see Example 10.1 for educational and social history). Although she had a history of depression and several medical problems, she had been doing well in recent years, maintaining an independent and active lifestyle.

About a year before the present evaluation, she had developed an unsteady gait and experienced several falls. At the urging of her son, she moved from her home to a retirement facility; she was unhappy about this move, had difficulty finding activities that she enjoyed, and told her son that she wished she could die in her sleep.

About a week before this assessment, she was found in her room in a stuporous state

EXAMPLE 10.1

Background

Seventy-four-year-old Caucasian woman.

Retired clinical social worker; has not worked for 10 to 15 years, but keeps license active.

B.A. degree in social work, M.A. degree in counseling psychology.

Married for 30 years, widowed for 18 years.

Since husband died, has lived alone but is socially active; had been involved in volunteer work until a year before this assessment.

Medical history significant for recent episode of delirium; hypertension, congestive heart failure, chronic atrial fibrillation, and syncope; status post pacemaker surgery; multiple falls within past year; lumbar disc disease; history of atypical sclerosis, Bell's palsy, and carpal tunnel syndrome.

Workup for delirium (CT scan, blood studies, urinanalysis, toxic drug screen) negative. Episode of depression 16 years ago; treated with Elavil, which she continued to take on and off until recently.

Medications at the time of assessment included nortriptyline, digoxin, verapamil, Dyazide, Premarin, and Colace.

Presenting problems

Had been hospitalized for one week at a medical center for increasing somnolence and confusion before the present psychiatric admission; precipitating factors unclear, but improper use of medications considered likely.

Referred for psychiatric evaluation to assess possible depression and to continue monitoring of mental status.

Behavior during testing

Cooperative, but with complaints of fatigue. Slowed speech and mild lethargy. Sensitive and guarded about possible cognitive deficits. Difficulty remembering dates and sequences of personal events (e.g., work history, retirement).

Test findings

Mini-Mental State Examination (MMSE): 25

Neurobehavioral Cognitive Status Exam: Mild impairment on orientation; severe impairment on memory; within normal limits on other scales.

Wechsler Adult Intelligence Scale—Revised (WAIS-R)	Age-scaled score	Percentile
Vocabulary	19	99
Information	14	91
Block Design	11	63
Digit Symbol	8	25

	Raw score	Percentile/ rating
Wechsler Memory Scale—Revised (WMS-R)		
Logical Memory, immediate	18	40
delayed	0	2
Visual Reproduction, immediate	24	46
delayed	6	14
Boston Naming Test (60 items)	59	80
Controlled Oral Word Association Test	38	56
Hamilton Depression Rating Scale	7	Normal

Qualitative aspects of performance

Unable to benefit from cues or multiple choices on the delayed recall of items from the NCSE; confabulation during recall of paragraphs.

Interpretation

Greatest impairment is in recall of new material. Adequate attention and verbal abilities; nonverbal abilities within normal limits for age, but significantly below verbal skills. Results suggest an early dementia; may be vascular in origin in light of medical history, but Alzheimer type dementia cannot be ruled out.

and was admitted to a medical hospital for observation. The precipitants of this episode were unclear. A series of laboratory tests to screen for specific causes of delirium produced negative results. However, continued discussion with the patient suggested that self-medication with amitriptyline (Elavil) may have contributed to the confusion. She had taken this drug periodically for nearly 20 years, beginning with an earlier episode of depression. In recent years, she had had the prescription refilled by her internist and regulated the dose and schedule on her own, taking more on days when she felt tired or sad. Although she denied that she had attempted suicide, her recall of recent events was quite poor.

After several days in the hospital, she was seen by a geriatric internist who noted that she continued to be lethargic and to have some problems with orientation, perhaps as a lingering effect of medication. A neurological consultant felt there was evidence of dementia, including impairment of recent memory, language errors, difficulty in changing cognitive sets, and mildly deficient insight and planning.

Because of continued questions about her mental status, she was transferred to a psychiatric unit for monitoring of cognitive symptoms and for assessment of the possibility of depression. In an initial examination, she was noted to have depressed mood, constricted affect, and prominent complaints of fatigue. Her speech was slow, with decreased volume. She was oriented to place, name, and date and recalled two of three objects after a brief delay. Her digit span was also within normal limits (6 forward,

4 backward), and she completed serial 7's with no errors. However, her memory for incidents within the past year was poor. She denied any suicidal ideation, changes in sleep or appetite, trouble concentrating, or psychomotor slowing. However, she continued to express a desire to "go to sleep and not wake up" and felt that her dysphoria and anhedonia were worse than usual.

Amitriptyline was discontinued because of her past history of misuse and the high potential of this drug for producing confusional symptoms (see Chapter 6). However, because she still had some symptoms of depression, nortriptyline was prescribed at a starting dose of 25 mg per day, gradually increasing to 75 mg per day. She reported subjective improvement in mood and became more sociable over the remaining two weeks in the hospital. However, throughout her stay, she continued to have memory impairment, sometimes forgetting conversations with staff, aspects of her treatment, or the daily routine.

Neuropsychological assessment was performed about a week after admission to the psychiatric unit. At this time, she was slightly dysphoric, with some restriction of affect. Her speech was still slow, and she continued to be lethargic. Unsteadiness of gait was also observed.

The patient was cooperative with testing and worked with good effort on the cognitive tasks. However, she was very sensitive about performances in which she felt she had done poorly and generally denied any cognitive problems. Her ability to give historical information was still impaired. She had problems remembering the dates and sequence of both recent and remote events (e.g., she could not remember when she had become a social worker or when she retired).

Test performance (see Example 10.1 for specific scores) was appropriate for age and background on measures of verbal intelligence, confrontation naming, and verbal fluency. Her scores on Block Design and tests of immediate recall (Logical Memory and Visual Reproduction) were somewhat lower, but still within normal limits. By contrast, on all measures of delayed recall, performance was clearly impaired. On the NCSE, for example, which tested for retention of a list of four words after a delay of about 10 minutes, she could not recall any of the items and, instead, intruded the word *ball* (perhaps retained from earlier testing with the MMSE). When given category cues, she retrieved one additional item correctly but gave two erroneous answers, and when given multiple-choice alternatives, she made two false-positive errors. She could recall nothing of either of the Logical Memory passages after a 30-minute delay; when given cues about the first story, she confabulated a response, stating that a woman had found her children dead and that the police had been of no help to her.

The poor performance on delayed recall was clearly below expectations for age. In addition, depressive symptoms were not severe enough to account for this level of impairment. Other possible causes that were considered included residual effects of amitriptyline overdose or early dementia, and retesting in six to eight months was recommended.

Arrangements were made for the patient to have weekly psychotherapy visits in a geriatric outpatient program to deal with issues of loneliness and inactivity and to monitor her use of medications. In the course of these visits, continued memory problems were observed; she had difficulty recalling what had been discussed from session to session, often made several phone calls a day to verify her next appointment, and had persistent problems locating her therapist's office.

A follow-up evaluation was arranged through an outpatient program specializing in dementia. In conjunction with this assessment, she was given a second series of neuropsychological tests, approximately seven months following the testing described above. Only a summary report was available from this evaluation, and on some tests, raw scores were not provided. Therefore, only a rough comparison can be made with initial testing. Nonetheless, the similarity in the pattern of test outcomes is quite striking.

On the MMSE, a perfect score of 30 correct was reported, a result suggesting some improvement in global mental status, and scores on Digit Span were identical to those obtained during the earlier inpatient stay (6 forward, 4 backward). Performance on tests of verbal intelligence and language also continued to be high (WAIS-R Vocabulary was at the 75th percentile for age, a score of 57 out of 60 was obtained on the Boston Naming Test, and verbal fluency was said to be at the 80th to 84th percentile for age). On WMS Logical Memory, a score of 13 was obtained on immediate recall, which was above expectations for age (see Table A.1 in the Appendix). However, on delayed testing, only 2.5 items were retrieved, a result suggesting a continued problem in retention of information over time. Similarly, on the Rey-Osterrieth Complex Figure Test, only 3.5 elements of the figure were reproduced after a three-minute delay, which is at the 1st percentile or lower based on the norms provided by Van Gorp *et al.* (1990; cf. Chapter 4). Block Design performance had declined slightly (to the 25th percentile for age), while Digit Symbol performance was similar to that observed on prior testing (25th percentile). Although she was able to complete both forms of the Trail Making Test, completion times (76 seconds for Trail A, > 4 minutes for Trail B) exceeded expectations for age and background (see Table A.7 in the Appendix).

Retest results were interpreted as consistent with mild dementia, and depressive symptoms were again considered too mild to explain the observed impairments (Hamilton Depression Rating Scale score = 10). Additional diagnostic evaluations (magnetic resonance imaging scan, neurology consultation) were ordered, and with the patient's consent, the possibility of a move to a board-and-care facility was being explored. The prospects for closer family involvement were not promising, since the patient had only a single close relative, whose work required extensive travel outside the country.

In this example, retest evaluation provided somewhat clearer evidence of dementia than the initial evaluation. The persistence of impairments on neuropsychological tests and the increasing evidence of everyday memory impairment strengthened the impression of clinically significant memory loss. In addition, follow-up testing suggested the beginnings of impairment in some other cognitive functions (e.g., visual spatial performance and executive functions). While mild symptoms of depression continued, they did not appear to explain the extent of everyday problems with cognitive function.

In light of the history of hypertension and cardiovascular disease, multi-infarct dementia (MID) was considered a likely diagnostic possibility in this case. However, there were no areas of infarction on the magnetic resonance imaging (MRI) and no focal neurological signs or symptoms. The possibility of early dementia of Alzheimer type

(DAT) could not be excluded. In fact, the increased rate of forgetting, relative prominence of memory loss, and occasional blatant errors of intrusion were all consistent with DAT. For this individual, however, distinguishing between DAT and MID was less important than in some other cases, since there was a clear need to control cardiovascular risk factors, whether or not these were the cause of cognitive decline.

DEMENTIA WITH EXCESS DISABILITIES

The second example (10.2) concerns an individual whose cognitive problems were exacerbated by illness in the family, frequent relocation, and high doses of neuroleptic medication.

The patient was an 81-year-old man who had worked most of his adult life on an assembly line in an automotive factory. He was in good physical health but, in the last four years, had undergone many stressful life changes. According to his daughters, he had been functioning well until his wife had been placed in a nursing home because of advanced Alzheimer's disease. The patient stayed in his own home for a while but became increasingly lonely and isolated; he visited his wife in the nursing home less and less frequently, since she no longer recognized him. At his children's urging, he had moved first to a retirement home, which he didn't like, and then to a board-and-care home. It was here that he began to have noticeable problems. He developed a belief that one of his daughters was trying to take his money and often argued loudly with her when she came to visit. Staff described him as very anxious and as tending to "fly off the handle" with little provocation. Problems worsened when he moved to a second board-and-care home, and finally, he was admitted to a psychiatric hospital for evaluation of his symptoms. It was at this facility that he first received a diagnosis of dementia and was started on a course of treatment with neuroleptic medications (first with Haldol, later with Prolixin). He was discharged to a locked nursing home, where he received Prolixin in increasingly greater doses. His daughter, concerned about his increasing stiffness and somnolence, removed him from the home and requested a reevaluation at a program specializing in dementia. This led to the recommendation that neuroleptics be discontinued, and that a more complete inpatient assessment be performed to yield a better sense of his level of function off medications.

During the latter evaluation, the patient had no problems with paranoia or agitation, was pleasant and sociable with other people, and managed his personal care without difficulties. He continued to exhibit some psychomotor retardation and some slowness and paucity of speech.

Neuropsychological testing was begun eight days after admission. The patient was cooperative with testing and showed good persistence on the various tasks. He was cordial with the examiner and generally denied depressive symptoms.

The MMSE score of 19 out of 30 indicated mild impairment of cognitive function, with problems observed in orientation, serial 7's, and delayed recall. On the WAIS-R, scores were below average on most subscales compared to norms for 70- to 74-year-olds.

The patient's best performance was on Comprehension, suggesting good preservation of practical intelligence. Low scores on Vocabulary, Information, and Similarities may be explained in part by this individual's background as a manual laborer and his limited outside interests. Language tests yielded scores consistent with verbal intellectual level (i.e., in the low normal or borderline impaired range) based on norms that take age and educational background into consideration (Borod *et al.*, 1980; Montgomery, 1982; see Tables A.5 and A.6 in the Appendix).

Interestingly, scores on performance subscales were not generally lower than verbal subscale scores; in fact, given that the patient was 81 years old, several performance scores may be considered within normal limits for age. On Block Design, he failed the second and third items but completed the fourth correctly and was subsequently able to do two of the nine-block designs correctly when allowed to work slightly beyond the standard time limit.

Prorated IQ scores based on the WAIS-R norms for ages 70 to 74 years were 78, 80, and 79, for Verbal IQ, Performance IQ, and Full IQ, respectively; however, if the extended age norms of Ryan *et al.* (1990) are used (see Chapter 4), prorated IQs increase to 87, 86, and 86, respectively. Therefore, in this case, use of the WAIS-R norms led to an impression of greater impairment than norms that would have been better suited to the individual's age and educational background.

Tests of attention yielded variable results. Digit Span was the low point of his WAIS-R profile; the patient was able to repeat six digits forward but could not repeat even two- or three-digit strings correctly in reverse order. On a number cancellation test, he showed good persistence and made no errors but required 2½ minutes to complete a single page. Performance on Trail A was within normal limits based on norms from Davies (1968), but the patient could not understand the task requirements for Trail B.

Performance was also variable on memory tests. On the Object Memory Evaluation, scores were well within expectations for people in their 80s (Fuld, 1981), suggesting some ability to learn and retain new information, despite distraction and delay. However, on Logical Memory, very few facts were retained from either story, and on Associate Learning, the patient was unable to learn any of the hard word pairs. He made frequent intrusion errors in his responses to these items, usually giving a synonym or a semantic association (e.g., for *school*, "teacher"; for *obey*, "behave"). On the multiple-choice version of the Visual Retention Test, he correctly recognized only 6 of 16 items, which is in the impaired range based on age norms provided by Montgomery (1982; cf. Chapter 4).

The test results provide some evidence of cognitive impairment, but they also show areas of strength. Areas of difficulty included memory for meaningful and novel information and complex attentional functions. Verbal information and naming abilities were possibly impaired, but for this individual, work history and lack of intellectual interests need to be considered as contributing factors. Areas of strength included practical knowledge, learning and recall of rote information, and simple attention. In addition, nonverbal intellectual functions were fairly well preserved, particularly when his obvious psychomotor slowing is taken into account.

EXAMPLE 10.2

Background

Eighty-one-year-old Caucasian man.

High school education; had been employed on the assembly line in an auto factory; retired for approximately 25 years.

First marriage ended in divorce; current spouse diagnosed as having Alzheimer's disease, placed in a nursing home four years ago.

Lived alone for a time after his wife was institutionalized but became increasingly despondent; moved to a board-and-care home and, later, to a retirement home, where he became anxious, angry, and delusional.

Admitted to a psychiatric hospital and treated first with haloperidol (Haldol) and later with fluphenazine (Prolixin); discharged to a locked nursing facility, where he continued to receive Prolixin combined with trihexyphenidyl (Artane).

Dissension within the family about the patient's condition and ability to function outside an institutional setting.

Medical history largely negative; had surgery for a hernia many years ago; vague history of peptic ulcer disease, treated with antacids; recent history of rib fracture; only active medical problems are dermatological (abscess, skin rash).

Computerized tomography (CT) scan showed mild diffuse cerebral atrophy; blood count, blood chemistries, urinalysis, and tests for syphilis negative.

No medications at the time of assessment; however, had been receiving Prolixin and Artane until two weeks before admission.

Presenting problem

Admitted to a geropsychiatric inpatient facility for assessment of the severity of cognitive and emotional problems under medication-free conditions.

Behavior during testing

Polite and cooperative. Understood test instructions. Highly motivated but had occasional problems with sustained attention. Mood was euthymic, and there was no evidence of agitation, hallucinations, or paranoid ideation. There were some residual signs of Parkinsonism (e.g., pronounced psychomotor slowing, mild difficulty initiating speech, limited facial expressiveness).

Test findings

Mini-Mental State Examination: 19

WAIS-R	Scaled score (70–74 years)	Percentile
Information	5	5
Digit span	4	2

Vocabulary	7	16
Comprehension	10	50
Similarities	6	9
Picture Completion	7	16
Block Design	7	16
Object Assembly	8	25
Digit Symbol	5	5
	Raw score	Percentile/ rating
WMS		
Logical Memory, immediate	1.5	5
Associate Learning, immediate	6.5	16
Object Memory Evaluation		
Storage	39	37
Retrieval	32	37
Repeated Retrieval	20	50
Ineffective Reminders	7	50
Delayed Recall	8	Normal
Visual Retention Test (multiple choice, max = 16)	6	2
Boston Naming Test (60 items)	32	16
Controlled Oral Word Association Test	17	5
Trail Making Test		
Form A	120 seconds	10–25
Form B	Unable to perform	Impaired
Number cancellation	Accurate but slow	Low normal

Qualitative aspects of performance

Psychomotor slowing and paucity of speech. On Block Design, quality of performance improved as the number of items increased. Errors of intrusion on novel paired associates (synonyms or semantic associations).

Interpretation and recommendations

Cognitive profile characterized by difficulty with attentional processes, concreteness, and inflexibility; limited vocabulary; and poor fund of general information. Performance on verbal intelligence subtests may be consistent with occupational background and limited outside interests. Psychomotor slowing and speech hesitancy suggest some continued neuroleptic toxicity. Memory and visuospatial performances raise doubts about cortical dementia (e.g., Alzheimer's disease). Was discharged to home of daughter. Recommended continuing off drugs, reassessment after six months to a year, and psychotherapy or support group attendance to deal with personal and family issues.

Results of neurological evaluation were largely negative, although some residual Parkinsonian symptoms, attributed to effects of Prolixin, were still observed. The CT scan was interpreted as showing atrophy, but there were no indications of infarction or periventricular lucencies.

For this individual, too, reassessment in several months was recommended, to allow symptoms to be reexamined after he had had more time off neuroleptic medications. He went home to live with one of his daughters, although there continued to be disagreement within the family about his ability to manage his own affairs or to live successfully outside a nursing-home setting.

This case is something of a puzzle from the standpoint of neuropsychological test findings, because of inconsistencies observed in certain areas of testing. The balance of evidence suggests a mild dementia, probably of the Alzheimer type. However, the complicated history had undoubtedly reduced the patient's functioning far below the level explained by his dementia.

COGNITIVE IMPAIRMENT AND PARKINSON'S DISEASE

The third patient (Example 10.3), a 67-year-old woman, provides a good example of the types of cognitive impairments that can be observed in an elderly person with early Parkinson's disease.

The event that precipitated psychiatric assessment was an episode of visual hallucinations that began about a week before admission. The patient reported seeing people in her house engaging in routine activities (e.g., watching television, putting on her clothes, or getting into her bed). These visions always appeared in the early evening, and the people did not speak or attempt to communicate. She had had two similar episodes several months earlier, each lasting about four days; symptoms remitted spontaneously in both cases.

The patient was aware that her visions were unusual and wondered if there might be "something neurological" that was causing these experiences. She denied feelings of sadness or dysphoria and had none of the vegetative symptoms normally associated with depressive disorder. Family members described the patient as a sociable and pleasant person without any history of thought disorder or mood disturbance.

Upon admission, there were several signs of motor disturbance apparent. Gait was slow, and there was immobility of facial expression. Speech was very soft in volume and monotonic. Neurobehavioral consultants diagnosed early Parkinson's disease but recommended that treatment with anti-Parkinson medications be delayed.

The patient had some mild complaints about her memory and felt that these difficulties had been getting worse in recent months. Therefore, neuropsychological testing was requested to provide some objective data on memory function. In addition, during a medical hospitalization two years earlier, the patient had received cognitive testing which suggested significant impairment. Only a brief summary of these findings was available, and quantitative scores were noted for only a few tests. The conclusion from this examination was that there was evidence of "diffuse brain dysfunction due to aging and severe verbal and visual memory impairment." However, this level of performance seemed inconsistent with the patient's current functioning as described by her family and as observed by hospital staff.

On the Vocabulary and Similarities subtests from the WAIS, the patient achieved high-average scores, consistent with her educational background. On performance subtests, scores were lower, particularly on tasks that required speeded psychomotor responses. She understood the Digit Symbol task easily and worked accurately, although slowly. On Block Design, she was relatively organized in her approach to constructing the designs and correctly completed two additional designs over the time limits. Her prorated scores for Verbal IQ (VIQ) and Performance IQ (PIQ) were 108 and 85, respectively. The present VIQ was higher than the score of 96 that had been reported two years earlier, and PIQ was not significantly below the earlier estimate of 91.

On verbal memory testing, scores were in the low-normal to borderline-impaired range for age. On the Shopping List Test, where she was asked to memorize 10 grocery items (see Chapter 4), recall improved steadily across trials, and after a delay of 15 minutes, the patient was still able to recall 9 items. On verbal paired-associate learning (Inglis, 1959; see Chapter 4), she had mild initial difficulty with intermediate pairs (e.g., *cup-plate*). She found novel pairs (e.g., *sponge-chimney*) considerably harder but, after seven presentations, correctly learned two of three pairs. This is a slower rate of learning than is usually observed in people of her age and background (La Rue *et al.*, 1986a; cf. Chapter 4), but a basic ability to learn and retain new information was still evident. There were no errors of intrusion on either of the verbal memory tasks.

Nonverbal memory performance was considerably lower. On the Visual Retention Test, the patient correctly copied only the first and third designs based on immediate recall. As the difficulty of items increased, she made frequent errors of omission and distortion, combined with occasional misplacements and rotations. Whether this performance reflected memory *per se*, or difficulties with visuoconstruction, could not be determined since the test was not readministered in direct-copy form.

The most striking deficits were noted on relatively demanding tests of cognitive flexibility. On the Wisconsin Card Sort Task (see Chapter 4), the patient had difficulty discerning the initial category and could not shift accurately between categories. On Trail B, she was not able to grasp the concept of alternating between number and letter sequences. She was very perplexed about her difficulties with this task and asked the examiner to try to help her learn what was required. Despite 45 minutes of instruction, demonstration, and practice, the patient was still unable to perform the alternation for more than one or two segments at a time.

This pattern of test results fits very well with what is commonly observed in early stages of Parkinson's disease (see Chapter 8). There was a disproportionate impairment of executive functions relative to other cognitive losses. Verbal intelligence was well preserved, and verbal memory was only slightly lower than expectations for age and education. Visuospatial and visuoconstructive deficits were apparent, but these were fairly mild and were most noticeable when speed of response was required.

EXAMPLE 10.3

Background

Sixty-seven-year-old Caucasian woman.

B.A. degree and some graduate courses.

Homemaker; began to work as a teacher's aide at age 57, following her husband's death; continued this until a few months before the present evaluation.

Active lifestyle (exercise class, organist for church).

Medical history significant for a long-standing sleep disorder; possible angina; possible hypothyroidism; postural hypotension; no prior psychiatric or neurological illness.

Received extensive medical workup for possible angina attacks two years before present testing; findings were negative for cardiac or cerebrovascular disease; CT scan and EEG were within normal limits, although psychological testing suggested "general brain dysfunction."

Medical assessment during the present hospital admission found no evidence of hypothyroidism or cerebrovascular disease. However, a diagnosis of early Parkinson's disease was made. Brain CT scan was normal, but there was mild generalized slowing on EEG.

Medications were limited to aspirin (for joint pain) and chloral hydrate (for insomnia).

Presenting problems

Visual hallucinations (three episodes, each lasting a few days, occurring 1 week, 6 months, and 18 months prior to the present assessment).

Memory complaints; mild problems since husband's death 10 years earlier; "gradually getting worse."

Behavior during testing

Cooperative, motivated, persistent; appropriate use of humor.

Psychomotor slowing; low-volume, monotonic speech.

Test findings

Mini-Mental State Examination: 26

WAIS	Age-scaled score	Percentile
Vocabulary	14	91
Similarities	12	75
Digit Span	9	37
Block Design	6	9
Picture Completion	9	37
Digit Symbol	7	16

	Raw score	Percentile/ rating
Paired Associate Learning Test		
Mediate pairs	13	16
New pairs	4	5
Visual Retention Test		
Total correct	2	<1
Total errors	22	<1
Shopping List Test	5 to 9 items recalled per trial	Low normal
	9/10 recalled after delay	Normal
Digit cancellation	Accurate but slow	Low normal
Trail Making Test—Part B	Unable to do	Impaired
Wisconsin Card Sort Test	Unable to shift categories	Impaired

Qualitative aspects of performance

Was able show some learning of novel paired associates with more trials; no intrusion errors on either of the verbal learning and memory tasks. On the Visual Retention Test, most frequent errors were omissions and distortions, with occasional rotations and misplacements. Despite extensive coaching on Trail B, was unable to alternate sequences in a consistent way, and on the card-sorting task, frequently perseverated in making inaccurate classifications.

Interpretation and recommendations

Deficits consistent with Parkinson's disease. Cognitive flexibility and visuospatial functions are impaired, while verbal intelligence is intact and verbal memory is only mildly deficient for age and background. No decline in intelligence or memory performance from testing performed two years earlier. Involvement of posterior association cortex is suggested by visuospatial performance and visual hallucinations. Reassurance was provided about memory problems, and information was given to both patient and family about Parkinson's disease and home care services.

Performance had not clearly declined over the two-year period since she had last received cognitive testing. In fact, verbal intellectual scores were higher than those observed at the earlier testing, and verbal memory could hardly be described as "severely impaired." On the earlier testing, the patient had been described as resistant to intellectual assessment. On this more recent evaluation, however, she was very cooperative, highly motivated, and interested in understanding why she had performed as she did. Her improved motivation and greater comfort in testing may have contributed to her relatively sound performance in many areas.

The patient was reassured about her memory problems and was encouraged to return to her activities outside the home. She was given information about Parkinson's disease, and both she and her family were encouraged to make plans for future situations when she might need more assistance in day-to-day affairs. Continuing follow-up care was arranged through a neurobehavioral specialist.

DEPRESSION AND MID

The last example (10.4) involves mixed symptoms of depression and dementia. In this type of case, effects of depression cannot be firmly distinguished from those produced by brain impairment. However, repeated testing, combined with other clinical data, can sometimes help to clarify the clinical picture.

The patient was a 74-year-old retired physician who had recently moved so that he could be closer to his daughters. He had begun to show signs of depression about three years earlier; these problems had worsened significantly in the past year, despite psychotherapy and several trials with antidepressant medications. He had had two earlier episodes of serious depression, 10 and 14 years earlier and on both occasions had shown a good response to treatment with medications and electroconvulsive therapy (ECT).

Several stressful events had occurred in the patient's life within the past year. His wife had died unexpectedly about six months before this assessment, and that loss had been shortly preceded by his retirement from medical practice. Finding it hard to live on his own, he had moved to be nearer his daughters; however, both were busy with their professions and families, and neither was able to give him the time or attention for which he had hoped.

About two weeks before this assessment, the patient had been hospitalized for congestive heart failure. At that time, he was felt to be severely depressed and was encouraged to consider a more thorough assessment of his psychiatric symptoms.

When he first came to the psychiatric unit, his mood was depressed and sad, and his affect was constricted. His thoughts were coherent and logical, but he had some difficulty relating details of his recent history. There was severe psychomotor retardation and a profound loss of interest and initiative. His daughters described him as very dependent emotionally and socially and as often requiring their assistance in making decisions. They felt that he had declined intellectually and were reluctant to assume continuing responsibility for his care.

Because of the family's reports of decline and the patient's problems in relating his history, a referral was made for neuropsychological testing. He was cooperative with this assessment, but on the last testing, when he was about to leave the hospital, he was particularly sad and withdrawn. He tended to work quickly, was generally able to stay on task, and was not unusually anxious or self-critical about his performance. However, on several of the memory tests, his effort diminished sharply after a certain point. If prompted to try harder to remember, he was frequently able to provide additional accurate details.

On the MMSE, he was well oriented and made no errors on delayed recall. His poorest performance was on the attention/calculation items (serial 7's and spelling of a word backward). His copy of the interlocking pentagons was sloppy, but the basic outlines of the figures were preserved.

On the WAIS, verbal skills were generally in the very superior range, consistent with his education and occupation. Nonverbal intelligence was in the average range. Digit Span was much lower than other verbal skills, and Block Design was lower than other Performance scales. While attempting to construct the designs, he worked quickly but did not monitor the details of his constructions in an accurate way; when prompted to correct specific errors, he was not always able to do so and seemed to have difficulty judging how closely he was approximating the design.

On tests of learning and memory, moderate deficits were observed. He had some difficulty learning novel word pairs and frequently intruded answers from an earlier set of words. On the Object Memory Evaluation, Storage and Retrieval scores were roughly within the normal range, but consistency of retrieval was very poor. On the Visual Retention Test, he copied only 1 of the 10 designs correctly; a combination of errors was observed, including some perseveration of peripheral figures from one design to the next.

On other nonverbal tests (e.g., the Visual Organization Test and Coloured Progressive Matrices), his scores were roughly within normal limits for age but were lower than expected for his general intellectual level.

The Minnesota Multiphasic Personality Inventory (MMPI) suggested severe depression, nervousness, anxiety, lack of initiative, and poor self-esteem. Hypochondriacal tendencies were also observed. The pattern was that of a persistent worrier who was likely to blame himself for problems in life and to become preoccupied with personal deficiencies.

The MMPI findings reinforced the impression of severe psychiatric impairment. The cognitive findings were less clear. The strong performance on most intelligence subscales argues against a general loss of cognitive function, and the Storage and Retrieval scores on the Object Memory Evaluation suggest some continued ability to learn. However, nonverbal memory and the ability to retrieve information consistently were severely impaired, and on most nonverbal tasks, there was a tendency toward sloppiness and inaccuracy in monitoring details. Also, there were several instances of "organic" errors (e.g., intrusions on paired-associate learning). The CT scan indicated a possible small infarct in the region of the right basal ganglia, and on EEG, there was intermittent slow-wave activity in the frontal region. Overall, the impression was of MID with severe coexisting depression.

The patient refused to consider ECT, even though he had once responded well to this treatment, and his recent trials with antidepressants had not been very helpful. He was started on a low dose of trazodone, but when he experienced some cardiac arrythmia, this drug was discontinued. He was later treated with phenelzine but showed little improvement over a period of several weeks. When psychological testing was repeated, there was no improvement in depression noted on the MMPI, and if anything, cognitive performance was slightly worse (see Example 10.4 for specific scores).

Discouraged by the lack of benefit, the family made arrangements for the patient to

EXAMPLE 10.4

Background

Seventy-four-year-old Caucasian man.
Retired physician (internal medicine).
Widowed 6 months ago; recently moved to Los Angeles to be near his daughters.
Medical history significant for congestive heart failure and adult-onset diabetes; recently hospitalized for his heart condition.
CT scan showed possible small infarct in the right basal ganglia; mild diffuse slowing on EEG, with intermittent frontal slow-wave activity.
Symptoms of depression for 3 years, worsening since wife's death; outpatient therapy and antidepressant medications had been ineffective. Two previous episodes of depression, 10 and 15 years earlier.

Presenting problems

Dysphoric mood, anhedonia, decreased energy, psychomotor retardation; family reports that he cannot manage his own affairs (e.g., finances).

Behavior during testing

Cooperative; understood tasks easily. Concentration generally adequate. On memory tasks, tended to give up easily.

Test findings

Mini-Mental State Examination: 25

WAIS	Age-scaled score	Percentile
Vocabulary	15	95
Information	16	98
Comprehension	18	99
Similarities	17	99
Digit Span	8	25
Picture Completion	14	91
Digit Symbol	11	37
Block Design	6	9

	Raw score	Percentile/ rating
Object Memory Evaluation		
Storage	44	25
Retrieval	38	50
Repeated Retrieval	9	<1
Ineffective Reminders	5	9
Visual Retention Test		
Total correct	1	<1
Total errors	18	<1
Paired Associate Learning Test		
Mediate pairs	15	84

New pairs	10	42
Shopping List Test	Recalled 8/10 items by 4th trial	Low normal
Visual Organization Test	21.5	Low normal
Progressive Matrices	20	50
MMPI—Welsch code: 2″710′534-896/F/LK		

Test findings (1-month retest; on stable dose of Trazodone)

Visual Retention Test		
Total correct	2	<1
Total errors	14	<1
Paired Associate Learning		
Mediate pairs	13	16
New pairs	4	7
Shopping List Test	8/10 recalled by 4th trial	Low normal
MMPI: 2**07′1536894 LF-K		

Qualitative aspects of performance

Evidence of primacy and recency on verbal list learning; spontaneously recalled only a few items per trial but was able to provide more if prompted to try harder; occasional intrusions on second administration. On paired associate learning, had difficulty acquiring novel pairs and made frequent errors of intrusion. On the Object Memory Evaluation, there was little consistency in items recalled from one trial to the next. On Block Design and the Visual Retention Test, responded quickly and carelessly.

Interpretation and recommendations

Findings are consistent with a mild dementia. Attention is reduced, and visuospatial performance is lower than expected for age and background. Memory is also impaired relative to the patient's general intellectual level. These findings could be due to very severe depression. However, the types of errors made on memory and visuospatial tasks are more typical of organic brain disorder than depression alone. CT and EEG findings are also consistent with MID. Was encouraged to continue in outpatient treatment for depression and to arrange for a living situation that would provide some help with monitoring of medications and other basic activities.

move to a "retirement home" (actually a board and care). In a follow-up interview a year later, he was described by his daughter as unchanged; he continued to be depressed and lacking in initiative, depending on staff to dispense his medications and his family to handle his financial affairs. He had not received any additional treatment for depression since leaving the hospital.

As discussed in Chapter 11, older patients sometimes experience a dementia when they become depressed; in many cases, cognitive losses remit or improve substantially with antidepressant therapy. In the present example, since depression was persistent and severe, the possibility of a "depressive pseudodementia" cannot be completely excluded. Nonetheless, the lack of benefit from antidepressant therapy, combined with the CT scan results and errors made on testing, strengthen the case for a diagnosis of MID.

This example illustrates the frustration that can result when treatments have little benefit. The patient was discouraged about not feeling better, and the family was left with difficult decisions about placement; staff wondered (with hindsight) whether they had made the right decision to continue with medications for the depressive symptoms. In many cases, however, remarkable improvements occur with treatment for depression, even when a mild dementia is suspected (e.g., see Example 12.3). These successes help to put the present case in better perspective and illustrate why it is important to attempt to intervene in such confusing and difficult cases.

SUMMARY AND CONCLUSIONS

Four examples have been presented in which the history and clinical presentation suggest a diagnosis of dementia. None of these examples is free of complicating factors that may explain or contribute to cognitive losses. Instead, they were selected to represent the types of cases for which neuropsychological testing can be helpful diagnostically and in planning for continuing care.

In the first example, excessive medication may have contributed to the patient's memory losses and to her declining self-care. However, memory impairments persisted and some other functions worsened over subsequent months, lending support to diagnosis of early dementia. In the second example, medication effects and psychosocial stressors exacerbated cognitive problems, rendering an individual with mild dementia totally dependent on others for his care. In the third example, cognitive impairments were felt to be related to Parkinson's disease. The configuration of cognitive deficits differed from that of the first two cases, with cognitive flexibility impaired to a greater degree than learning and memory. In the final example, severe depression and several recent losses compounded the effects of a mild multi-infarct dementia, leading to persistent impairments in cognition and motivation that proved difficult to change with treatment.

These examples illustrate the interplay between clinical history, medical diagnostic procedures, and neuropsychological testing in arriving at a working diagnosis and show how repeat evaluations can be used to assess the persistence or reversibility of impairments. They also exemplify the wide range of recommendations that can stem from diagnostic assessments. Even though dementia was suspected in each of these examples, active treatment was recommended in three out of four instances, in the form of either psychotherapy or medications. In terms of living arrangements, recommendations followed the principle of providing for patient safety at the least restrictive level of care. In the first case, the initial recommendation was for the person to continue living in her retirement hotel with close psychotherapeutic follow-up and supervision of medications; only when her condition failed to improve after several months was the possibility of a board-and-care arrangement discussed. In the second case, the daughter's hope of having her father come to her home, instead of returning to the nursing home, was supported and encouraged by staff, since very few problems with behavior or self-care had been observed during the hospital stay. This type of individualized planning, with readjustments made as needed, can help to reduce the sadness and guilt that dementia caregivers are likely to experience when patients are no longer able to live entirely on their own.

11

Depression

Most people have had the experience of feeling "down" or uninterested in the daily routine. These feelings seldom interfere with work or social activities, and they usually resolve spontaneously within a few hours or days. In depressive illness, however, mood disturbance is more severe and persistent and may be accompanied by other physical, cognitive, or emotional changes.

Older people frequently suffer mild depression in conjunction with medical and social problems. These conditions do not usually cause sufficient cognitive problems to warrant neuropsychological assessment. By contrast, in severe depression, it is not unusual for the person to have subjective or objective evidence of cognitive loss.

This chapter summarizes clinical features of depression in later life and briefly reviews current findings on neurobiology, epidemiology, and treatment options. Neuropsychological findings are examined in two parts, first in the "typical" case, where cognitive loss is fairly mild, and second, in the more unusual presentation known as *depressive pseudodementia* or *dementia syndrome of depression*.

BACKGROUND

Clarification of Terms

Diagnostic classification systems draw a distinction between depressive symptoms, which are experienced to a degree by normal adults, and depressive disorders, where mood disturbance is persistent and pervasive. Depressive disorders can be major or minor, depending on the severity of symptoms, and can be primary or associated with other psychiatric, neurological, or medical conditions. Within the category of major depression, distinctions are drawn between unipolar illness, where depressive episodes are interspersed with periods of normal mood, and bipolar illness, where depression alternates with periods of elevated mood.

This chapter is concerned primarily with major depression. The behavioral characteristics of this disorder, as specified in the revised third edition of the *Diagnostic and Statistical Manual* (DSM-III-R; American Psychiatric Association, 1987), are as follows:

1. depressed mood;
2. markedly diminished interest or pleasure in all, or almost all, activities;
3. significant undesired weight loss or gain or a decrease or increase in appetite;
4. insomnia or hypersomnia;
5. psychomotor agitation or retardation;
6. fatigue or loss of energy;
7. feelings of worthlessness or excessive guilt;
8. diminished ability to think or concentrate, or indecisiveness;
9. recurrent thoughts of death or suicidal ideation, a suicide plan, or suicide attempt. (p. 222)

Five or more of these symptoms must be present for at least two weeks, and either depressed mood or loss of interest must be observed most of the day, nearly every day.

A variety of exclusionary criteria also apply. That is, in major depression, symptoms cannot be due to an organic factor or simple bereavement and cannot be superimposed on other psychiatric disorders (e.g., schizophrenia or delusional disorder).

Patients who meet the preceding criteria and have a history of manic episodes are diagnosed with bipolar disorder, depressed phase. Those with no history of elevated mood have major depression, also called *unipolar depression*.

Diagnostic Procedures

The most important tools for diagnosing depression are clinical interview and history. For research-level diagnosis, structured interviews such as the Schedule for Affective Disorders and Schizophrenia (SADS; Spitzer & Endicott, 1977), the Structured Clinical Interview for the DSM-III-R (SCID; Spitzer & Williams, 1986), or the Comprehensive Assessment and Referral Evaluation (CARE; Gurland & Wilder, 1984) are very helpful. The SADS, in particular, has been strongly recommended for use with older patients (see review by Gallagher, 1986).

Certain medical screening tests may be indicated if physical illness or medications are suspected as a cause of depression (see Blazer, 1989; Spar & La Rue, 1990). Computerized tomography (CT) or magnetic resonance imaging (MRI) scans can be used to exclude brain tumor or stroke; blood tests and urinalysis can screen for other specific causes, including infection, anemia, thyroid dysfunction, and calcium, potassium, or glucose abnormalities. Medications also need to be evaluated, since a variety of drugs have been associated with depression, including analgesics, antihypertensives, chemotherapy drugs, and psychotropic agents (Blazer, 1989; Spar & La Rue, 1990).

Clinical Features and Course

Diagnostic criteria allow for variability in the presentation of depression, since the prominence of specific symptoms differs for individuals and episodes. Dysphoric mood or loss of interest is required for the diagnosis, but other features (e.g., sleep and appetite changes, psychotic symptoms, and cognitive complaints and impairment) are only variably observed.

In general, manifestations of depression appear to be quite similar in younger and older adults. However, there may be age trends in the overall severity of depression and in the clustering of specific features.

Blazer and Williams (1980) noted that "Much of what is called 'depression' in the elderly may actually represent decreased life satisfaction and periodic episodes of grief secondary to the physical, and economic difficulties encountered by aging individuals" (p. 442). Gurland (1976) made a similar point, suggesting that older people may be especially prone to transient depressions that are "distressing" but "not incapacitating" (p. 290).

Compared to younger depressives, older patients may show greater global cognitive impairment during depressive episodes, and at times, these impairments may be severe enough to suggest an organic dementia. This problem is discussed in detail below (see "Dementia Syndrome of Depression").

Somatic complaints are also more prominent in older depressives than in younger individuals. In part, these result from the higher rates of illness in the aged. On occasion, however, somatic complaints may serve as depressive equivalents, taking the place of mood disturbance (so-called masked depression), or these complaints may be amplified out of proportion to the underlying physical state.

Depression Rating Scales

Several standardized interviews and questionnaires have been developed to measure depression severity. These scales are helpful in screening for depression and in monitoring symptoms over time. Only a few of these scales have been developed with older patients in mind, but several have now been validated for use with older adults (for reviews, see Gallagher, 1986; Yesavage, 1986).

The Beck Depression Inventory (BDI; Beck *et al.*, 1961) is a 21-item, multiple-choice survey which includes items evaluating mood, sense of pessimism and guilt, social withdrawal, sleep disturbance, loss of energy, and weight and appetite. It has acceptable reliability and validity when used with older patients (Gallagher, Nies, & Thompson, 1982; Gallagher, Breckenridge, Steinmetz, & Thompson, 1983) and is particularly helpful for monitoring psychological symptoms of depression. A 13-item short form of the BDI (Beck & Beck, 1972) can be used with medically ill older patients or others who have limited tolerance of formal questioning (Scogin, Beutler, Corbishley, & Hamblin, 1987).

Another self-rated instrument, the Geriatric Depression Scale (GDS), was specifically developed for older patients (Yesavage *et al.*, 1983a). The GDS consists of 30 items presented in yes-no format (see Table 11.1). Mood is surveyed quite extensively, and there are additional items assessing cognitive complaints and social behavior. The GDS has eliminated most somatic items ("Do you often get restless and fidgety?" and "Do you feel full of energy?" are the closest approximations). It has relatively high sensitivity and specificity in identifying clinically diagnosed depression in older inpatient and outpatient samples (Norris, Gallagher, Wilson, & Winograd, 1987; Rapp, Parisi, Walsh, & Wallace, 1988b).

Self-rated scales may be inappropriate for some older patients. For example, in a

TABLE 11.1. The Geriatric Depression Scale (GDS)[a]

Choose the best answer for how you felt over the past week.	
1. Are you basically satisfied with your life?[b]	yes/**no**
2. Have you dropped many of your activities and interests?[b]	**yes**/no
3. Do you feel that your life is empty?[b]	**yes**/no
4. Do you often get bored?[b]	**yes**/no
5. Are you hopeful about the future?	yes/**no**
6. Are you bothered about thoughts you can't get out of your head?	**yes**/no
7. Are you in good spirits most of the time?[b]	yes/**no**
8. Are you afraid that something is going to happen to you?[b]	**yes**/no
9. Do you feel happy most of the time?[b]	yes/**no**
10. Do you often feel helpless?[b]	**yes**/no
11. Do you often get restless and fidgety?	**yes**/no
12. Do you prefer to stay at home, rather than going out and doing new things?[b]	**yes**/no
13. Do you frequently worry about the future?	**yes**/no
14. Do you feel you have more problems with memory than most?[b]	**yes**/no
15. Do you think it is wonderful to be alive now?[b]	yes/**no**
16. Do you often feel downhearted and blue?	**yes**/no
17. Do you feel pretty worthless the way you are now?[b]	**yes**/no
18. Do you worry a lot about the past?	**yes**/no
19. Do you find life very exciting?	yes/**no**
20. Is it hard for you to get started on new projects?	**yes**/no
21. Do you feel full of energy?[b]	yes/**no**
22. Do you feel that your situation is hopeless?[b]	**yes**/no
23. Do you think that most people are better off than you are?[b]	**yes**/no
24. Do you frequently get upset over little things?	**yes**/no
25. Do you frequently feel like crying?	**yes**/no
26. Do you have trouble concentrating?	**yes**/no
27. Do you enjoy getting up in the morning?	yes/**no**
28. Do you prefer to avoid social gatherings?	**yes**/no
29. Is it easy for you to make decisions?	yes/**no**
30. Is your mind as clear as it used to be?	yes/**no**

[a]Critical answers are in bold print. From Yesavage, Brink, Rose, Lum, Huang, Adey, and Leirer (1983a, pp. 37–49). Adapted by permission.
[b]See text for discussion of the short form (items marked by *b*).

study with older medical outpatients, Toner, Gurland, and Teresi (1988) found that 35% were unable to complete a self-rated depression scale (28% because of visual problems, 9% because of illiteracy, 34% because of lack of motivation or wanting the scale read to them). The Hamilton Depression Rating Scale (HAMD; Hamilton, 1967), or other observer-rated measures, can be used in these cases. The HAMD is a 23-item instrument that was originally designed as an outcome measure for drug studies of depression. Thus, it is weighted for the type of variables medications are able to alter (i.e., sleep, weight change, psychomotor speed, and other biological concerns), although it also taps depressive mood, anxiety, guilt, loss of libido, paranoia, obsessional symptoms, and suicidal ideation. The HAMD has been extensively used in clinical research with older adults, where it has been shown to be sensitive to changes in depressive symptoms. A structured interview guide has been developed for the HAMD (Williams, 1988), which may help to increase reliability in busy clinical settings.

Changes over Time

Depression is usually an episodic condition that remits with treatment or the passage of time; often, there are recurrent episodes over the course of a lifetime. Many elderly patients respond well to standard treatments for depression (see "Approaches to Treatment," below). For others, however, depression can be a persistent and disabling condition. In a one-year follow-up of older patients who were treated for major depression, Murphy (1983) found that about 35% had stayed well, 19% had relapsed, and 29% had remained continuously ill, despite continued treatment (cf. Blazer, 1989; Blessed & Wilson, 1982). Patients who have lengthy or severe initial episodes, or complicating health and social problems, are most likely to have persistent depression (Murphy, 1983).

Epidemiology

Prevalence

Depression is considered the second most common mental disorder in old age, exceeded only by dementia. As with other neuropsychiatric conditions, specific prevalence estimates vary, reflecting differences in sample characteristics, criteria for case identification, and methods of evaluation (see discussions by Blazer *et al.*, 1987; Gurland, 1976). Studies using symptom-rating scales generally report higher frequencies of depression than those using clinical interview. Also, as noted in Chapter 1, rates of depression are much higher among hospitalized older adults and residents of nursing homes than among older people residing in the community (see Table 1.2).

The percentage of older people in the community who meet diagnostic criteria for major depression appears to be quite low, with estimates ranging from less than 1% to as high as 4% to 6%; by contrast, less severe forms of depression are quite common, with estimates ranging from 2% to 26% (Blazer & Williams, 1980; Blazer *et al.*, 1987; Regier *et al.*, 1988). In acute care medical hospitals, 15% to 25% of older patients meet criteria for major depression (Rapp *et al.*, 1988a; Small & Fawzy, 1988), and in nursing homes, prevalence estimates for major depression range from 12% to 25%, and for minor depression, from 30% to 50% (Hyer & Blazer, 1982; Parmelee, Katz, & Lawton, 1989; Rovner *et al.*, 1986).

Risk Factors

Age. Old age itself has been proposed as a risk factor for depression, but evidence for this supposition is equivocal (see review by Newmann, 1989). Early studies tended to find higher rates of depression in people over 65 years of age compared to young and middle-aged adults (Gurland, 1976), but several recent studies have reported an opposite age trend (e.g., Regier *et al.*, 1988). Older people may be more prone to mild depression than younger adults, and less prone to certain severe depressive syndromes.

Gender. Among young and middle-aged adults, depression tends to affect women more often than men. This trend is also observed in many studies of older adults (e.g., Krause, 1986; Regier *et al.*, 1988). The causes of gender differences in depression are unclear (see reviews by Nolen-Hoeksema, 1987; Weissman & Klerman, 1977). Genetic and endocrine factors may play a role, but psychological and social factors (e.g., differential life stress, vulnerability to stress, or modes of coping with changes in mood) generally appear to be more important.

Medical Illness. Physical disease is an important contributor to depression at all ages. However, research suggests a particularly strong connection in older people. Blazer and Williams (1980) reported that almost 15% of a large random sample of older adults in the community had "substantial depressive symptomatology," and in nearly one-half of this group, depressive symptoms were related to medical illness. When community-resident elderly were followed longitudinally (Phifer & Murrell, 1986), those with poorer initial health or who became ill in the interim were more likely to develop depression than those in better health. Hospitalization for depression in old age is often preceded by surgery or worsening of a medical condition, particularly in men who became depressed for the first time after age 60 (Roth & Kay, 1956), and in a one-year follow-up of older depressed patients, those with major chronic health problems were significantly more likely to relapse or to remain continuously ill than those with less severe health problems (Murphy, 1983).

In another longitudinal study, Turner and Noh (1988) compared predictors of depression among three adult age groups (18 to 44 years, 45 to 64 years, and 65 years and above). Physical disability measures (pain and functional limitation) were significantly related to depression in the oldest age group, but not in the two younger groups. By contrast, stressful life events were more closely linked to depression in the young than in the old. Social support and a sense of mastery were significant contributors at all ages.

Social Correlates. Relationships between depressive and stressful events are complex and likely to be mediated by a variety of other factors. In their longitudinal study of depressive symptoms in older adults, Phifer and Murrell (1986) found few relationships between stressful life events and development of depression. The only exceptions were for health problems and loss of loved ones, where increased depression was observed. When social support was available, the risk of depression following health and loss events was much reduced. The buffering effect of social support, and of intimate relationships in particular, has been noted in many other studies as well (see Chapter 1).

Bereavement clearly influences mood, but only a small percentage of older people become severely depressed when a spouse or other loved one dies (see Chapter 1). By contrast, with physical disability, it may be harder to make an acceptable social adjustment. Many older people with physical problems must move to retirement or nursing homes, and these relocations may add to psychological distress. In one recent study, particularly high rates of depressive symptoms were observed in older people who had recently moved to nursing or retirement homes compared to established residents (Parmelee *et al.*, 1989).

Family History. Twin studies and family history investigations show that depression tends to cluster within families (Gershon, 1983). Allen (1976) found an average concordance rate for unipolar depression of 11% in dizygotic twins and 40% in monozygotic twins. In a case-control family history study, Weissman, Kidd, and Prussoff (1982) found rates of depression to be two to five times higher in relatives of depressed patients than in relatives of controls. Single-gene hypotheses, chromosomal hypotheses, and polygenic models have been proposed to explain these outcomes, but no one model is clearly supported at this time. When the first episode of depression occurs late in life (i.e., age 50 or beyond), there may be less genetic influence than in depressions that start at earlier ages (Blazer, 1989).

Neurobiology

Many different theories have been proposed to explain how depression develops, including cognitive, psychodynamic, and behavioral models. Neurobiological interpretations are considered here, since these may relate more directly to neuropsychological test findings.

Biochemical Theories

Since the efficacy of antidepressant medications first became apparent in the 1950s, there has been extensive research aimed at identifying neurochemical bases of depression. The literature on this topic is large and complex and has been extensively reviewed elsewhere (for reviews aimed at nonmedical professionals, see Byrne & Stern, 1981; McNeal & Cimbolic, 1986).

Depression has been associated with a decrease in brain catecholamines (norepinephrine and dopamine, particularly norepinephrine; see Bunney & Davis, 1965; Schildkraut, 1965) or indolamine neurotransmitters (especially serotonin, or 5-HT; see Amsterdam & Mendels, 1980; Glassman, 1969) and to increased activity of the cholinergic neurotransmitter system (see Gershon & Shaw, 1961; Janowsky, 1980). Other theories emphasize interactions between the amine neurotransmitter systems (Dumbrille-Ross & Tang, 1983; Mendels, Stinnett, Burns, & Frazer, 1975) or propose different subgroups of patients whose mood disturbance is more dependent on one neurotransmitter system than another (e.g., Maas, 1975).

Most commonly prescribed antidepressant medications increase the activity of catecholamines in the brain (see Chapter 2 and Figure 2.2), either by preventing the breakdown of norepinephrine (NE) by monoamine oxidase (MAO; as with monoamine oxidase inhibitors), or by blocking the uptake of NE released into the synapse (most tricyclic antidepressants). Many of these drugs also affect availability of 5-HT in the brain. By contrast, drugs that simply reduce acetylcholine levels are usually ineffective in treating depression.

Another neurochemical model suggests that in depression, disturbances in the limbic system may lead to disregulation of the hypothalamic-pituitary-adrenal axis, which in turn, leads to abnormal production of neuroendocrines (e.g., cortisol, thyroid-stimulating hormone, growth hormone, or prolactin). The relationship between neuroendocrine changes and neurotransmitter changes is unclear, although a variety of links with NE and 5-HT receptor activity have been proposed. The neuroendocrine hypothesis spawned a popular clinical measure, the dexamethasone suppression test (DST), which is sensitive to abnormal cortisol regulation (Carroll, Feinberg, Greden, Tarika, Albala, Hasket, James, Kronfol, Lohr, Steiner, de Vigne, & Young, 1981). While a number of studies have suggested that the DST may help to identify patients who can benefit from treatment with tricyclics, other studies, including some with elderly patients, have not found this test to be helpful (e.g., Spar & La Rue, 1983).

Because elderly depressed patients respond to the same types of treatments as younger depressives, neurochemical theories of late-life depression have been similar to those proposed for younger patients (see Blazer, 1989; Spar & La Rue, 1990). However, because aging does affect brain concentrations of all of the major neurotransmitters implicated in depression (see Chapter 2), dosages of antidepressant medications usually need to be altered for older patients.

Neurobehavioral Models

Neurobehavioral interpretations of depression are more descriptive than explanatory. These models draw analogies between behavioral findings in depression and the effects of focal brain impairments.

A right-hemisphere hypothesis has been advanced, where in depression, the balance of cortical activity is believed to shift from the left to the right hemisphere, the result being an abnormally high level of activity in the right hemisphere. Flor-Henry (1979) reviewed some of the older data in support of this hypothesis, including electrophysiological and neuropsychological studies (cf. Weingartner & Silberman, 1982). Stroke patients with lesions in the anterior regions of the left hemisphere appear particularly liable to depression (see Robinson, 1986; Starkstein & Robinson, 1989), and on cognitive testing, depressed patients often perform poorly on "right-hemisphere" tasks (e.g., Performance as opposed to Verbal subtests from the Wechsler Adult Intelligence Scale; see Fromm-Auch, 1983). However, as noted in Chapter 3, problems with Performance subtests frequently result from diffuse brain injuries as well as right-hemisphere impairments. To further confuse the lateralization issue, there are several studies that show superior performance of depressed patients relative to controls on right-hemisphere tasks (Handel, Albert, Kaplan, Moss, & Hurwitz, 1985; Silberman, Weingartner, Stillman, Chen, & Post, 1983b). These outcomes have been interpreted as suggesting either enhanced right-hemisphere processing in depression or compensation by the right hemisphere for the relative deactivation of the dominant left hemisphere.

Cummings and Benson (1983) classify depression-related cognitive impairments as a mild form of subcortical dementia in which disruption of the frontal circuit is a prominent neuropsychological feature (see Chapter 8 for additional discussion of subcortical dementia). Like certain patients with frontal lesions or early PD, depressed patients tend to perform poorly on effortful learning and memory tasks and on measures that require speed or flexibility of cognitive processing (see "Neuropsychological Findings," below). In addition, there are several studies that demonstrate improvement in effortful memory processes in depression with medications that increase arousal and activation (e.g., Murphy & Weingartner, 1973; Reus, Silberman, Post, & Weingartner, 1979; Siegfried, Jansen, & Pahnke, 1984).

Studies of cerebral metabolism and blood flow have sometimes provided support for focal brain impairment in depression, but there are many inconsistencies. For example, a recent study evaluating cerebral blood flow (Silfverskiold & Risberg, 1989) found a normal overall blood flow in depression. Regional flow patterns were described as "close to identical" for patients and controls, and only minor and statistically insignificant flow changes were noted when depression improved. By contrast, a recent positron emission tomography (PET) study (fluoro-D-glucose technique) found some evidence for regional asymmetry (Baxter, Schwartz, Phelps, Mazziotta, Guze, Selin, Gerner, & Sumida, 1989). Prior to treatment, glucose metabolic rates were reduced for patients with either unipolar or bipolar major depression in both the left and right prefrontal cortex. With treatment, metabolic rates increased in the left, but not the right, prefrontal cortex, a finding suggesting that depression may entail a left prefrontal abnormality.

Approaches to Treatment

The same types of therapy that are used in treating depression in younger patients commonly produce good results in older adults as well. Detailed discussions of treatment for geriatric depression can be found in Blazer (1989), Gallagher and Thompson (1983), Knight (1986), Spar and La Rue (1990), and Smyer, Zarit, and Qualls (1990). A few studies are mentioned below to illustrate the extent of improvement that can be expected.

Psychotherapy

Thompson, Gallagher, and Breckenridge (1987) compared the effects of individual behavioral, brief psychodynamic, and cognitive therapies for older adults diagnosed with major depressive disorder. At a six-week interim evaluation using an extensive battery of symptom-rating scales (including the BDI, GDS, and HAMD), treated patients had improved significantly relative to wait-list controls; there was no indication of spontaneous improvement in the untreated control condition. At the end of three to four months of active therapy, 70% of the treated subjects had improved substantially and 52% were judged to be in remission. There were no significant differences between the therapy modalities.

This study did not describe the medical status of participants, and it is reasonable to question whether such a high a degree of efficacy would be obtained for physically ill depressed individuals. An investigation that addressed this question was that of Jarvik, Mintz, Steuer, and Gerner (1982), who compared the effectiveness of two forms of group psychotherapy, cognitive-behavioral and psychodynamic, for elderly depressed patients who had medical contraindications for antidepressant medication. At 26 weeks of treatment, an average improvement in HAMD scores of 30% was observed, compared with a 19% decrement on this symptom index in a placebo control condition. Twelve percent of these patients were in remission from depression at this point in treatment.

Somatic Therapies

Antidepressant medications can also be effective in treating geriatric depression. For example, in a companion investigation of the psychotherapy study noted above, Jarvik and colleagues (1982) studied the efficacy of two tricyclic antidepressants, imipramine and doxepin, in a double-blind placebo-controlled study in elderly outpatients with major depression. A 50% improvement in HAMD scores was observed at 26 weeks for the drug-treated patients, and 45% of the subjects were in remission at this treatment point. A bimodal distribution was observed, with subjects either responding well to the drug early in treatment or failing to show an appreciable response at any point in the investigation.

Several good reviews (e.g., Bernstein, 1984; Davidson, 1989; Halaris, 1986–1987; Spar & La Rue, 1990) are available which provide guidelines for the use of various antidepressants and outline the most common side effects and contraindications. Since treatment with antidepressants entails some risk for older patients (e.g., possible anticholinergic effects, orthostatic hypotension, and cardiac conduction disturbances), careful monitoring is very important.

For very severe geriatric depression, electroconvulsive therapy (ECT) can be an effective treatment option (e.g., Godber, Rosenvinge, Wilkinson, & Smithies, 1987;

Kramer, 1987), although certain complications of this treatment (e.g., cardiorespiratory difficulties, falls, and severe confusion) may be special problems in older patients (Burke, Rubin, Zorumski, & Wetzel, 1987).

NEUROPSYCHOLOGICAL FINDINGS

Depressed patients frequently complain of memory loss and poor concentration, and on neuropsychological testing, it is not unusual to find some evidence of cognitive impairment (for reviews, see Caine, 1986; Johnson & Magaro, 1987; Marcopulos, 1989; W. R. Miller, 1975; Niederehe, 1986). In most cases, cognitive changes are less debilitating than dysphoric mood or other depressive symptoms. However, in older, severely depressed patients, about one in five experience serious cognitive loss ("depressive pseudodementia" or "dementia syndrome of depression").

In the following discussion, findings for mildly depressed patients are only briefly mentioned, since significant cognitive impairments are rare at this level of illness. Results for severely depressed patients are examined in more detail; in this group, there is greater evidence of cognitive loss, but usually, global mental status is still well preserved. Factors that influence cognitive losses are discussed, and findings are summarized in the form of a neuropsychological "depressive profile." Very severe cognitive disturbance in depression is considered in a separate section (see "Dementia Syndrome of Depression," below), since it is not clear whether these deficits are similar to, or distinct from, the usual depressive pattern.

Mild to Moderate Depression

In depressed outpatients or community volunteers, only mild cognitive loss should be expected, even on sensitive tests (e.g., Blau & Ober, 1988; Hassinger & La Rue, 1986; Niederehe, 1986; Niederehe & Yoder, 1989; Reisberg, Ferris, Georgotas, de Leon, & Schneck, 1982b; Rush, Weissenburger, Vinson, & Giles, 1983).

For example, in a study of older outpatients with major depression who were given a memory battery similar to the Wechsler Memory Scale (WMS), 41% performed above the expected level for age, 32% scored at or near the mean, and only 27% scored a standard deviation below expected levels (Reisberg *et al.*, 1982b). On the California Verbal Learning Test, Blau and Ober (1988) found a slight reduction for mildly depressed community subjects on the first free-recall trial, but by the fifth trial, there was no difference compared to controls. Depressed patients were described as showing a "slow start" on the memory task, but in general, the pattern and level of performance were similar to those of normals. Niederehe (1986) also found very few significant differences on experimental tests of episodic and semantic memory for either younger (20 to 45 years) or older (55 to 80 years) depressives compared to healthy controls (cf. Niederehe & Yoder, 1989). Depressed patients adopted a more conservative response bias on recognition tests and had more complete (as opposed to partial) omissions in narrative recall. However, their overall performance on verbal list learning, tests of remote recall, and nonverbal memory tasks (e.g., the Visual Recognition Test and Facial Recognition Test) was at or near normal levels. Finally, in a study with younger depressives, Rush, Weissenburger, Vinson, and Giles (1983) found no impairment relative to norms on tests of short-term visual memory, verbal list learning, mental time sharing, or response inhibition (Stroop Color-Word Interference Test); the only significant deficit was on the Trail Making Test, where endogenous depressives had an increased completion time.

Severe Depression

Generally, it is only among inpatients that the level of cognitive problems reaches practical significance. With these patients, it may be the overall level of functional impairment that influences cognitive loss, rather than the severity of depressive symptoms *per se* (see "Clinical Correlates of Cognitive Impairment," below), and in elderly patients, factors such as medications, poor physical health, or disruption of routine can contribute to the reduced test scores.

Scope of Impairment

Table 11.2 provides an example of the level of cognitive performance that may be expected in depression in elderly inpatients in contrast to healthy aging and mild dementia of Alzheimer type (DAT). Subjects were participants in the UCLA Family Study of Dementia (cf. La Rue *et al.*, 1986a), who were screened to exclude medical complications or mixed diagnostic status. Depressed patients had unipolar major depression (DSM-III; American Psychiatric Association, 1980) and relatively severe levels of depressive symptoms (mean HAMD score = 25.2 ± 3.7). All had some complaints about memory, but none was sufficiently impaired to raise a question of pseudodementia. Depressed patients performed as well as healthy controls on the Mini-Mental State Examination (means = 26.6 and 27.4, respectively), and all had negative neurodiagnostic findings for dementia.

The three groups were matched with respect to age and education, but as indicated in the table, mental status scores and general intellectual level were much lower for patients with DAT than for the depressed or healthy groups.

Examination of test findings suggests a slight general lowering of performance in depressed patients compared to controls. This effect can be seen in very sick patients of all sorts and is not necessarily a result of depression. On the Wechsler Adult Intelligence Scale (WAIS), depressed patients scored within the general normative levels expected for their age and educational background. Although their performance was lower overall than that of controls, subtest profiles were similar.

When patterns of test outcomes are compared, the clearest areas of difference for depressed patients and controls were on certain tests of learning and recall (the Object Memory Evaluation and the Visual Retention Test) and visuospatial processing (WAIS

TABLE 11.2. Cognitive Test Findings in Depression Compared to DAT and Healthy Aging[a]

Cognitive measure	Normal aging	Depression	DAT
Mini-Mental State Examination	27.4 (2.6)	26.6 (2.5)	13.3 (3.7)**
WAIS (age-scaled scores)			
Vocabulary	14.4 (2.1)	12.1 (1.9)*	9.9 (1.6)**
Comprehension	14.8 (2.3)	12.2 (4.7)	7.1 (3.3)**
Similarities	15.8 (2.9)	12.6 (1.8)*	7.7 (2.1)**
Digit Span	13.9 (1.4)	10.5 (2.9)*	9.4 (1.7)
Digit Symbol	14.3 (2.2)	9.7 (2.6)*	4.8 (3.8)**
Block Design	12.2 (1.9)	9.6 (2.7)*	4.1 (3.7)**
Verbal IQ (VIQ)	125.2 (12.2)	113.4 (13.3)	89.6 (10.9)**
Performance IQ (PIQ)	116.9 (7.3)	93.1 (11.8)*	71.1 (13.4)**
Full IQ (FIQ)	122.9 (10.2)	104.6 (11.5)*	80.9 (10.1)**
Object Memory Evaluation[b]			
Storage	9.7 (0.3)	8.6 (1.1)	3.7 (2.5)**
Retrieval	9.2 (0.6)	6.9 (1.4)*	2.2 (1.8)**
Repeated Retrieval	8.6 (1.2)	5.3 (1.6)*	1.1 (1.0)**
Ineffective Reminders	0.0 (0.1)	1.3 (0.9)	6.8 (2.7)**
Category Retrieval	52.4 (11.5)	37.0 (10.9)*	19.1 (8.5)**
Extralist intrusions	0.1 (0.3)	0.0 (0.0)	1.2 (3.0)
Paired Associate Learning Test			
Mediate pairs—total correct	14.1 (1.1)	13.5 (2.1)	6.5 (4.7)**
Intrusion errors	0.1 (0.3)	0.5 (0.7)	4.2 (5.1)**
Omission errors	0.3 (0.7)	0.9 (1.3)	3.4 (4.1)
New pairs—total correct	10.5 (4.1)	6.1 (4.5)	2.8 (1.9)
Intrusion errors	0.1 (0.4)	0.8 (1.2)	3.5 (3.1)**
Omission errors	2.1 (2.1)	5.9 (4.0)	6.0 (2.9)
Visual Retention Test			
Total correct	5.5 (1.3)	3.1 (1.9)*	1.9 (2.0)
Total errors	7.0 (2.5)	13.5 (3.8)*	19.9 (6.2)**
Omissions	1.2 (1.2)	4.0 (2.3)	7.9 (4.8)**
Distortions	3.1 (1.7)	4.7 (2.9)	5.8 (2.7)
Perseverations	0.9 (1.1)	1.1 (0.9)	2.5 (2.3)
Rotations	1.2 (1.1)	1.1 (1.1)	0.1 (0.3)
Misplacements	0.5 (0.7)	1.6 (1.3)	1.7 (1.6)
Size errors	0.1 (0.3)	0.8 (1.1)	0.8 (1.1)
Visual Organization Test	22.1 (3.8)	18.8 (4.3)	13.8 (7.1)
Coloured Progressive Matrices	30.4 (4.1)	20.2 (3.9)*	20.7 (6.8)

[a]See Chapter 4 for test descriptions and references. Table values are mean scores with standard deviations in parentheses. Portions of these data were previously presented in La Rue, D'Elia, Clark, Spar, and Jarvik (1986a, pp. 72–73). Reprinted by permission.

[b]Storage scores are from Trial 5; Retrieval, Repeated Retrieval, and Ineffective Reminders are mean scores averaged across all trials (maximum = 10).

*$p < .05$, normal aging vs. depression.

**$p < .5$, depression vs. DAT.

Performance subtests and Coloured Progressive Matrices). On memory tests, depression-related impairments were in the mild to moderate range compared to clinical age norms (see Chapter 4), with the greatest problems noted in nonverbal recall and in consistent retrieval of items from a list (see "Learning and Memory," below).

Compared to patients with DAT, the depressed group performed much better on tests of verbal information (Comprehension, Vocabulary) and verbal learning and recall. On Digit Span, both groups had mild impairment relative to controls. On the Visual Retention Test, neither depressed nor demented patients were able to copy many designs correctly, but DAT patients made more numerous and flagrant errors. On Coloured Progressive Matrices, depressed and demented patients were equally, and relatively severely, impaired.

These findings illustrate a general similarity in the pattern of cognitive performance in normal aging and depression. In both cases, relatively poor performance can be expected on visuospatial tasks, measures of abstract reasoning, and tests requiring spontaneous recall of new facts or details. The combination of aging and depression produces poorer performance overall than normal aging alone, but the relative strength of different skills is unchanged. In DAT, deficits are generally more severe than in depression, and a greater range of abilities is impaired (see Chapter 7).

The following sections take a closer look at specific cognitive areas, examining the quantitative and qualitative impact of depression in clinical tests. Effects of moderating variables and treatment effects are discussed at the end of this section.

Attention

On simple tests of attention and concentration such as Digit Span or Mental Control, some studies report slight impairment in depression (e.g., Breslow, Kocsis, & Belkin, 1980; Stromgren, 1977; cf. Table 11.2), but many others do not (e.g., Friedman, 1964; Fromm & Schopflocher, 1984; Gass & Russell, 1986; Gilleard, 1980; Kopelman, 1986; Reisberg *et al.*, 1982b; Richards & Ruff, 1989; Wechsler, 1987; Whitehead, 1974). Tasks that require clerical accuracy (e.g., number cancellation or figure tracing; see Neville & Folstein, 1979; Raskin, Friedman, & DiMascio, 1982) or sustained concentration (e.g., the Continuous Performance Test; see Byrne, 1977; Frith, Stevens, Johnstone, Deakin, Lawler, & Crow, 1983) are more sensitive to depression effects, but the magnitude of impairment is still quite mild. Greater deficits can be expected on tests that require shifting or flexibility of attention (e.g., Trail B; see Caine, 1981), and many elderly depressives cannot complete such tasks without extensive prompting (see "Problem Solving and Executive Functions," below).

Learning and Memory

Primary Memory. Primary memory is intact or only mildly impaired in depression. As noted above, Digit Span deficits are sometimes observed and, when present, may contribute to a mild general lowering of neuropsychological performance. On list-learning tasks, most depressed patients perform well in recalling items of which they have recently been reminded or on immediate recall of short lists of words (Gibson, 1981; Hart *et al.*, 1987a; Henry, Weingartner, & Murphy, 1973).

Secondary Memory: Learning and recall. Tests of secondary memory usually require conscious effort, and since effortful processing is an area of weakness for depressed patients (see Cohen, Weingartner, Smallberg, Pickar, & Murphy, 1982; Roy-Byrne, Weingartner, Bierer, Thompson, & Post, 1986; Weingartner, Cohen, Murphy, Martello, & Gerdt, 1981a), relatively severe impairments can be expected on these tasks. In some cases, it can be quite difficult to distinguish between depression-related memory impairments and those produced by organic dementing disorders.

On immediate Logical Memory on the WMS, three studies have reported very low mean scores (4.0 ± 3.3 to 5.3 ± 3.3) for older depressed inpatients (Gilleard, 1980; Piersma, 1986; Whitehead, 1973). These levels of performance are below expectations for age (see Table A.1 in the Appendix) and do not differ greatly from the levels expected in mild DAT (see Table 7.3). Kopelman (1986) also studied inpatients, but excluded those who were thought to have pseudodementia; although the mean Logical Memory score (9.3) was in the normal range, 5 of 16 depressives (31%) performed as poorly as patients with DAT, remembering fewer than seven items on immediate recall (cf. Hart *et al.*, 1987a).

On paired associate learning tests, moderate deficits can be expected for inpatients, especially on novel word pairs (Fromm & Schopflocher, 1984; Kopelman, 1986; La Rue *et al.*, 1986a; Piersma, 1986; Stromgren, 1977; Whitehead, 1973). In our study (La Rue *et al.*, 1986a), older depressives had no difficulty learning intermediate strength associations (e.g., *gold-lead*); on the novel pairs (e.g., *knife-trumpet*), they performed worse than healthy controls but better than patients with mild DAT (see Table 11.2). A few depressed patients could not learn the novel pairs, and as a result, this task did not distinguish the depressed and demented groups as well as some other measures.

Nonverbal learning and recall are particularly weak areas of performance for depressed inpatients (e.g., Crookes & McDonald, 1972; Fromm & Schopflocher, 1984; Richards & Ruff, 1989). On WMS Visual Reproduction, Piersma (1986) and Gilleard (1980) reported mean scores for elderly depressed inpatients of 3.61 (± 2.7) and 3.5 (± 2.7), respectively. On the Visual Retention Test, deficits can be expected on both the total correct and the total error scores (see Table 11.2). In our study, all of the healthy elderly subjects copied at least three designs correctly, compared to only 60% of the depressed patients and 30% of DAT patients. Therefore, on these tests, too, considerable overlap can be expected between depression and organic dementias.

List-learning tasks sometimes provide a better discrimination between depression and DAT. For example, on verbal free recall, depressed patients usually have a normal serial position curve (i.e., with primacy as well as recency; see Gibson, 1981), whereas in DAT, primacy is often lacking or reduced below normal levels (e.g., Miller, 1975; cf. Chapter 7). On the Object Memory Evaluation, we found deficits in depressed patients on the Retrieval and Repeated-Retrieval measures, but not on Storage or Ineffective

Reminders (see Table 11.2). Retrieval scores classified 100% of depressed and demented patients and 90% of normals and provided better diagnostic discrimination than Paired-Associate Learning or Visual Retention. A similar pattern was reported on the verbal Selective Reminding Test (Hart *et al.*, 1987a). However, a later investigation (La Rue, 1989) raised some doubts about finding a specific "depressive pattern" in routine inpatient testing. Subjects were consecutively referred for cognitive assessment and were not preselected to exclude medical illness or medications. In this study, depressed patients fell below normal expectations on all of the measures from the Object Memory Evaluation, particularly in the young-old group (60 to 79 years). Overall, performance was much higher in the depressed group than in patients with DAT, but was not distinguishable from the scores observed in multi-infarct dementia (MID) or Parkinson's disease (PD).

Recognition versus recall. Since recognition memory requires less effort than recall, depressed patients may be expected to perform better on recognition than recall. Whether normal levels of recognition are observed appears to depend on task difficulty. Experimental studies using difficult recognition tasks often find some impairment for patients with serious depression (e.g., Golinkoff & Sweeney, 1989; Miller & Lewis, 1977; Watts, Morris, & MacLeod, 1987). On easier clinical tasks, performance is much closer to normal levels. For example, in studies with elderly patients, normal recognition scores have been reported on both the California Verbal Learning Test (Blau & Ober, 1988) and the Selective Reminding Test (Hart *et al.*, 1987a). On these measures, recognition is tested for only a small set of items that have been presented multiple times; therefore, high scores may reflect a ceiling effect.

Delayed recall and recognition. Several studies have reported normal rates of forgetting in depression (e.g., Cronholm & Ottosson, 1961; Hart, Kwentus, Taylor & Harkins, 1987b; Kopelman, 1986; Sternberg & Jarvik, 1976; Whitehead, 1973). On delayed Logical Memory, for example, Kopelman (1986) observed a 73% retention rate for elderly depressed inpatients, compared to 82% for healthy volunteers and only 9% for patients with DAT (see Chapter 7); all of the depressed patients recalled at least 50% of the material after delay, while none of the DAT patients was able to perform at this level (cf. Whitehead, 1973). On the Object Memory Evaluation, younger depressed inpatients (60 to 79 years) recalled an average of 6.7 ± 2.6 items after delay, and older patients (80 to 90 years), 4.4 ± 2.8 items (La Rue, 1989); these scores were well above the means for patients with DAT, but slightly below the normative levels reported by Fuld (1981).

Patterns of errors. Clinical lore suggests an excessive rate of omissions ("don't know" answers) in depression compared to dementia (cf. Cummings & Benson, 1983; Wells, 1979), but research has not confirmed this trend (cf. La Rue *et al.*, 1986a; Whitehead, 1973; Young, Manley, & Alexopoulos, 1985). Instead, it is the absence of intrusions or other "organic" errors that appears to be diagnostically important (see Chapters 4 and 7). Depressed patients make very few errors of intrusion during paired-associate learning (La Rue *et al.*, 1986a; Whitehead, 1973) or list learning (La Rue *et al.*, 1986a; Loewenstein *et al.*, 1989c; see Table 11.2). On recognition testing, false-positive errors are much rarer in depression than in DAT (Miller & Lewis, 1977). On tasks that require copying of designs from memory (e.g., the Visual Retention Test), depressed patients have relatively low rates of certain errors that are common for brain-damaged patients (e.g., size errors, rotations, or perseverations; Crookes & McDonald, 1972; La Rue *et al.*, 1986a), but they frequently omit figures or distort details (see Table 11.2).

Cuing and encoding enhancement. In a series of experimental studies, Weingartner *et al.* (1981a) concluded that depressed patients fail to use spontaneous encoding operations that facilitate later recall. On tasks which present information in an optimally structured form (e.g., word lists organized by semantic category), they perform very well; however, when they are required to impose structure, deficits can be expected. Sensitivity to organization distinguishes depression from DAT, where learning, even of organized and meaningful information, tends to be poor (see Chapter 7).

D'Elia (personal communication, August 15, 1987), has developed a clinical procedure patterned after Weingartner's experimental tests. Two sets of 16 nouns are presented, one with items organized by semantic category and the other with items in a random order. Preliminary findings with elderly inpatients confirm the trend reported in the laboratory; that is, depressed patients perform significantly better on recalling the organized list, while patients with DAT perform at similar levels under both procedures.

The Controlled Learning with Delayed Recall procedure (Grober & Buschke, 1987) may also be helpful in separating depression-related memory loss from DAT. On this test, stimuli are presented in small groups so that a high level of acquisition is insured, and semantic cues are provided during learning and recall. Under these conditions, even severely depressed patients would be expected to perform well. However, no data have been reported to confirm this prediction.

Incidental learning. Testing for incidental recall is an additional procedure that may help to separate depression-related memory impairment from DAT. In a study with older depressives, Hart *et al.* (1987c) first administered the WAIS Digit Symbol test according to standard instructions; immediately afterward, without forewarning, subjects were asked to draw the Digit Symbol pairs from memory. Depressed patients did as well as healthy controls on total recall of symbols, reproducing an average of 6.1 of the 10 symbols compared to 6.9 for the normal group. By contrast, DAT patients recalled an average of only 1.7 symbols. On recall of specific Digit Symbol pairs, depressed patients had greater difficulty than controls; however, 12 of 15 depressed subjects remembered at least two pairs, compared to none of the 15 DAT patients.

Tertiary (Remote) Memory. In autobiographical recall, depressed patients retrieve negative events more quickly and in greater detail than positive ones (e.g., Lloyd & Lishman, 1975; Williams & Scott, 1988). For emotionally neutral material (e.g., public events), findings are equivocal. In younger depressives, Frith *et al.*, (1983) found reduced performance relative to controls on a task requiring recognition of famous personalities from past decades. However, Kopelman (1986) found minimal problems for older depressed inpatients on brief tests of remote personal memory and recall of general public events.

Language

Verbal communication of depressed patients is remarkable for negative themes, reduced rates of spontaneous speech, and protracted verbal response times (see W. R. Miller, 1975, for a review). Speech pauses correlate with severity of depression and diminish in response to treatment (Hoffman, Gonze, & Mendlewicz, 1985).

On brief aphasia-screening tests, depressed patients usually have minimal impairment (e.g., Fromm & Schopflocher, 1984). Language comprehension is reportedly intact (Caine, 1981), but the paucity of verbal elaboration can lead to impairments on some types of language tests (e.g., picture description).

Deficits in verbal fluency and confrontation naming have sometimes been reported (King, Caine, Salzman, & Conwell, 1988). With younger depressives, Wolfe, Granholm, Butters, Saunders, and Janowsky (1987) found reduced fluency in bipolar depression, but not in unipolar depression. In elderly samples, depressives perform better on verbal fluency than patients with DAT (King *et al.*, 1988; La Rue, 1989; cf. Table 11.2) but may do as poorly as patients with MID or PD (La Rue, 1989).

Most depressed patients score within normal limits on verbal subtests of the WAIS and WAIS-R. On Vocabulary, they can usually provide a higher quality of responses (e.g., perfect synonyms vs. vague descriptions) than patients with DAT (Houlihan *et al.*, 1985); however, they may lose points for failing to expand upon partial-credit responses. On Similarities and Comprehension, answers may be concrete and lacking in elaboration compared to those of normal adults.

Visuospatial Ability

On simple mental status items which require the copying of geometric designs, depressed patients usually score within normal limits for age (Caine, 1981; King *et al.*, 1988). However, on more demanding visuoperceptual and visuoconstructive tasks, deficits have been documented for both younger and older depressed patients (e.g., Flor-Henry, 1979; Fromm & Schopflocher, 1984; Taylor & Abrams, 1987; Taylor, Greenspan, & Abrams, 1979; cf. Heaton *et al.*, 1978; Lezak, 1983).

In a factor-analytic study, Fromm and Schopflocher (1984) found that depressed patients were most clearly distinguished from controls on a "processing and retrieval of visuospatial material" dimension composed of scores on the Tactual Performance and Category tests from the Halstead-Reitan Neuropsychological Battery and a test of memory for designs. This factor and a short-term memory factor were the only aspects of cognitive performance that consistently improved with treatment for depression.

Raskin *et al.* (1982), who also studied depressed inpatients, found impairments relative to controls on several psychomotor and perceptual tasks requiring speed, fine eye–hand coordination, and/or accuracy (e.g., tracing a circle as exactly as possible or placing dots within a target), and on visual tasks that required shifting of attention or cognitive flexibility (e.g., the Stroop Color-Word Interference Test). Patients over the age of 40 performed particularly poorly on these tests relative to controls, a result leading to the speculation that older patients, who are already beginning to experience declines in these areas, have the greatest vulnerability to negative cognitive effects of depression.

On intelligence testing, depressed patients often perform worse on WAIS Performance as opposed to Verbal subtests (see Table 11.2). This difference does not appear to be due entirely to psychomotor retardation, since rescoring of data (i.e., eliminating bonus points for speed and giving credit for correct responses achieved over time limits) does not eliminate the relative deficits of depressed patients (Dean, Gray, & Seretny, 1987).

On drawing and design-copying tasks, depressed patients often omit portions of a figure or misplace details (Caine, 1981). However, they preserve the general outlines of the figure and generally do not make the more flagrant errors (e.g., perseveration, "closing in," or segmentation) that are sometimes observed in organic dementia (Albert & Kaplan, 1980).

Problem Solving and Executive Functions

A final important area of difficulty for depressed patients concerns reasoning, problem solving, and executive functions. Complaints of indecision are common in depression, and many depressed patients seem unable to manage everyday tasks which require judgment and reasoning.

Silberman, Weingartner, and Post (1983a) compared younger (mean age = 38 years) depressed inpatients and controls on a concept identification task. A series of geometric figures varying in different attributes was presented, and the subject's task was to infer which attribute was "correct" based on feedback from the examiner. Several depressed patients (6 out of 13) had greater difficulty than controls in narrowing down the set of possible solutions (poor "focusing") and tended to perseverate on disconfirmed hypotheses; the remainder performed normally. There was a trend toward more severe depression in the patients with reasoning problems, a finding that agrees with earlier findings by Braff and Beck (1974), who studied performance on series completion tasks and proverb interpretation.

Raskin *et al.* (1982) found that depressed patients provided more concrete responses on proverb interpretation than normal controls; this tendency was most pronounced for depressed patients over the age of 40. Savard, Rey, and Post (1980) noted a similar trend in performance on the Category Test. When tested prior to treatment, both younger and older depressed patients made more errors than controls; retesting showed a reduction in error scores for depressed patients, but all older patients (age $\geqslant$ 40 years, all with bipolar illness) still scored in the impaired range, even when depression was in remission. The investigators suggested that aging and depression may share overlapping neural substrates, and that combined effects of these changes may lead to "major and additive" cognitive impairment (see below for additional discussion of age effects).

Very low scores are often observed on Coloured Progressive Matrices, which tests nonverbal reasoning (see Table 11.2); the Stroop Color-Word Interference Test, which requires selective attention and inhibition of overlearned responses (e.g., Raskin *et al.* 1982); and Trail B, which requires attentional shifting (Caine, 1981). In our clinical work with older depressed inpatients, we have found that only a minority are able to perform Trail B accurately within time limits expected for age. Many refuse to complete the task, protesting that it is too difficult. Others make errors in alternation, particularly at the middle to later stages of the sequence.

Clinical Correlates of Cognitive Impairment

The studies summarized above suggest general trends in performance that can be expected in severe depression. However, some depressed individuals have negligible cognitive problems, despite severe depression. The reasons for this variability are poorly understood at this time, but several possible moderating factors have been considered.

Some studies have reported that the negative impact of depression on cognition is magnified in old age (e.g., Caine, 1981; Fromm & Schopflocher, 1984; Raskin, 1986; Raskin *et al.*, 1982; Savard *et al.*, 1980), but others have found no evidence of age × depression interactions (*e.g.*, Niederehe, 1986; Niederehe & Yoder, 1989). Similarly, although significant correlations have sometimes been observed between scores on depression-rating scales and cognitive performance (Cohen *et al.*, 1982; Fromm & Schopflocher, 1984; Henry *et al.*, 1973; Raskin, 1986; Siegfried *et al.*, 1984; Sternberg & Jarvik, 1976; Stromgren, 1977; Whitehead, 1974), other studies have found no relationship between these variables (Coughlan & Hollows, 1984; Friedman, 1964; Hemsi, Whitehead, & Post, 1968; Kopelman, 1986; La Rue, Spar, & Hill, 1986b; Niederehe, 1986; Reisberg *et al.*, 1982; von Ammon-Cavanaugh & Wettstein, 1983). Among inpatients, global ratings of psychiatric dysfunction (e.g., the Global Assessment Scale; Endicott, Spitzer, Fleiss, & Cohen, 1976) may be more closely related to test performance than are depression ratings *per se* (La Rue *et al.*, 1986b).

Certain behavioral features associated with depression have also been proposed as moderators of cognitive change. For example, depressed patients commonly experience feelings of fatigue and show decreased motivation in everyday tasks; a subjective sense of poor concentration or failing memory is also very common (Raskin & Rae, 1981; Watts & Sharrock, 1985). When approached for testing, they may protest that they are too tired or unwell to participate, and during assessment, they may persist in saying that they are unable to do a task despite relatively adequate performance (Friedman, 1964). Cognitive test findings can be adversely affected because of these "noncognitive" complications, but it is unclear how much of the observed impairments should be attributed to these factors. One study (Hayslip, Kennelly, & Maloy, 1989) confirmed that administration of a lengthy and demanding test battery in a single setting is likely to exaggerate deficits observed in older depressed patients. However, another study

(Richards & Ruff, 1989) with younger depressives found that motivating instructions designed to counteract poor effort had little effect on neuropsychological performance; these investigators concluded that it is doubtful that cognitive effects of depression can be explained by a simple notion of decreased motivation. Likewise, most studies show only a weak relationship between subjective memory complaints and memory performance (e.g., Kahn, Zarit, Hilbert, & Niederehe, 1975; Niederehe & Yoder, 1989; Popkin, Gallagher, Thompson, & Moore, 1982; see Gilewski & Zelinski, 1986, for a review).

Treatment Effects

Cognitive deficits in depression are generally believed to be reversible, and although few data are available, the time course of cognitive improvement is often assumed to parallel changes in dysphoric mood or other depressive symptoms. In younger adults, several studies have found improvement in cognitive function following antidepressant therapy (e.g., Sternberg & Jarvik, 1976; Stromgren, 1977). However, for elderly patients, there are fewer data that support this effect (see Siegfried *et al.*, 1984, for an exception), and it is not unusual for cognitive impairments to persist beyond the end of acute therapy (e.g., Fromm & Schopflocher, 1984; Fromm-Auch, 1983; Hemsi *et al.*, 1968; Savard *et al.*, 1980).

Adverse effects of antidepressant therapies also need to be considered. Detrimental effects of tricyclic antidepressants (especially amitriptyline) on learning and memory have been demonstrated in carefully controlled investigations (e.g., Branconnier, deVitt, Cole, & Spera, 1982; Burns, Moskowitz, & Jaffe, 1986; Cole & Schatzberg, 1980; Katz, Greenberg, Barr, Garbarino, Buckley, & Smith, 1985). By contrast, naturalistic studies that have correlated cognitive performance with levels of antidepressants taken at the time of testing have generally found no clear associations (e.g., Heaton & Crowley, 1981; La Rue, 1989; La Rue, Goodman, & Spar, 1992a; Marcopulos & Graves, 1987).

The negative effects of ECT on memory functions are well documented (Heaton & Crowley, 1981), and usually, diagnostic neuropsychological testing should be delayed for four to six months after treatment. Nonetheless, some seriously depressed patients actually improve in memory performance following treatment with ECT (Hemsi *et al.*, 1968; Stromgren, 1977).

A Neuropsychological Profile for Depression

Table 11.3 summarizes some of the behaviors and outcomes that can be expected during testing of older depressed patients.

The patient's behavior during testing is an important diagnostic feature. There should be obvious indications of depressed mood and/or anxiety, accompanied by protests of incapacity or a more passive withdrawal from the demands of the testing (e.g., minimal spontaneous speech, giving up easily on difficult tasks, or "drifting off" into private thoughts). When encouraged to try harder or to provide more complete

TABLE 11.3. Summary of Neuropsychological Test Findings in Geriatric Depression[a]

I. Typical presentation
  Depressed mood or pervasive loss of interest, accompanied by
  A. Mild memory deficit.
  B. Mild to moderate visuospatial impairment.
  C. Reduced abstraction and cognitive flexibility.
II. Behavior during testing
  Self-critical of performance; may underestimate ability or reject positive comments from the examiner.
  Complaints of fatigue or physical distress, often accompanied by an objective loss of stamina.
  Complaints of poor concentration, but usually can attend to tasks if encouraged.
III. Most informative tests
  A. List-learning tests
    1. Storage, recognition, and rate of forgetting close to normal.
    2. Mild to moderate impairments in recall.
    3. Low rate of intrusion errors.
    4. Benefit from cuing and encoding enhancement.
  B. Intelligence testing
    1. WAIS Verbal IQ close to normal levels.
    2. WAIS Digit Span $\leq$ other verbal subtests.
    3. Mild to moderate impairment on WAIS Performance subtests, due primarily to slowing, carelessness, or refusal to complete the test.
IV. Findings that rise a question about the diagnosis
  Depressive symptoms mild or questionable.
  Problems in language comprehension.
  Severe memory deficit.
V. Cautions
  Cognitive loss may be linked more closely to global dysfunction than to severity of depression *per se*.
  Depression often coexists with organic brain disorder.
  10% to 20% of patients have cognitive problems that are hard to distinguish from DAT or other organic dementias.

[a]From La Rue *et al.* (1992b, p. 655). Adapted by permission.

answers, many depressed patients are able to provide additional correct information; by contrast, patients with dementia often confabulate or make additional errors when "pushed" to perform. Depressed patients are also more likely to show some benefit from cues or strategies provided by the examiner.

Some depressed patients have no clear objective deficits, even in the areas most susceptible to depressive impairment (e.g., secondary memory, visuospatial processing). For most, however, test scores will be slightly below expectations for age and background. Severe impairments should be absent or restricted to certain measures (e.g., difficult free-recall tasks or tests of speeded psychomotor integration). Intrusions, confabulation, and perseveration errors are usually rare.

Use of age-adjusted tests is imperative for reducing the risk of misdiagnosing DAT or other organic disorders in older, severely depressed patients. In general, a benefit-of-the-doubt approach should be taken in interpreting cognitive problems in these individuals, especially if deficits are in the mild to moderate range. In some cases, cognitive problems persist during in the initial weeks of antidepressant therapy, and retesting after several months may be needed to disclose the full benefits of treatment.

Examiners should be alert to signs of medication toxicity in patients on antidepressants (e.g., drowsiness, fluctuations in alertness or attention, sudden disorientation, marked psychomotor changes) and should avoid testing on days when major changes are made in medications; however, in patients without evidence of toxicity, who are on low dosages of psychoactive drugs, or who are stabilized on an effective medication, findings can be considered valid for most diagnostic and treatment purposes.

DEMENTIA SYNDROME OF DEPRESSION

Between 10% and 20% of depressed older adults have cognitive problems severe enough to rival the deficits produced by organic dementia (McAllister, 1983; Rabins, 1983). This combination of cognitive and affective symptoms has been referred to as *depressive pseudodementia* (Caine, 1981; Wells, 1979), *dementia syndrome of depression* (Folstein & McHugh, 1978), or *depression with cognitive impairment* (e.g., Caine, 1986). In this discussion, the term *dementia syndrome of depression* (DSD) is used to underscore the severity of cognitive symptoms and to draw a distinction between these impairments and the milder cognitive problems that are typically observed in depression (Tables 11.2 and 11.3).

The fact that psychiatric disease may be accompanied by severe cognitive problems has been recognized for many years (see Kiloh, 1961; Madden, Luhan, Kaplan, & Manfredi, 1952). Anxiety disorders, dissociative disorders, schizophrenia, and paranoid states have all been shown to produce dementia in specific cases (for examples, see Caine, 1981; Kiloh, 1961; Wells, 1979). Among the elderly, however, depression is the most common cause of psychiatrically based dementia (Wells, 1979, 1983), and as a result, DSD has attracted considerable attention among clinicians and researchers.

Recognition of DSD is complicated by the fact that patients with organic dementia can also develop depression (for cases examples, see Caine, 1986; McAllister & Price, 1982; Reifler, Larson, & Hanley, 1982; cf. Chapters 7 through 9). Thus, combinations of cognitive and depressive symptoms can have many different underlying causes. In general, DSD and organic dementia should not be considered mutually exclusive (Caine, 1986; Marcopulos, 1989; Stoudemire, Hill, Kaplan, Hill, Morris, Cohen-Cole, & Houpt, 1988).

Recognizing DSD

The cardinal feature of DSD is clinically significant cognitive disturbance that coincides with a depressive episode and that remits or improves substantially when depressive symptoms abate. DSD can be clearly identified only on a *post hoc* basis, that is, when cognitive performance returns to normal as depression lifts. This complicates treatment decisions, since clinicians would usually treat DSD more aggressively than organic dementia with depressive features.

To encourage clinicians to screen for DSD, Wells (1979, 1983) and others (e.g., Cummings, 1989) have presented lists of features that may help to distinguish this disorder from DAT and other organic dementias. History can provide some clues to etiology, and the patient's behavior during interview and testing may reveal additional discriminating features (see Table 11.4).

These guidelines are based primarily on case examples and have not been validated in prospective studies. Evidence for certain of the distinguishing features appears equivocal at best. For example, frequent "don't know" answers during cognitive testing are not specific to DSD, since DAT patients also make many omission errors (see "Patterns of Errors," above, and Chapter 7). Also, it is now recognized that there are many patients with DAT who are distressed by their losses or who experience significant depressive symptoms (see Chapter 7). In general, therefore, guidelines such as those in Table 11.4 are more useful for raising the question of DSD than for confirming its presence.

Clinical Research on DSD

There have been only a few systematic studies of DSD. Criteria for defining DSD have varied, and sample sizes have usually been small. Nonetheless, examining these investigations provides some interesting clues about risk factors, reversibility with treatment, and long-term prognosis.

Clinical Characteristics of Patients with DSD

Depressed patients with severe cognitive losses are probably a heterogeneous group. Some may have true DSD, while others may be in the early stages of an organic dementia. In addition, it is not clear yet whether DSD patients represent a distinct subtype in the depressed population or merely the lowest segment of the cognitive distribution.

DSD versus Typical Depression. An early examination of DSD was provided by Post (1966). The sample consisted of 68 elderly patients hospitalized for depression, including 11 (16%) who scored well below the "organic cutoff" on a verbal learning and memory test. Patients were randomly assigned to treatment conditions (ECT or imipramine) and retested at the end of three months. Post described the memory-impaired subjects as a discrete subgroup with the following characteristics: low verbal intelligence; intense, frequently delusional depression; "perplexity or marked thinking and memory difficulties, subjectively," and poor knowledge of recent events. Of these 11 patients, 6 (55%) improved with treatment and had normal learning scores prior to discharge. Post reported that "follow-up did not suggest that these patients differed

TABLE 11.4. Clinical Features of Dementia Syndrome of Depression Compared to Organic Dementia[a]

	Dementia syndrome of depression	Dementia
History and clinical course		
Family awareness of cognitive loss	Always aware.	Often unaware.
Onset of illness	Can be dated with some precision.	Can be dated only within broad limits.
Duration of symptoms before help is sought.	Short.	Long.
Rate of progression	Rapid.	Slow.
Prior psychiatric illness	Common.	Unusual.
Complaints and clinical behavior		
Complaints of cognitive loss	Severe and detailed.	Mild and vague.
Reaction to dysfunction	Emphasize disability, highlight failures.	Conceal disability, delight in accomplishments.
Effort to perform and to keep up with daily tasks	Minimal effort.	Struggle to perform; rely on notes, calendars, etc.
Distress communicated by patient.	Strong sense of distress.	Often appear unconcerned.
Affective change	Often pervasive.	Affect labile and shallow.
Social skills	Prominent early losses.	Often retained.
Congruity of behavior with severity of cognitive loss.	Incongruent.	Usually compatible.
Nocturnal accentuation	Uncommon.	Common.
Performance of cognitive tests		
Attention and concentration	Often well preserved.	Usually faulty.
"Don't know" answers	Typical.	Near-miss answers.
Orientation testing.	Frequent "don't know's."	Obvious errors.
Memory loss	Recent, remote equally impaired; gaps for specific periods or events.	Recent more impaired than remote; specific gaps uncommon.
Variability on performance	Marked, even across similar tasks.	Consistent for similar tasks.

[a]From Wells (1979, p. 898). Adapted by permission.

to any convincing extent from the general run of elderly depressives" (p. 16), but the interval and procedures used for follow-up were not specified.

La Rue *et al.* (1986b) also compared DSD patients to other older depressives. There were 55 depressed inpatients (mean age = 74 years) divided into cognitively impaired and cognitively intact subgroups (*n*'s = 12 and 43, respectively) based on pretreatment scores on the Mini-Mental State Examination (MMSE); a conservative cutoff of 20 or below was used for classification as cognitively impaired. Treatments included tricyclic antidepressants (desipramine or amitriptyline), trazodone, or phenelzine, with neuroleptics or anxiolytics prescribed as needed. Those who did not respond to the initial treatment were switched to an alternate medication or, occasionally, ECT. Patients were discharged from the hospital when adequate remission was attained, or when all treatments to which the patient would consent had been attempted. For the 12 cognitively impaired patients, and for a matched subgroup with intact cognition, follow-up evaluation was performed after discharge (mean = 22 months).

There were no differences between the subgroups in age, gender, initial levels of depression, or cognitive complaints. However, cognitively impaired patients were less well educated than cognitively intact subjects and, on initial clinical assessment, had greater global psychiatric impairment and more anxiety and agitation and were more likely to have depressive delusions (present for 42% vs. 9%, respectively).

Both groups showed an improvement in depression with treatment. However, cognitively impaired patients had to be hospitalized for a significantly longer period of time (mean = 57 vs. 40 days) and were more likely to require a combination of neuroleptic and antidepressant medications rather than antidepressants alone. On follow-up, the cognitively impaired subjects were doing as well as the cognitively intact group on measures of everyday function and psychiatric symptom ratings, and their MMSE scores had improved into the normal range. However, greater attrition was observed in the low-MMSE subgroup, leaving open the possibility that some patients declined.

Most recently, La Rue *et al.* (1992a) compared small groups of older depressed inpatients with impaired versus intact memory (*n* = 7 per group). Memory-impaired patients scored more than two standard deviations below the mean for age on all scores from the Object Memory Evaluation (Fuld, 1981; see Chapter 4), whereas memory-intact patients performed above the normative means. No differences were noted in age, gender, education, or depressive features recorded on admission (e.g., presence or absence of delusions, somatic features). However, memory-impaired subjects had been ill for a substantially longer period of time than those whose with intact memory performance (mean = 22 vs. 5 months). Five of the seven memory-impaired patients had been depressed for at least a year prior to testing, whereas six of seven memory-intact patients had been ill for four months or less. Reynolds, Perel, Kupfer, Zimmer, Stack, and Hoch (1987) reported a similar trend in another group of older depressed inpatients.

Considered together, these studies suggest that DSD patients may have certain distinguishing demographic and clinical characteristics compared to other depressed patients. Poorly educated patients, or those with "low intelligence," may be most likely to be perceived as having DSD. Delusional depressives, or those with severe anxiety or agitation, may be liable to severe cognitive problems, although these trends are not always observed. Protracted depressive illness is another potential risk factor for DSD.

This research also suggests a favorable short-term course for DSD; that is, with standard antidepressant therapies, many patients with this condition improve substantially in both depressive symptoms and cognitive performance. However, DSD patients may require lengthier and more aggressive treatment to overcome their depression, and it is not clear whether cognition improves at the same rate as other depressive features.

DSD versus DAT. Reynolds, Hoch, Kupfer, Buysse, Houck, Stack, and Campbell (1988) compared pretreatment clinical presentations of 14 patients with DSD and 28 diagnosed with DAT. DSD patients had all shown a positive response to treatment with antidepressant medications. Compared to the patients with DAT, those with DSD had initially presented with a milder level of global cognitive impairment (mean MMSE score of 23 as opposed to 17), more severe depressive symptomatology (mean HAMD score of 20 as opposed to 16), and fewer problems with everyday activities such as finding one's way around familiar streets. On the MMSE, DSD patients had as many problems as DAT patients on delayed recall, repetition of a phrase, and following the three-stage command, but they outperformed the demented group on orientation, registration, calculations, and language and visuographic items. On the HAMD, the DSD patients were rated as having more anxiety, insomnia, and loss of libido than those with DAT.

Rabins, Merchant, and Nestadt (1984) compared elderly inpatients with a dual diagnosis of dementia and major depression (presumably, DSD cases) to a matched group with dementia alone (n = 18 per group). All subjects scored 24 or lower on the MMSE. In contrast to the dementia-only patients, the depressed-demented subjects were more likely to have had a past history of depression and a subacute onset of illness, and to be suffering from delusions (present in 15 of 18 cases). All of the depressed-demented patients were described as showing "some improvement in their mood" with either tricyclic antidepressants or ECT, and 15 of 18 had improved MMSE scores on discharge (cf. Reynolds *et al.*, 1987). At a two-year follow-up, all of these 15 subjects were still cognitively intact, whereas 2 of the 3 who had not improved remained demented, and the third was deceased. No quantitative measures of depression were used in this study, and no details were given about treatment or response.

Reding, Haycox, and Blass (1985) studied a different population of patients with mixed depressive and cognitive symptoms. These subjects (n = 28) had initially been referred to a dementia clinic for evaluation of cognitive impairment, but after extensive diagnostic assessment, they were judged to have depression or dysthymic disorder (DSM-III criteria). Most scored in the normal range on a simple mental status examination and a dementia behavior-rating scale. All received either inpatient or outpatient treatment for depression, usually with antidepressant medications. Sixteen of these patients (57%) had become demented over a 30-month follow-up interval. Those who declined were said to be older than those who did not (specific ages were not given), and 13 of the 16 had subtle focal neurological or extrapyramidal signs. Regarding treatment, the investigators noted: "In each case of treatment failure, follow-up showed that the patient was suffering from depression plus a progressive dementing disorder" (p. 896), and that the patients who became demented "were often intolerant of antidepressants, showing increased confusion or somnolence at subtherapeutic dosages" (p. 896).

These studies suggest that, on the average, DSD patients are likely to be more depressed, but less cognitively and functionally impaired, than patients with DAT. The DSD patients usually show a clear benefit from antidepressant therapy, and they are unlikely to experience cognitive decline, at least for one or two years. However, when evaluation is prompted primarily by cognitive loss, or when there are neurological signs and symptoms, treatment with antidepressants may produce more side effects than improvements, and in many cases, a clear dementia may emerge within a year or two.

Long-Term Prognosis of DSD. Very few investigations have followed patients with mixed depressive and cognitive symptoms for a protracted time period. In the few pertinent studies, methods are poorly described, and results are contradictory.

Two investigations (Nott & Fleminger, 1975; Ron, Toone, Garralda, & Lishman, 1979) examined the long-term course (5 to 15 years) of younger inpatients who had initially been referred for treatment of depression, but who were subsequently diagnosed as having presenile dementia based on lengthy inpatient evaluations. Many of these subjects (31% in one study, 57% in the other) failed to show the progressive deterioration expected in dementia. With hindsight, it was concluded that a high proportion of the misdiagnosed subjects had probably been suffering from depression after all, even though their cognitive test performance and neurodiagnostic findings had been suggestive of dementia.

Ron *et al.* (1979) reported that 11 of 16 misdiagnosed individuals had received antidepressant therapy (typically tricyclics) while in the hospital and that "only half improved." This was similar to the response rate observed in the patients who later showed progressive dementia; cognitive performance was reportedly "unchanged" with treatment in both the misdiagnosed and the correctly diagnosed patients. Therefore, in this study, neither neuropsychological testing nor short-term improvement with antidepressants was helpful in identifying patients with DSD or in predicting their long-term course.

Another study has suggested that DSD may progress to a clear dementia over a period of years (Kral & Emery, 1989; see also Kral, 1983). However, this brief report provided almost no information about diagnostic procedures, cognitive assessment, or follow-up testing. The sample consisted of 44 elderly patients with clinical diagnoses of depressive pseudodementia. Evaluations had been prompted by "the patient's rather sudden loss of his or her usual interests, slowing in speech and actions, difficulties concentrating and particularly loss of memory and even orientation in time and place. The care-takers feared the beginning of senile dementia." (p. 445). On psychiatric examination, however, patients were felt to be depressed and were treated "intensively" (generally with medications). In all cases, depression was said to have "cleared up" in a relatively short time, and "the cognitive failures also disappeared" (p. 446). Patients were subsequently examined at six-month intervals over a period of several years (mean = 8 years; range = 4 to 18). Outcomes were described as follows:

> During this long follow-up period a gradual change in the patients' condition could be detected. Their intellectual capacities deteriorated. The EEG became abnormal with gradual general slowing and, where CT scans were available, they too become abnormal, showing dilation of the ventricles and cortical atrophy. In cases where postmortems were permitted, the neuropathology revealed the typical markers of Alzheimer's disease: neuronal loss, fibrillary tangles, neuritic plaques. (p. 446)

With so little detail provided about the sample or procedures, it is difficult to know what to make of this study. Nonetheless, there is an interesting consistency between this study and that of Reding *et al.* (1985) in the manner in which subjects came to professional attention. In both cases, patients were brought in by relatives or professionals who were concerned that they were developing dementia. By contrast, in the long-term follow-up of Ron *et al.* (1979)—where a substantial percentage did *not* show progressive cognitive decline—patients were initially felt to be depressed and only later were judged to be demented based on test results and lack of benefit from specific treatments.

Neuropsychological Findings

Very little is known about the neuropsychological performance of DSD patients. In the studies described above, impairments on cognitive tests were used to identify DSD, but generally, classification has been based on a single measure, and other aspects of cognitive performance are not reported.

In case reports (e.g., Caine, 1981; Wells, 1979), different tests have been given to different patients, and results are only vaguely described. Because the data are so limited, it is not clear whether DSD patients exhibit the same neuropsychological pattern as other depressed patients, only to a more severe extent, or whether other types of cognitive functions (e.g., language or orientation) are likely to be compromised.

Caine (1981, 1986) has suggested that cognitive impairments in DSD tend to be of a subcortical as opposed to a cortical type. However, this hypothesis is based on a small number of cases ranging widely in age (15 to 77 years), whose overall level of impairment was unspecified. One patient (out of 11) was noted to have deficits in praxis and gnosis, and another was described as having a Verbal IQ deficit that remitted with treatment. Elsewhere, Caine (e.g., King *et al.*, 1988) has commented on the heterogeneity of cognitive impairments in elderly depressed patients.

In another case series, Wells (1979) noted that all nine patients who were given neuropsychological evaluations performed poorly on tests usually used to measure organic dysfunction. He suggested that inconsistency in performance from test to test is the strongest indication of the psychiatric etiology of cognitive problems in these patients.

Ron *et al.* (1979) and Nott and Fleminger (1975) did not find cognitive testing to be helpful in preventing misdiagnoses of DSD patients. In fact, it was partly on the basis of psychological testing that these patients received a dementia diagnosis, which long-term follow-up failed to substantiate. However, in the Ron *et al.* investigation, only intelligence testing was performed (with DSD patients scoring at the low end of the normal range on both Verbal and Performance IQ), and in the Nott and Fleminger study, it is unclear which tests were used.

In our first study of depressives with cognitive impairment (La Rue *et al.*, 1986b), where an MMSE score of 20 or less was used in defining DSD, impairments were observed in all aspects of the mental status exam; however, particularly poor scores were seen on attention/calculation, delayed three-item recall, and design copying (cf. Reynolds *et al.*, 1988). None of the DSD patients could recall three items after a delay, only 2 of 12 could correctly perform serial 7's or backward spelling, and only 3 of 12 were accurate in copying a design. On the Object Memory Evaluation (La Rue, 1989), memory-impaired depressives could not be distinguished from DAT patients on the basis of subtest profiles; on this measure, DSD patients had as severe an impairment in storage and retrieval as patients with mild DAT (cf. Post, 1966).

In our experience, DSD patients tend to be difficult test cases. They are often extremely withdrawn and passive or highly distressed during the evaluation; encouragement, reducing the difficulty of the exam, or arranging for very brief sessions does not greatly change their ability to cope with the process. Examiners are usually concerned that the results may underestimate the patient's ability and tend to attribute poor outcomes to problems with motivation. These clinical observations are often the primary reason for suspecting DSD (cf. Wells, 1979), but whether or not they have predictive value remains to be determined.

SUMMARY AND CONCLUSIONS

Depression affects older adults in much the same way as it does younger people. However, it is in older patients that the cognitive sequelae of depression have attracted the greatest attention.

Depressed patients often worry about their cognitive abilities, and in older individuals, there is the additional fear that their illness may be the beginning of DAT. In many cases, testing can help to allay some of these concerns, at least for treating physicians and family members, if not for the patients themselves.

In about four cases out of five, depression has a fairly mild and circumscribed impact on cognition. Effortful learning and memory processes are undermined, response speed is slowed, and there are reductions in reasoning and executive functions. These changes are similar to those observed in normal aging but, when added to aging changes, can sometimes produce impairment in everyday cognitive function.

A minority of older depressives have generalized cognitive losses (DSD). Poorly educated patients, delusional or agitated patients, or those who have been continuously ill for a lengthy time may be especially liable to these problems. Patients with severe cognitive problems may require a lengthier or more aggressive course of treatment to recover from a depressive episode. Eventually, however, cognitive problems can be expected to remit if mood can be effectively treated.

It is still very difficult to distinguish DSD from mild organic dementia, and neuropsychological tests can be helpful only in certain cases. Testing can discriminate the typical presentation of depression from DAT, but in DSD, there is more overlap in cognitive symptoms. As more prospective studies of DSD are performed, additional means of distinguishing these disorders can be expected.

12

Depression

Case Examples

Older depressed patients can come to the attention of neuropsychologists in several ways. Some are self-referred because of concerns about cognitive loss; others are encouraged to get an evaluation by their families so that their worries can be put in better perspective. For those with more severe cognitive losses, testing is often requested to assess the possibility of dementia syndrome of depression (DSD).

The following examples span the range of complaints and impairments that one is likely to see in severe geriatric depression. In two cases, the evaluation was prompted by subjective complaints. In the other, there is objective evidence for cognitive impairment in addition to severe depression.

SUBJECTIVE COGNITIVE IMPAIRMENT: I

Most depressed patients have at least mild complaints about memory loss or poor concentration, and for a few, cognitive changes are the focal point for their subjective sense of illness and distress. Example 12.1 concerns a 60-year-old Afro-American woman whose chief complaint was severe loss of recent memory. She had had one previous episode of major depression 20 years earlier. She also had multiple physical complaints and had been on disability from her work as a nurse because of chest pain and breathing problems.

In the year before this assessment, she had suffered from a variety of depressive symptoms, including feelings of dysphoria and loneliness, problems sleeping, frequent

EXAMPLE 12.1

Background

Sixty-year-old Afro-American woman.

Eighth grade education; former licensed vocational nurse, on disability for past 15 years.

Divorced once; has been in second marriage for 19 years.

Hospitalized for depression 20 years ago; received amitriptyline as an outpatient for 10 years; hospitalized at a private psychiatric facility 4 months before this assessment because of memory loss and depression; EEG and CT scan were normal for age, but neurologist felt that Alzheimer's disease was a possibility and psychological testing was said to be "consistent with a dementing process."

Medical history suggested possible angina, diverticulitis, gastritis, dysphagia, asthma, and arthritis; however, most of these complaints were not substantiated on examination by a specialist in geriatric medicine.

Had been taking multiple medications, including fluoxetine (Prozac) and trazodone (Desyrel) for depression, digoxin, hydrochlorothiazide, and nitroglycerin for a heart condition; cimetidine for gastric symptoms; ibuprofen for arthritic pain; and beclomethasone inhaler for possible asthma.

Presenting problems

Complaints of severe short-term memory loss, dysphoria, mood lability, insomnia, crying, and feelings of isolation for a year before this assessment.

Behavior during testing

Very talkative and friendly during the examination, showed good persistence on most tasks; not excessively anxious or self-critical about her performance.

Test findings

Neurobehavioral Cognitive Status Examination: Impaired calculations and memory; other scales normal for age.

WAIS-R:	Age-scaled scores	Percentile
Vocabulary	9	37
Information	9	37
Similarities	11	63
Digit Span	8	25
Digit Symbol	7	16
Block Design	6	9
Picture Completion	6	9
Object Assembly	11	63

	Raw score	Percentile/ rating
WMS-R		
Logical Memory, immediate	20	40
delayed	16	37
Visual Reproduction, immediate	30	57
delayed	26	46
Mental Control	3	7
Object Memory Evaluation		
Storage	40	1
Retrieval	36	25
Repeated Retrieval	23	25
Ineffective Reminders	5	7
Delayed Recall	8	Normal
Verbal Fluency (2 minutes, naming within categories)	49	95
Trail Making Test		
Part A	66 seconds	25
Part B	159 seconds	25–50

Qualitative aspects of performance

No errors of intrusion on tests of verbal learning and recall; errors on Visual Reproduction consisted of omissions and minor distortions. Slowed rate of storage of new information on the Object Memory Evaluation, but was able to retrieve items from storage and to retain them after a delay. Performance on Digit Symbol and Block Design was accurate but slow; completed two additional block designs slightly beyond time limits. Patient indicated lifelong problems with calculations, which she attributed to limited education.

Interpretation and recommendations

Performance was generally at or above the levels expected for age and background; slight reduction in nonverbal intellectual skills, especially on novel tasks, but nonverbal learning and recall is intact; mild slowing on speeded tasks. The patient's generalized complaints of memory loss in everyday life are out of proportion to her performance on tests and clinical interviews; the subjective memory loss is thus most likely part of a broader pattern of depressive and somatic complaints. Reassurance was provided about cognitive abilities and arrangements were made for psychotherapy and medication follow-up.

crying spells, anxiety, and a loss of interest in her usual activities. She found it increasingly difficult to remember recent information and experiences and felt that she could not control her emotions and behavior. It was principally because of her memory loss and emotional lability that she sought psychiatric treatment. About four months before the current testing, she had been hospitalized at a private psychiatric facility. The diagnostic workup there produced conflicting information about the presence of a possible dementia. The electroencephalogram (EEG) and computerized tomography (CT) scan were normal, but the neurologist raised a question of Alzheimer's disease, and psychological testing was reportedly consistent with a dementia. Other consultants, including a psychiatrist and another psychologist, felt that her symptoms might be due to depression and recommended a more thorough evaluation by geriatric specialists.

During the subsequent admission at a different hospital, the geriatric medicine consultant made note of the patient's multiple medical complaints and long list of medications. Examination and review of records provided little evidence of arthritis, asthma, or ulcer disease, and the recommendation was made to taper off or discontinue most current medications. Psychiatric interview confirmed the presence of depression and also noted problems with concentration, tangential and circumstantial thinking, and mild recent memory impairment.

Neuropsychological testing was requested to clarify cognitive strengths and weaknesses and to provide an opinion about whether current deficits were consistent with depression. Testing was divided into three 1-hour sessions spanning a period of a week; the patient was taking a low dose of doxepin during this time. She was friendly with the examiner and talked freely and at length about her current problems. She complained about dysphoria, conflicts with family members, and problems in learning and recalling new things; however, when encouraged to begin the testing, she was readily able to focus and sustain her attention on the tasks. She was less anxious about the testing than expected and was not unusually self-critical about her performance.

The Neurobehavioral Cognitive Status Examination (NCSE; see Chapter 4) was administered to give an overview of level of performance in different cognitive areas. She was accurate in her orientation to place and time and had no difficulty with the screening items for attention, language, visuoconstruction, and reasoning. She had mild difficulties with mental calculation, and on the memory task (recalling four words after a delay of 10 minutes), she remembered none of the items on her own but recalled two with category cues and recognized a third.

On the Wechsler Adult Intelligence Scale—Revised (WAIS-R), Verbal subscale scores were within the range expected for her age and education. Scores on the Performance subscales were somewhat lower, with the exception of Object Assembly. On Picture Completion, the patient focused on obvious, but nonessential, missing elements (e.g., the leash for the dog on the beach or a person playing the violin). On Block Design, performance was accurate but slow (she completed two additional designs correctly beyond time limits). On Digit Symbol, there were no difficulties comprehending instructions or following the sequence, but rate of completion was slow. In general, this performance is quite consistent with expectations for a seriously depressed individual. There was evidence of slowing that was especially apparent on novel tasks.

However, verbal intelligence was well preserved, and there were no errors suggestive of brain impairment. Performance on the Trail Making Test also provided little support for organic dementia. The patient readily comprehended the instructions and made no errors on either Part A or B. Completion time was at the 25th percentile for age on Part A and between the 25th and 50th percentiles for Part B according to the norms provided by Davies (1968; see Table A.7 in the Appendix).

Wechsler Memory Scale—Revised (WMS-R) scores were generally consistent with the patient's verbal intelligence. On Logical Memory, she occasionally elaborated or interpreted story details; however, there were no intrusions of irrelevant information and no confusion of details between the two stories. Also, there was little loss of information on delayed recall. Visual Reproduction performance was surprisingly strong in light of the lower WAIS-R Performance subtest scores; the overall outline of each figure was correctly reproduced, and there were no rotation errors or perseverations. On the Object Memory Evaluation, the rate of entering items into storage was below expectations, but by the fifth trial, all 10 items had been stored; retrieval and consistent retrieval were in the low-average range, and delayed recall was normal. Verbal fluency was very strong for the patient's overall intellectual level, suggesting adequate access to semantic memory.

Performance on the Mental Control items from the WMS-R suggested some problems in concentration, but these difficulties were not severe enough to preclude an adequate performance on tests of learning and recall. There were also some inconsistencies in the scores observed across similar tests. On the NCSE, for example, the patient had difficulty remembering a list of four words, but on subsequent (and more difficult) memory tests, less impairment was observed. The latter finding may reflect increasing comfort with the examiner or testing process or some improvement in clinical condition during the week of testing.

The results of cognitive testing did not bear out the patient's complaints of severe memory loss, nor did they agree with the earlier psychological report suggesting dementia. The discrepancy between subjective and objective findings is not unexpected in depression, but the difference in conclusions raised by psychological examiners is harder to explain. There may have been some improvement in the level of depression since the earlier testing; alternatively, the prior conclusions may have been based on tests or norms that were less suited to the patient's age and abilities.

SUBJECTIVE COGNITIVE IMPAIRMENT: II

Example 12.2 also involves severe subjective memory loss in an individual with recurrent depression. However, this patient had an exceptionally high premorbid baseline, which increased the odds that an early dementia may have gone undetected.

The patient was a former university professor who had retired from full-time teaching four years before this assessment. He had continued his professional involvement on a part-time basis and had traveled extensively. He was single and lived alone but was socially active with former students and with friends.

EXAMPLE 12.2

Background

73-year-old Caucasian man.
Retired university professor.
Never married; has lived alone in the same home for many years.
Excellent physical health; no current medications.
Usually very active; travels frequently and continues professional involvement.
History of multiple depressive episodes, including a mild depressive phase in middle age treated with psychotherapy, and two more severe episodes (8 years and 1 year ago), both requiring hospitalization. Full recovery from earlier episodes but incomplete recovery from episode which began last year.
Had been taking phenelzine (Nardil) for several months, but is currently in a 2-week drug-washout phase.

Presenting complaints

Severe dysphoria, loss of interest in his work and social pursuits, complaints of memory loss and poor concentration: "I've been floating around this past year, unable to get my bearings. . . . I live one day at a time . . . feel there is no future . . . feel as if there is some type of degeneration in my brain."

Behavior during testing

Cooperative and gracious; worked with good effort, but frequently criticized his own performance.

Test Findings

WAIS-R:	Age-scaled scores	Percentile
Vocabulary	15	95
Similarities	13	84
Digit Span	12	75
Digit Symbol	16	98
Block Design	11	63
	Raw score	Percentile/ rating
WMS		
Logical Memory, immediate	7	25
delayed	5	34
Visual Reproduction, immediate	5	43
delayed	5	56
Verbal List Learning (max. = 16)		
Random list, 2nd trial	7	Low normal
Categorized list, 2nd trial	11	Normal
Incidental Recall (Digit Symbol items):	5 symbols, 2 pairs	Low normal
Boston Naming Test (60 items)	51	30
Controlled Oral Word Association Test	50	84

Qualitative aspects of performance

No confusion in recall between stories; no perseverations, rotations, or size errors on design recall; only one intrusion during verbal list learning; no loss of set on verbal fluency, but occasional repetition of items.

Interpretation

Performance mildly impaired for age and background on immediate nonverbal recall; other aspects of performance were within normal limits for exceptional older adults. Good retention on delayed recall and incidental recall, as well as enhancement of list learning by semantic organization, argues against a dementia. Reassurance was provided about cognitive abilities and arrangements were made for outpatient treatment for depression.

He was severely disturbed by his change in mood and functional level and described his problems in great detail. He stated that formerly he had been very productive and active, but now, "My whole world seems different somehow." He had stopped attending social events, saying, "My house feels like a tomb, but it's worse when I go out." He also complained of a loss of interest and motivation ("I do nothing . . . live one day at a time . . . feel there is no future").

In addition to these changes in mood, interest, and sociability, he also perceived a marked decline in his ability to think and remember. These problems were so severe subjectively that he felt as if there was some "degeneration" in his brain and feared that he might be developing dementia.

The patient had had several past episodes of depression. As a young man, he had spent some time in psychotherapy because of mild depressive symptoms. At age 65, he had been hospitalized for five months because of severe depression; he had been treated primarily with intensive psychotherapy and reported that he had recovered "back to my old self." About a year before this testing, he had become depressed again and had been hospitalized for six to seven weeks; with a series of antidepressant medications, he had made a partial recovery but had never returned to his baseline since the start of that episode. He had continued antidepressant medications since discharge but had become increasingly discouraged by his failure to improve and was currently seeking additional assistance with his problem.

During the interview prior to testing, he talked at length about his symptoms of depression and his strong desire to recoup his zest for work and entertainment. He had some difficulties relating his personal history and recent events. For example, he first gave his age as 72 and then corrected himself, giving his age as 73 and providing his birth date. He also had some problems relating when he had recently been hospitalized, first describing it as a year before, then two years before, and then providing the date.

He easily comprehended test instructions and showed good persistence on the various tasks. However, he often criticized his performance and apologized for not being able to do as well as he should.

His scores on WAIS-R subtests were all at or above expectations for age. Vocabulary was the high point of the Verbal profile, as would be expected in light of his education and occupation. His definitions were prompt and succinct, and for many items, he provided exact synonyms. Similarities and Digit Span were slightly lower, a result suggesting a slight reduction in abstraction and attention relative to his general fund of word knowledge. On Digit Symbol, he worked with surprising speed and accuracy and obtained an age-scaled score that was well above average. By contrast, on Block Design, he was doubtful of his ability to perform and critical of his attempts. With encouragement, he was able to complete the first six designs correctly within the allotted times but had difficulty with Item 7 and asked to discontinue.

Language testing provided little evidence of impairment. On the Boston Naming Test, he named 51 of 60 items quickly and accurately and gave relevant semantic associations for most of the others. This is a low-average performance for healthy, well-educated older adults (Van Gorp *et al.*, 1990; see Table A.5 in the Appendix). On the Controlled Oral Word Association Test, he named 50 relevant words within three minutes. This is above expectations, even for much younger adults (Albert *et al.*, 1988; cf. Table A.6 in the Appendix). His production declined slightly across the three letters, from 20 words to 13, and on the last letter, he made two repetition errors (in each case asking, "Did I already say that?").

On the WMS Logical Memory, his immediate recall score was slightly, but not significantly, below the means reported for well-educated older adults (Abikoff *et al.*, 1987; Albert *et al.*, 1988). He did not confuse elements between the two stories and had no serious extrastory intrusions. Somewhat greater problems were noted on Visual Reproduction. He produced a fairly accurate copy of the first design, but on the second, he distorted the pattern, producing four small squares inside each quadrant of the larger square. On the third design, he reproduced one figure fairly accurately but omitted most of the other. His total score of 5 was slightly below the age norms reported by Van Gorp *et al.* (1990) but was at the mean reported by Haaland *et al.* (1983; see Table A.4 in Appendix). There were no rotations, perseverations, or size or misplacement errors.

On both of the preceding tests, he retained a high proportion of information on delayed recall (71% for Logical Memory; 100% for Visual Reproduction). This argues against a memory impairment of the type observed in dementia of Alzheimer type (DAT; see Chapter 7). There were two other indications that learning and memory were essentially intact. On incidental recall of WAIS Digit Symbol pairs, he correctly reproduced five of the nine symbols, which is clearly above the levels noted in mild DAT (Hart *et al.*, 1987c). Similarly, on two list-learning tasks, he showed a rapid improvement in the rate of learning when items were organized by semantic category instead of randomly (cf. Weingartner *et al.*, 1981a; Chapter 11).

Overall, this patient's memory performance was consistent with expectations for depression (see Chapter 11) and was quite dissimilar, qualitatively and quantitatively, to the typical performance of patients with early DAT. Other findings also supported this impression; that is, fluency and naming were intact, and there were no serious problems on any of the intelligence subtests. In fact, the very strong performance on Digit Symbol was better than usual for older patients with serious depression.

On positron emission tomography (PET) scanning, there was no evidence of hypometabolism in the temporal or parietal regions, as might be expected in early DAT (see Chapter 7), nor were there any patchy cortical or subcortical reductions suggesting multi-infarct dementia (MID; see Chapter 9). Therefore, from this perspective also, there was little evidence for a dementia.

The patient appreciated the feedback from the testing but still believed that his memory was impaired. He accepted the fact that this impairment might be due to depression and was anxious to begin treatment with some other antidepressant medication.

DEMENTIA SYNDROME OF DEPRESSION

The final example (12.3) illustrates the dramatic improvement in cognition and day-to-day functioning that can sometimes be observed with treatment for depression. The overall level of psychiatric and cognitive deficit was initially very severe, and as is often the case with such patients, the possibility of underlying brain disease could not be excluded. However, the observed improvements indicated that some of the apparent dementia was due to the depression.

The patient, a 78-year-old Afro-American woman, had been free of psychiatric problems until a year before this assessment. Family members first noticed that the patient was losing track of everyday events and activities; she became noticeably forgetful and was occasionally confused in her own neighborhood. Over time, these symptoms worsened, and others began to appear. She began to sleep less and became argumentative with her son; she stopped cooking and attending to her appearance and began hiding objects around her home. She became convinced that the television was watching her, believed that her house was wiretapped, and began speaking with nonexistent people. She also developed visual hallucinations of ants and fleas and, believing that her food was poisoned, often refused to eat. In the days just before admission, she had thrown objects at the television and threatened family members.

There had been some stressful events in the patient's life that may have contributed to her decline. One of her sons had returned to live with her about a year before admission, causing some strains and readjustments for both. A favorite cousin developed cancer and also came to live with the patient; when the cousin died about six months later, the patient became noticeably more confused and delusional. The patient herself had been diagnosed with cancer of the breast more than 20 years earlier and, six months before (about the time of her cousin's death), had been told that the cancer had progressed and that she would need radiation therapy. She refused this treatment, as well as mastectomy, and generally denied that she had any illness.

At the time of admission, the patient refused to answer most questions and offered no information spontaneously. Her affect was flat and she would not maintain eye contact. She appeared to be having auditory hallucinations and also appeared very frightened. Her ability to attend and concentrate was markedly reduced, and she would not attempt cognitive testing.

EXAMPLE 12.3

Background

Seventy-eight-year-old Afro-American woman.
Worked as a beautician and homemaker; 9th-grade education.
Son, aged 34, recently moved in to help with her care.
Negative history for psychiatric illness.
Medical history significant for breast cancer diagnosed 15 years ago; currently taking tamoxifen but has refused other workup or treatment.

Presenting problems

Increasing forgetfulness and confusion for about 1 year.
Sleep disturbance and increased irritability for several months.
About 2 months prior to admission, developed paranoid delusions about her food being contaminated, often refusing to eat; auditory and visual hallucinations; wandering in neighborhood; violent toward son.

Behavior during testing (initial evaluation)

Either apathetic to the point of being unresponsive to questions or negativistic and hostile. On some days, would refuse assessment; on others, would abruptly terminate sessions. Depressed mood and blunted affect. Did not recognize examiner across sessions.

Test findings (initial evaluation)

Mini-Mental State Examination: 16

	Raw score	Percentile/rating
WMS		
Logical Memory, immediate	3.5	16
Object Memory Evaluation		
Retrieval, Trial 1	3	<1
Visual Retention Test		
Multiple choice (max. = 16)	4	<1
Direct copy (max. = 10)	0	Impaired
Boston Naming Test (60 items)	34	16
Verbal fluency (1 minute, proper names)	5	<1

Qualitative aspects of performance

Confabulation during recall of stories; gross naming errors and perseveration on confrontation naming; many repetitions of items on fluency task; gross distortions on design copying.

Behavior during testing (retest, following ECT)

Friendly and very verbal. Rapport easily established; motivation and persistence adequate. Remembered examiner across sessions.

Test findings (retest)

WAIS-R	Age-scaled score	Percentile
Vocabulary	9	37
Comprehension	9	37
Digit Symbol	5	5
Block Design	4	2
Visual Retention Test		
Direct copy	4	Impaired
Boston Naming Test	44	40

Qualitative aspects of performance
Ability to attend to tasks considerably improved. Less severe distortions noted in design copying and on confrontation naming.

Interpretation

Marked treatment-related improvement in clarity of thought and selected cognitive abilities; suggests initial problems were partly due to dementia syndrome of depression. Residual visuospatial impairments suggest that mild organic deficits may also be present. Discharged to sheltered living arrangement on low-dose antidepressant medication; retesting in 4 to 6 months was recommended to evaluate recovery of memory and changes in other cognitive functions.

She was initially treated with haloperidol to alleviate psychotic symptoms. As the delusions and hallucinations decreased, her depression became more apparent. She admitted that her mood was depressed and showed little interest in activities or social contact. She still had poverty of speech but, at times, spoke of "losing the contest." She felt that others were laughing at her and became tearful when asked about her family. Sleep and appetite continued to be poor. She was started on nortriptyline, but when her psychotic symptoms returned, this was discontinued and replaced with phenelzine. Little improvement was noted over a period of weeks, and eventually, she and her family agreed to electroconvulsive therapy (ECT). After a course of 12 treatments (9 unilateral and 3 bilateral), her mood and affect improved dramatically. She became very sociable and helpful to other patients and expressed a keen sense of humor. Her appetite improved and she began to gain weight, but her sleep continued to be poor. Her mental status was generally clear, but she showed some confusion and memory loss after the last three treatments.

Cognitive testing had been started about three weeks into the hospitalization, after psychotic symptoms had decreased, but before there had been any improvement in mood or activity level. The goal of this testing had been to clarify the severity of cognitive impairment, so that decisions could be made about continuing treatment for depression.

It proved very difficult to develop enough rapport to complete a valid assessment.

Testing was attempted on several occasions. At times, the patient was unresponsive to questions of any kind. At other times, she would agree to attempt the tasks but was very apathetic in both her verbal and her nonverbal behavior. She frequently made statements that suggested severe demoralization (e.g., "What's the use . . . I've lost anyway," or "I shouldn't be here . . . I should be dead"). On her best days, her motivation was low, and she tended to give up very easily.

Test findings indicated severely diminished performance in all areas. On the Mini-Mental State Examination (MMSE), she could not name the date, month, hospital, or state; she could recall the list of three words immediately but, after a brief delay, remembered none of the words, even with cues or multiple-choice alternatives. She would not attempt concentration or calculation items and produced a grossly inaccurate copy of the interlocking pentagons. On the Boston Naming Test, there was a low rate of accurate responses and there were multiple perseverative errors. On WMS Logical Memory, she initially recalled a few relevant bits of information, but when she was encouraged to remember more, her remarks were distorted in a manner consistent with her depression. For example, for the first story, she remarked, "Hungry people . . . everybody's hungry nowadays," and for the second, "The story was about everybody . . . the boat sank." On the Visual Retention Test, her copies were grossly distorted, and on the multiple-choice version of this test, she performed at only a chance level. Even when compared to norms for older persons with little education (e.g., Borod *et al.*, 1980, for Boston Naming; Hulicka, 1966, for Logical Memory), these performances were all in the impaired range, numerically and qualitatively.

Some additional testing was performed near the end of ECT. No memory tests were given, since it would be difficult to interpret any impairments observed in this area because of ECT side effects. However, less adverse impact would be expected on intelligence and higher cortical functions.

At this later evaluation, the patient's attitude toward the examiner and the testing process was greatly improved. She was friendly and very verbal; she showed good persistence on tasks and remembered the examiner when she encountered her on later days. The retest data showed verbal intelligence to be intact; scores on nonverbal subtests were lower but were out of the profoundly impaired range. There was also considerable improvement both on the Boston Naming Test and on copying of designs from the Visual Retention Test.

Despite the improvements observed, the patient still had some cognitive problems that affected her ability to function. She remembered most people on the ward and had learned the general routine, but still she confused details of her schedule and would occasionally have problems finding her room. Therefore, some degree of dementia may well have been present. The CT scan showed no sign of brain metastases, cerebrovascular lesions, or prominent atrophy. The EEG showed only mild, nonfocal slowing. Therefore, no specific etiology for dementia was suggested. Her medications (including tamoxifen, Naprosyn, and lithium carbonate at the time of discharge), residual effects of ECT, and systemic effects of cancer must all be considered as contributing factors.

On follow-up, approximately one year later, there had been no worsening of cognitive problems, but the patient still had not received treatment for her cancer. She was still not able to live independently, but her level of self-care continued to be higher than it had been before the psychiatric hospitalization. There had been some recurrence of depression and paranoia, but these problems improved with an increase in antidepressant medication.

In this case, neuropsychological testing played an important role in interpreting the patient's apparent lack of awareness and other cognitive problems. There had been serious doubts on the part of the patient's family about the value of ECT, especially if the patient was developing dementia. By confirming the severity of depression and interpreting the cognitive problems in light of the depression, neuropsychological input helped to tip the balance in favor of treatment. At the very least, psychiatric treatment had given this person another year of reasonable comfort and ability to care for herself, even if it had not eliminated all disabilities.

SUMMARY AND CONCLUSIONS

As the examples in this chapter illustrate, neuropsychological testing can help to put a depressed person's concerns about cognitive function in better perspective and can indicate whether an individual's problems are consistent with the deficits that typically accompany depression.

In the first and second examples, subjective concerns about cognitive loss were so distressing that they prompted the search for professional help. Testing did not substantiate significant cognitive impairments, although mild problems, consistent with depression, were observed (e.g., reduced attention and problems with effortful learning). In the third example, serious cognitive deficits were present, but these problems improved considerably as other depressive symptoms remitted. This case qualified as an example of DSD, since cognitive losses were objectively apparent and severe enough to interfere with basic aspects of everyday living.

The negativity and pessimism that accompany depression can limit a person's ability to benefit from positive feedback about memory or other abilities; however, objective information about cognitive function can be of great use to professionals treating depressed patients. In the first two cases, feedback about the basic adequacy of cognitive functions helped to shape psychotherapeutic interactions and increased expectations for a positive treatment outcome. In the third case, testing provided an additional rationale for continuing treatment, despite the failure of some earlier treatment attempts. Positive outcomes are not always seen in cases of combined dementia and depression (e.g., compare with Example 10.4), and at present, there is no way of predicting when beneficial effects will occur. However, the attention that has been paid to DSD has greatly increased the prospects that a serious attempt at treatment will be made in these difficult cases, and as more is learned about the factors that account for DSD, the process of treatment is likely to become more specific and more effective.

Appendix

Age Norms for Selected Neuropsychological Tests

TABLE A.1. Age Norms for Wechsler Memory Scale: Logical Memory

Study	Sample	Group (age)	Mean	*SD*
Wechsler (1945)	"Normal subject"; mean IQ = 102.	20–29 (*n* = 50)	9.28	3.10
		40–49 (*n* = 46)	8.09	2.52
Albert *et al.* (1988)	Community-resident men participating in a longitudinal aging study; screened to exclude neurological and psychiatric illness and common medical problems such as hypertension; mean education = 15 years.	30–39 (*n* = 16)	10.63	3.70
		50–59 (*n* = 20)	9.60	2.64
		60–69 (*n* = 21)	10.29	3.21
		70–80 (*n* = 23)	8.17	3.49
Haaland *et al.* (1983)	Healthy volunteers screened to exclude common medical problems such as hypertension; no prescription medications; mean education = 14 years.	65–69 (*n* = 49)	7.40	2.50
		70–74 (*n* = 74)	6.70	2.60
		75–79 (*n* = 40)	5.90	2.50
		80 and above (*n* = 13)	6.10	1.70
Van Gorp *et al.* (1990)	Volunteers from an affluent retirement community (Leisure Village); generally healthy by self-report; mean education = 14 years.	58–65 (*n* = 28)	9.75	2.40
		66–70 (*n* = 45)	8.47	2.65
		71–75 (*n* = 57)	9.27	3.15
		76–85 (*n* = 26)	8.05	2.19
Abikoff *et al.* (1987)	Volunteers recruited from business or community organizations or medical center employees; mean education = 12–14 years; no information about health.	18–29 (*n* = 39)	11.18	5.34
		30–39 (*n* = 33)	13.79	5.82
		40–49 (*n* = 24)	12.79	3.31
		50–59 (*n* = 30)	11.73	4.73
		60–69 (*n* = 32)	9.88	4.84
		70–83 (*n* = 28)	9.11	4.52
Hulicka (1966)	Younger adults were hospitalized veterans; older groups included hospitalized patients, long-term care residents, and members of seniors clubs; excluded subjects with diagnoses of psychotic disorder or organic brain damage; mean education = 8–10 years; age groups equated for Vocabulary.	30–39 (*n* = 53)	7.99	2.95
		60–69 (*n* = 70)	7.34	2.90
		70–79 (*n* = 46)	7.35	3.83
		80–89 (*n* = 25)	6.80	3.19
Klonoff and Kennedy (1966)	Canadian male veterans; in community group, most subjects had good global health ratings (from internist) and were moderately or very active; in the custodial care group, health ratings were poor for a majority, and most were "minimally active" or "inactive"; in both groups, a majority of subjects had unskilled/semiskilled occupational backgrounds.	Community: 80–92 (*n* = 115)	5.72	2.91
		Custodial: 80–93 (*n* = 115)	3.56	2.86
			% with defective scores compared to 60- to 64-year-olds	
Benton *et al.* (1981)	Volunteers from seniors groups and retirement homes; no history of psychiatric, neurological, or major medical illness by self-report; mean education = 13 years; mostly women.	65–69 (*n* = 28)	4%	
		70–74 (*n* = 62)	3%	
		75–79 (*n* = 35)	3%	
		80–84 (*n* = 37)	11%	

TABLE A.2. Age Norms for Wechsler Memory Scale: Associate Learning Subtest

Study	Sample	Group (age)	Mean	*SD*
Wechsler (1945)	"Normal subject"; mean IQ = 102.	20–29 (*n* = 50)	15.72	2.81
		40–49 (*n* = 46)	13.91	3.12
Hulicka (1966)	Mixed sample, with oldest including hospital and long-term care patients as well as community volunteers; mean education = 8–10 years; see Table A.1.	30–39 (*n* = 53)	15.48	3.48
		60–69 (*n* = 70)	11.94	4.53
		70–79 (*n* = 46)	10.98	4.78
		80–89 (*n* = 25)	9.98	3.28
Klonoff and Kennedy (1966)	Veterans; most with unskilled or semiskilled occupational backgrounds; in custodial care group, most had fair to poor health; see Table A.1.	Community residents, 80–92 (*n* = 115)	10.15	3.80
		Custodial care group, 80–93 (*n* = 115)	6.74	4.54
			% with defective scores compared to 60- to 64-year-olds	
Benton *et al.* (1981)	Volunteers from senior groups and retirement homes; healthy by self-report; mean education = 13 years; see Table A.1.	65–69 (*n* = 28)	0%	
		70–74 (*n* = 62)	0%	
		75–79 (*n* = 35)	6%	
		80–84 (*n* = 37)	11%	

TABLE A.3. Age Norms for the Selective Reminding Test

A. Ruff *et al.* (1988)[a]

Gender and age (years)		Long-term storage[b] Education (years) ≤ 12	13–15	≥ 16	Consistent long-term retrieval[b] Education (years) ≤ 12	13–15	≥ 16
Women							
16–24	*M*	120.0	125.9	128.8	100.8	114.9	123.4
	SD	14.1	10.8	11.5	27.4	15.5	16.0
25–39	*M*	114.8	120.0	126.3	92.3	103.6	114.7
	SD	13.5	14.4	12.7	26.9	30.4	24.4
40–54	*M*	116.4	119.2	111.2	89.0	96.3	79.5
	SD	11.4	15.3	16.3	24.7	36.9	27.2
55–70	*M*	102.1	95.8	108.4	65.2	71.4	74.1
	SD	20.4	22.1	32.8	31.3	36.8	33.4
Men							
16–24	*M*	104.0	110.0	121.9	74.4	84.9	113.5
	SD	27.7	14.3	17.5	41.5	33.2	24.2
25–39	*M*	110.5	110.4	114.0	83.5	89.9	97.0
	SD	16.5	25.6	17.9	28.8	35.8	28.8
40–54	*M*	104.5	105.7	104.1	78.9	82.9	69.9
	SD	24.0	17.5	19.5	39.1	29.4	30.6
55–70	*M*	81.6	88.2	92.8	49.7	60.2	63.9
	SD	26.5	22.7	24.9	21.0	32.4	30.3

B. Banks *et al.* (1987)[c]

Age (years) and gender	*N*	Long-term storage[b] *M*	*SD*	Consistent long-term retrieval[b] *M*	*SD*
65–75					
Women	37	83.27	22.47	60.08	16.81
Men	23	57.82	22.13	39.26	23.26

C. Masur *et al.* (1989)[d]

Age (years)	*N*	Long-term storage[e] *M*	*SD*	Consistent long-term retrieval[e] *M*	*SD*
70–85	360	39.63	11.84	21.34	11.82

[a]Community-resident volunteers with a negative history for neurological and psychiatric illness; no information provided about physical health status; subgroup *n*'s ranged from 15 to 20.
[b]Maximum = 144; based on 12-item list and 12 recall trials.
[c]Community-resident volunteers; free of neurological or psychiatric illness by self-report; mean education = 15 years.
[d]Volunteers participating in a longitudinal aging study; normal scores on mental status examination; residential status unclear; relatively low level of education (63% ≤ 12 years; 30% < 9 years).
[e]Maximum = 72; based on 12-item list and 6 recall trials.

TABLE A.4. Age Norms for Wechsler Memory Scale: Visual Reproduction

Study	Sample	Group (age)	Mean	*SD*
Wechsler (1945)	"Normal subject"; mean IQ = 102.	20–29 (*n* = 50)	11.00	2.73
		40–49 (*n* = 46)	8.35	3.17
Van Gorp *et al.* (1990)	Leisure Village residents; healthy by self-report; mean education = 14 years; see Table A.1.	58–65 (*n* = 28)	9.60	2.76
		66–70 (*n* = 45)	8.67	3.81
		71–75 (*n* = 57)	7.79	2.99
		76–85 (*n* = 26)	4.09	2.26
Haaland *et al.* (1983)	Very healthy volunteers; mean education = 14 years; see Table A.1.	65–69 (*n* = 49)	6.00	2.10
		70–74 (*n* = 74)	5.10	2.00
		75–79 (*n* = 40)	4.90	2.00
		80 and above (*n* = 13)	3.30	2.00
Hulicka (1966)	Combination of hospital patients, custodial care residents, and community volunteers; 8–10 years of education; see Table A.1.	30–39 (*n* = 53)	10.09	3.01
		60–69 (*n* = 70)	6.03	3.72
		70–79 (*n* = 46)	4.95	3.42
		80–89 (*n* = 25)	4.00	2.38
Klonoff and Kennedy (1966)	Veterans; many with physical health problems; unskilled or semiskilled occupations; see Table A.1.	Community: 80–92 (*n* = 115)	3.76	2.70
		Custodial: 80–93 (*n* = 115)	2.78	2.37

TABLE A.5. Age Norms for the Boston Naming Test

Study	Sample	Group (age)	Mean	*SD*	Range
	A. 85-item version				
Albert *et al.* (1988)	Community-resident men participating in a longitudinal aging study; in excellent health and highly educated; see Table A.1.	30–39 (*n* = 16)	80.69	2.77	
		50–59 (*n* = 20)	80.75	2.47	
		60–69 (*n* = 21)	79.95	3.06	
		70–80 (*n* = 23)	74.57	5.75	
Nicholas *et al.* (1985)	Community residents recruited through advertising; all right-handed; screened to exclude neurological disorder, sensory deficit, bilingualism; mean education = 13–15 years; equal numbers of men and women in each age group.	30–39 (*n* = 38)	75.9	6.4	56–85
		50–59 (*n* = 38)	75.7	6.7	59–83
		60–69 (*n* = 38)	73.6	6.8	55–83
		70–79 (*n* = 38)	67.6	8.4	52–80
Borod *et al.* (1980)	Nonhospitalized controls recruited by advertising; reported free of neurological disease, learning disability, and alcoholism; education varied with age; 68% of oldest group had ≤ 12 years of education.	25–39 (*n* = 42)	76.5	5.9	60–85
		40–49 (*n* = 18)	76.3	7.8	60–84
		50–59 (*n* = 31)	75.6	7.3	50–84
		60–69 (*n* = 31)	70.3	11.7	18–81
		70–85 (*n* = 25)	63.2	16.2	17–81
	B. 60-item short form				
Van Gorp *et al.* (1990)	Leisure Village residents; self-reports of good health; mean education = 14 years; see Table A.1.	58–65 (*n* = 28)	55.50	4.53	
		66–70 (*n* = 45)	55.47	3.94	
		71–75 (*n* = 57)	53.88	5.73	
		76–85 (*n* = 26)	51.00	6.36	

TABLE A.6. Age Norms for Controlled Oral Word Association Test

Study	Sample	Group (age)	Mean	*SD*
Albert *et al.* (1988)	Community-resident men participating in a longitudinal study; in excellent health and highly educated; see Table A.1.	30–39 (*n* = 16)	49.19	9.11
		50–59 (*n* = 20)	46.05	9.41
		60–69 (*n* = 21)	45.33	11.56
		70–80 (*n* = 23)	39.65	10.44
Montgomery (1982)	Community-resident volunteers; Canadian; history negative for psychiatric or neurological illness; "reasonable" health; mean education = 12.4 years.	65–74 (*n* = 50)	41.12	12.41
		75–89 (*n* = 35)	36.97	11.60
Rosen (1980)	Nursing-home residents with normal mental status; history negative for psychiatric or neurological illness; mean education = 11.7 years.	*M* = 83.6 (*n* = 10)	27.90	
			% with defective scores compared to 60- to 64-year-olds	
Benton *et al.* (1981)	Volunteers from seniors groups and retirement homes; healthy and well educated; see Table A.1.	65–69 (*n* = 28)	4%	
		70–74 (*n* = 62)	2%	
		75–79 (*n* = 35)	6%	
		80–84 (*n* = 37)	11%	

TABLE A.7. Age Norms for the Trail Making Test

Study	Sample	Group (age)	Part A Mean	Part A SD	Part B Mean	Part B SD
Van Gorp *et al.* (1990)	Leisure Village residents; self-reports of good health; mean education = 14 years; see Table A.1.	58–65 (n = 28)	41.5	7.4	84.4	24.6
		66–70 (n = 45)	43.2	14.9	105.2	43.4
		71–75 (n = 57)	50.1	12.9	97.8	30.4
		76–85 (n = 26)	59.7	15.9	153.1	62.6
Bak and Greene (1980)	Community-resident volunteers; described as "healthy and active"; mean education = 14 years.	50–62 (n = 15)	32.5	12.6	81.7	30.8
		67–86 (n = 15)	41.6	10.3	109.0	38.4
Bornstein (1985)	Volunteers recruited from "a variety of sources" such as seniors groups; Canadian; no information about health; mean education = 12 years.	40–59 (n = 97)	29.9	10.4	75.5	35.6
		60–69 (n = 97)	36.7	10.3	92.7	32.5
Kennedy (1981)	Employees of a Canadian mental health center with diverse jobs; mean Quick Test score = 128.5; mean education = 12 years.	50–59 (n = 30)	37.7	19.0	96.0	39.2
		60–69 (n = 30)	35.2	12.4	95.0	34.6
Goul and Brown (1970)	Male hospital patients; no history of neurological illness; education range = 6–13 years; in hospital at least 3 months prior to testing.	50–59 (n = 17)	45.3	13.6	103.2	43.3
		60–72 (n = 9)	68.9	21.2	158.8	49.5

Study	Sample	Group (age)	Percentile	Time Part A	Time Part B
Davies (1968)	"Normal subjects"; recruited from a medical research sample in England; no information about health or education.	50–59 (n = 90)	90	25	55
			75	29	75
			50	38	98
			25	49	135
			10	67	177
		60–69 (n = 90)	90	29	64
			75	35	89
			50	48	119
			25	67	172
			10	104	282
		70–79 (n = 90)	90	38	79
			75	54	132
			50	80	196
			25	105	292
			10	168	450

References

Abikoff, H., Alvir, J., Hong, G., Sukoff, R., Orazio, J., Solomon, S., & Saravay, S. (1987). Logical Memory subtest of the Wechsler Memory Scale: Age and eduction norms and alternate-form reliability of two scoring systems. *Journal of Clinical and Experimental Neuropsychology*, *9*, 435–448.

Adams, R. D., & Victor, M. (1989). *Principles of neurology* (4th ed.). New York: McGraw-Hill.

Aharon-Peretz, J., Cummings, J. L., & Hill, M. A. (1988). Vascular dementia and dementia of the Alzheimer type: Cognition, ventricular size, and leuko-araises. *Archives of Neurology*, *45*, 719–721.

Albert, M. L. (Ed.). (1984). *Clinical neurology of aging*. New York: Oxford University Press.

Albert, M. S. (1981). Geriatric neuropsychology. *Journal of Consulting and Clinical Psychology*, *49*, 835–850.

Albert, M. S., & Kaplan, E. (1980). Organic implications of neuropsychological deficits in the elderly. In L. W. Poon & J. L. Fozard (Eds.), *New directions in memory and aging* (pp. 403–432). Hillsdale, NJ: L. Erlbaum.

Albert, M. S., & Moss, M. B. (Eds.). (1988). *Geriatric neuropsychology*. New York: Guilford Press.

Albert, M. S., & Stafford, J. L. (1988). Computed tomography studies. In M. S. Albert & M. B. Moss (Eds.), *Geriatric neuropsychology* (pp. 211–227). New York: Guilford Press.

Albert, M. S., Butters, N., & Brandt, J. (1981). Patterns of remote memory in amnesic and demented patients. *Archives of Neurology*, *38*, 495–500.

Albert, M. S., Heller, H. S., & Milberg, W. (1988). Changes in naming ability with age. *Psychology and Aging*, *3*, 173–178.

Alekoumbides, A., Charter, R. A., Adkins, T. G., & Seacat, G. F. (1987). The diagnosis of brain damage by the WAIS, WMS, and Reitan Battery utilizing standardized scores corrected for age and education. *International Journal of Clinical Neuropsychology*, *9*, 11–28.

Alexopoulos, G. S., Abrams, R. C., Young, R. C., & Shamoian, C. A. (1988). Cornell Scale for Depression in Dementia. *Biological Psychiatry*, *23*, 271–284.

Allen, G. S., Burns, R. S., Tulipan, N. B., & Parker, R. A. (1989). Adrenal medullary transplantation to the caudate nucleus in Parkinson's disease. *Archives of Neurology*, *46*, 487–491.

Allen, M. G. (1976). Twin studies of affective illness. *Archives of General Psychiatry*, *33*, 1476–1478.

Alzheimer, A. (1987). About a peculiar disease of the cerebral cortex. L. Jarvik & H. Greenson, trans. *Alzheimer Disease and Associated Disorders*, *1*, 7–8. (Originally published 1907).

American Psychiatric Association. (1980). *Diagnostic and statistical manual of mental disorders* (3rd ed.) (*DSM-III*). Washington DC: Author.

American Psychiatric Association. (1987). *Diagnostic and statistical manual of mental disorders* (3rd ed., rev.) (*DSM-III-R*). Washington DC: Author.

Amsterdam, J. D., & Mendels, J. (1980). Serotonergic function and depression. In J. Mendels & J. D. Amsterdam (Eds.), *The psychology of affective disorders* (pp. 57–71). New York: Karger.

Anderson, T. B. (1984). Widowhood as a life transition: Its impact on kinship ties. *Journal of Marriage and the Family*, *46*, 105–114.

Anschutz, L., Camp, C. J., Markley, R. P., & Kramer, J. J. (1987). Remembering mnemonics: A three-year follow-up on the effects of mnemonics training in elderly adults. *Experimental Aging Research*, *13*, 141–143.

Anthony, J. C., La Resche, L., Niaz, U., Von Korff, M., & Folstein, M. (1982). Limits of the "Mini-Mental State" as a screening test for dementia and elirium among hospital patients. *Psychological Medicine*, *12*, 397–408.

Anthony, W. Z., Heaton, R. K., & Lehman, R. A. W. (1980). An attempt to cross-validate two actuarial systems for neuropsychological test interpretation. *Journal of Consulting and Clinical Psychology*, *48*, 317–326.

Antonucci, T. (1985). Personal characteristics, social support, and social behavior. In R. Binstock & E. Shanas (Eds.), *Handbook of aging and the social sciences* (pp. 94–128). New York: Van Nostrand Reinhold.

Appell, J., Kertesz, A., & Fisman, M. (1982). A study of language functioning in Alzheimer patients. *Brain and Language*, *17*, 73–91.

Arbuckle, T. Y., Gold, D., & Andres, D. (1986). Cognitive functioning of older people in relation to social and personality variables. *Psychology and Aging*, *1*, 55–62.

Arenberg, D. (1968). Concept problem solving in young and old adults. *Journal of Gerontology*, *23*, 279–282.

Arenberg, D. (1978). Differences and changes with age in the Benton Visual Retention Test. *Journal of Gerontology*, *33*, 534–540.

Arenberg, D. (1982a). Changes with age in problem solving. In F. I. M. Craik & S. Trehub (Eds.), *Aging and cognitive processes* (pp. 221–236). New York: Plenum Press.

Arenberg, D. (1982b). Estimates of age changes on the Benton Visual Retention Test. *Journal of Gerontology*, *37*, 87–90.

Atchley, R. C. (1975). Adjustment to loss of job at retirement. *International Journal of Aging and Human Development*, *6*, 17–27.

Atchley, R. C. (1989). A continuity theory of normal aging. *The Gerontologist*, *29*, 183–190.

Atkinson, L., Bowman, T. G., Dickens, S., Blackwell, J., Vasarhelyi, J., Szep, P., Dunleavy, B., MacIntyre, R., & Bury, A. (1990). Stability of Wechsler Adult Intelligence Scale—Revised factor scores across time. *Psychological Assessment: A Journal of Consulting and Clinical Psychology*, *2*, 447–450.

Axelrod, S., & Cohen, L. D. (1961). Senescence and embedded-figure performance in vision and touch. *Perceptual and Motor Skills*, *12*, 283–288.

Babchuk, N. (1978). Childlessness and social isolation among the elderly. *Journal of Marriage and the Family*, *42*, 277–281.

Babikian, V., & Ropper, A. H. (1987). Binswanger's disease: A review. *Stroke*, *18*, 2–12.

Backman, L. (1985). Further evidence for the lack of adult age differences on free recall of subject-performed tasks: The importance of motor action. *Human Learning*, *4*, 79–87.

Backman, L., & Nilsson, L.-G. (1985). Prerequisites for lack of age differences in memory performance. *Experimental Aging Research*, *11*, 67–73.

Baddeley, A. D. (1986). *Working memory*. New York: Oxford University Press.

Bahrick, H. P., Bahrick, P. O., & Wittlinger, R. P. (1975). Fifty years of memory for names and faces: A cross-sectional approach. *Journal of Experimental Psychology: General*, *104*, 54–75.

Bak, J. S., & Greene, R. L. (1980). Changes in neuropsychological functioning in an aging population. *Journal of Consulting and Clinical Psychology*, *48*, 395–399.

Ball, S. S., Marsh, J. T., Schubarth, G., Brown, W. S., & Strandburg, R. (1989). Longitudinal P300 latency changes in Alzheimer's disease. *Journal of Gerontology: Medical Sciences*, *44*, M195–200.

Baltes, P. B., & Schaie, K. W. (1974). Aging and IQ: The Myth of the twilight years. *Psychology Today*, *7*, 35–40.

Baltes, P. B., Reese, H. W. & Nesselroade, J. R. (1977). *Life-span developmental psychology: Introduction to research methods*. Monterey, CA: Brooks/Cole.

Baltes, P. B., Sowarka, D., & Kliegl, R. (1989). Cognitive training research on fluid intelligence in old age: What can older adults achieve by themselves? *Psychology and Aging, 4*, 217–221.

Banks, P. G., Dickson, A. L., & Plasay, M. T. (1987). The verbal selective reminding test: Preliminary data for healthy elderly. *Experimental Aging Research, 13*, 203–206.

Barbeau, A. (1984). Etiology of Parkinson's disease: A research strategy. *Canadian Journal of Neurological Sciences, 11*, 24–28.

Barbeau, A., Sourkes, T. L., & Murphy, G. F. (1962). Les catecholamines dans la maladie de Parkinson. In J. de Ajuriaguerra (Ed.), *Monoamines et systeme nerveux central* (pp. 247–262). Paris: Masson.

Barbeau, A., Roy, M., Cloutier, T., Plasse, L., & Paris, S. (1986). Environmental and genetic factors in the etiology of Parkinson's disease. *Advances in Neurology, 45*, 299–306.

Barclay, L. L., Zemcov, A., Blass, J. P., & Sansone, J. (1985). Survival in Alzheimer's disease and vascular dementias. *Neurology, 35*, 834–840.

Barona, A., Reynolds, C., & Chastain, R. (1984). A demographically based index of premorbid intelligence for the WAIS-R. *Journal of Consulting and Clinical Psychology, 52*, 885–887.

Barr, M. L., & Kiernan, J. A. (1988). *The human nervous system: An anatomical viewpoint* (5th ed.). Philadelphia: J. B. Lippincott.

Bartus, R. T., Dean, R. L., III, Beer, B., & Lippa, A. S. (1982). The cholinergic hypothesis of geriatric memory dysfunction. *Science, 217*, 408–417.

Baxter, D. (1987). Clinical syndromes associated with stroke. In M. E. Brandstater & J. V. Basmajian (Eds.), *Stroke rehabilitation* (pp. 36–54). Baltimore: Williams & Wilkins.

Baxter, L. R., Schwartz, J. M., Phelps, M. E., Mazziotta, J. C., Guze, B. H., Selin, C. E., Gerner, R. H., & Sumida, R. M. (1989). Reduction of prefrontal cortex glucose metabolism common to three types of depression. *Archives of General Psychiatry, 46*, 243–250.

Bayles, K. A., & Kaszniak, A. W. (1987). *Communication and cognition in normal aging and dementia*. Boston: College-Hill.

Bayles, K. A., & Tomoeda, C. K. (1983). Confrontation naming impairment in dementia. *Brain and Language, 19*, 98–114.

Bayles, K. A., Tomoeda, C. K., & Boone, D. R. (1985). A view of age-related changes in language function. *Developmental Neuropsychology, 1*, 231–264.

Beatty, W. W., Salmon, D. P., Butters, N., Heindel, W. C., & Granholm, E. L. (1988). Retrograde amnesia in patients with Alzheimer's disease or Huntington's disease. *Neurobiology of Aging, 9*, 181–186.

Beck, A. T., & Beck, R. W. (1972). Screening depressed patients in family practice: A rapid technique. *Postgraduate Medicine, 52*, 81–85.

Beck, A. T., Ward, C. H., Mendelson, M., Mock, J., & Erbaugh, J. (1961). An inventory for measuring depression. *Archives of General Psychiatry, 4*, 561–571.

Beck, E. C., Swanson, C., & Dustman, R. E. (1980). Long latency components of the visually evoked potential in man: Effects of aging. *Experimental Aging Research, 6*, 523–542.

Becker, J. T. (1988). Working memory and secondary memory deficits in Alzheimer disease. *Journal of Clinical and Experimental Neuropsychology, 10*, 739–753.

Becker, J. T., Boller, F., Saxton, J., & McGonigle-Gibson, K. L. (1987). Normal rates of forgetting of verbal and non-verbal material in Alzheimer's disease. *Cortex, 23*, 59–72.

Beckman, L. J. (1981). Effects of social interaction and children's relative inputs on older women's psychological well-being. *Journal of Personality and Social Psychology, 41*, 1075–1086.

Bengtson, V. L., Reedy, M. N., & Gordon, C. (1985). Aging and self-conceptions, personality processes and social contexts. In J. E. Birren & K. W. Schaie (Eds.), *Handbook of the psychology of aging* (pp. 544–593). New York: Van Nostrand Reinhold.

Benson, D. F. (1979). Neurologic correlates of anomia. In H. Whitaker & H. A. Whitaker (Eds.), *Studies in neurolinguistics* (Vol. 4, pp. 293–328). New York: Academic Press.

Benson, D. F., Kuhl, D. E., Hawkins, R. A., Phelps, M. E., Cummings, J. L., & Tsai, S. Y. (1983). The fluorodeoxyglucose 18F scan in Alzheimer's disease and multi-infarct dementia. *Archives of Neurology*, *40*, 711–714.

Benton, A. L. (1974). *Revised Visual Retention Test* (4th ed.). New York: Psychological Corporation.

Benton, A. L., & Hamsher, K. de S. (1976). *Multilingual Aphasia Examination*. Iowa City: University of Iowa Press.

Benton, A. L., Hamsher, K. de S., & Stone, F. B. (1977). *Visual Retention Test: Multiple Choice I*. Iowa City: University of Iowa Hospitals and Clinics.

Benton, A. L., Van Allen, M. W., Hamsher, K., & Levin, H. S. (1978a). *Test of facial recognition*. Iowa City: University of Iowa Hospitals.

Benton, A. L., Varney, N. R., & Hamsher, K. de S. (1978b). Visuospatial judgment: A clinical test. *Archives of Neurology*, *35*, 364–367.

Benton, A. L., Eslinger, P. J., & Damasio, A. R. (1981). Normative observations on neuropsychological test performances in old age. *Journal of Clinical Neuropsychology*, *3*, 33–42.

Berezin, M. A. (1972). Psychodynamic considerations of aging and the aged: An overview. *American Journal of Psychiatry*, *128*, 33–41.

Berg, E. A. (1948). Simple objective technique for measuring flexibility in thinking. *Journal of General Psychology*, *39*, 15–22.

Berg, L. (1985). Does Alzheimer's disease represent an exaggeration of normal aging? *Archives of Neurology*, *42*, 737–739.

Berg, L. (1988a). The aging brain. In R. Strong, W. G. Wood, & W. J. Burke (Eds.), *Central nervous disorders of aging: Clinical intervention and research* (pp. 1–16). New York: Raven Press.

Berg, L. (1988b). Mild senile dementia of the Alzheimer type: Diagnostic criteria and natural history. *Mount Sinai Journal of Medicine*, *55*, 87–96.

Bernstein, J. G. (1984). Pharmacotherapy of geriatric depression. *Journal of Clinical Psychiatry*, *45*, 30–34.

Binstock, R. H. (1983). The aged as scapegoat. *The Gerontologist*, *23*, 136–143.

Birren, J. E., & Schaie, K. W. (Eds.). (1985). *Handbook of the psychology of aging* (2nd ed.). New York: Van Nostrand Reinhold.

Birren, J. E., & Schaie, K. W. (Eds.). (1990). *Handbook of the psychology of aging* (3rd ed.). New York: Academic Press.

Birren, J. E., & Zarit, J. (1985). *Concepts of health, behavior, and aging: Cognition, stress and aging* (pp. 1–18), Englewood Cliffs, NJ: Prentice-Hall.

Birren, J. E., Butler, R. N., Greenhouse, S. W., Sokoloff, L., & Yarrow, M. R. (1963). Interdisciplinary relationships: Interrelations of physiological, psychological and psychiatric findings in healthy elderly men. In J. E. Birren, R. N. Butler, S. W. Greenhouse, L. Sokoloff, & M. R. Yarrow (Eds.), *Human aging: A biological and behavioral study* (pp. 283–305). Washington, DC: U.S. Government Printing Office.

Bjorksten, J. (1968). The crosslinkage theory of aging. *Journal of American Geriatrics Society*, *16*, 408–427.

Blackburn, J. A. (1984). The influence of personality, curriculum, and memory correlates on formal reasoning in young adults and elderly persons. *Journal of Gerontology*, *39*, 207–209.

Blackburn, J. A., Papalia-Finlay, Foye, B. F., & Serlin, R. C. (1988). Modifiability of figural relations performance among elderly adults. *Journal of Gerontology: Psychological Sciences*, *43*, P87–89.

Blair, J. R., & Preen, O. (1989). Predicting premorbid IQ: A revision of the National Adult Reading Test. *The Clinical Neuropsychologist*, *3*, 129–136.

Blau, E., & Ober, B. A. (1988, January). *The effect of depression on verbal memory in older adults*. Paper presented at a meeting of the International Neuropsychological Society, New Orleans.

Blazer, D. G. (1989). Affective disorders in late life. In E. W. Busse &D. G. Blazer (Eds.), *Geriatric psychiatry* (pp. 369–401). Washington, DC: American Psychiatric Press.

Blazer, D. G., & Williams, C. D. (1980). Epidemiology of dysphoria and depression in an elderly population. *American Journal of Psychiatry*, *137*, 439–444.

Blazer, D., Hughes, D. C., & George, L. K. (1987). The epidemiology of depression in an elderly community population. *The Gerontologist*, *27*, 281–187.

Bleecker, M. L., Bolla-Wilson, K., Kawas, C., & Agnew, J. (1988). Age-specific norms for the Mini-Mental State Exam. *Neurology*, *38*, 1565–1568.

Blessed, G., & Wilson, I. D. (1982). The contemporary natural history of mental disorder in old age. *British Journal of Psychiatry*, *141*, 59–61.

Blessed, G., Tomlinson, B. E., & Roth, M. (1968). The association between quantitative measures of dementia and of senile change in the cerebral grey matter of elderly subjects. *British Journal of Psychiatry*, *114*, 797–811.

Blumenthal, J. A., Emery, C. F., Madden, D. J., George, L. K., Coleman, R. E., Riddle, M. W., McKee, D. C., Reasoner, J., & Williams, R. S. (1989). Cardiovascular and behavioral effects of aerobic exercise training in healthy older men and women. *Journal of Gerontology: Medical Sciences*, *44*, M147–157.

Boller, F., & Vignolo, L. A. (1966). Latent sensory aphasia in hemisphere-damaged patients: An experimental study with the Token Test. *Brain*, *89*, 815–831.

Boller, F., Mizutani, T., Roessmann, U., & Gambetti, P. (1980). Parkinson disease, dementia and Alzheimer disease: Clinicopathological correlations. *Annals of Neurology*, *7*, 329–335.

Boller, F., Passafiume, D., Keefe, N. C., Rogers, K., Morrow, L., & Kim, Y. (1984). Visuospatial impairment in Parkinson's disease. *Archives of Neurology*, *41*, 485–490.

Bondareff, W. (1985). The neural basis of aging. In J. E. Birren & K. W. Schaie (Eds.), *Handbook of the psychology of aging* (2nd ed., pp. 95–112). New York: Van Nostrand Reinhold.

Bornstein, R. (1985). Normative data on selected neuropsychological measures from a nonclinical sample. *Journal of Clinical Psychology*, *41*, 651–659.

Bornstein, R. A., Termeer, J., Longbrake, K., Heger, M., & North, R. (1989). WAIS-R cholinergic deficit profile in depression. *Psychological Assessment: A Journal of Consulting and Clinical Psychology*, *1*, 342–344.

Borod, J. C., Goodglass, H., & Kaplan, E. (1980). Normative data on the Boston Diagnostic Aphasia Examination, Parietal Lobe Battery, and the Boston Naming Test. *Journal of Clinical Neuropsychology*, *2*, 209–215.

Bosse, R., Aldwin, C. W., Levenson, M. R., & Ekerdt, D. J. (1987). Mental health differences among retirees and workers: Findings from the Normative Aging Study. *Psychology and Aging*, *2*, 383–389.

Botwinick, J. (1977). Intellectual abilities. In J. E. Birren & K. W. Schaie (Eds.), *Handbook of the psychology of aging* (pp. 580–605). New York: Van Nostrand Reinhold.

Botwinick, J. (1984). *Aging and behavior* (3rd ed.). New York: Springer.

Botwinick, J., & Storandt, M. (1974a). *Memory, related functions, and age*. Springfield, IL: Charles C Thomas.

Botwinick, J., & Storandt, M. (1974b). Vocabulary ability in later life. *Journal of Genetic Psychology*, *125*, 303–308.

Botwinick, J., & Storandt, M. (1980). Recall and recognition of old information in relation to age and sex. *Journal of Gerontology*, *35*, 70–76.

Botwinick, J., Storandt, M., & Berg, L. (1986). A longitudinal, behavioral study of senile dementia of the Alzheimer type. *Archives of Neurology*, *43*, 1124–1127.

Bowen, D. M., Benton, J. S., Spillane, J. A., Smith, C. C. T., & Allen, S. J. (1982). Choline acetyltransferase activity and histopathology of frontal neocortex from biopsies of demented patients. *Journal of Neurological Science*, *57*, 191–202.

Bowles, N. L., & Poon, L. W. (1985). Aging and retrieval of words in semantic memory. *Journal of Gerontology*, *40*, 71–77.

Bowles, N. L., Obler, L., & Albert, M. L. (1987). Naming errors in healthy aging and dementia of the Alzheimer type. *Cortex*, *23*, 519–524.

Braff, D. L., & Beck, A. T. (1974). Thinking disorder in depression. *Archives of General Psychiatry*, *31*, 456–459.

Braithwaite, V. A. (1986). Old age stereotypes: Reconciling contradictions. *Journal of Gerontology*, *41*, 353–360.

Branconnier, R. J., deVitt, D. R., Cole, J. O., & Spera, K. F. (1982). Amitriptyline selectively disrupts verbal recall from secondary memory of the normal aged. *Neurobiology of Aging*, *3*, 55–59.

Brandt, J., Spencer, M. McSorley, P., & Folstein, M. F. (1988). Semantic activation and implicit memory in Alzheimer Disease. *Alzheimer Disease and Associated Disorders*, *2*, 112–119.

Breitner, J. C. S., & Folstein, M. F. (1984). Familial Alzheimer's dementia: A prevalent disorder with specific clinical features. *Psychological Medicine*, *14*, 63–80.

Breslow, R., Kocsis, J., & Belkin, B. (1980). Memory deficits in depression: Evidence utilizing the Wechsler Memory Scale. *Perceptual and Motor Skills*, *51*, 541–542.

Bressler, R. (1987). Drug use in the geriatric patient. In L. L. Carstensen & B. A. Edelstein (Eds.), *Handbook of clinical gerontology* (pp. 152–174). New York: Pergamon Press.

Brinkman, S. D., & Braun, P. (1984). Classification of dementia patients by a WAIS profile related to central cholinergic deficiencies. *Journal of Clinical Neuropsychology*, *6*, 393–400.

Brody, H. (1955). Organization of the cerebral cortex: 3. A study of aging in the human cerebral cortex. *Journal of Comparative Neurology*, *102*, 511–556.

Bromley, D. B. (1957). Some effects of age on the quality of intellectual output. *Journal of Gerontology*, *12*, 318–323.

Brooks, D. J., & Frackowiak, R. S. J. (1989). PET and movement disorders. *Journal of Neurology, Neurosurgery, and Psychiatry, Special Supplement*, 68–77.

Brown, R. G., & Marsden, C. D. (1984). How common is dementia in Parkinson's disease? *Lancet*, *2*, 1262–1265.

Brown, R. G., & Marsden, C. D. (1986). Visuospatial function in Parkinson's disease. *Brain*, *109*, 987–1002.

Brown, R. G., Marsden, C. D., Quinn, N., & Wyke, M. A. (1984). Alterations in cognitive performance and affect-arousal state during fluctuations in motor function in Parkinson's disease. *Journal of Neurology, Neurosurgery and Psychiatry*, *47*, 454–465.

Brown, W. S., Marsh, J. T., & La Rue, A. (1983). Exponential electrophysiological aging: P3 latency. *Electroencephalography and Clinical Neurophysiology*, *55*, 277–285.

Brust, J. C. M. (1988). Vascular dementia is overdiagnosed. *Archives of Neurology*, *45*, 799–801.

Buell, S. J., & Coleman, P. D. (1979). Dendritic growth in the aged human brain and failure of growth in senile dementia. *Science*, *206*, 854–856.

Buhler, C. (1968). The general structure of the human life cycle. In C. Buhler & F. Massarik (Eds.), *In the course of human life*. New York: Springer.

Bunney, W. E., Jr., & Davis, J. M. (1965). Norepinephrine in depressive reactions: A review. *Archives of General Psychiatry*, *13*, 483–494.

Burger, P. C., & Vogel, F. S. (1973). The development of the pathologic changes in Alzheimer's disease and senile dementia in patients with Down's syndrome. *American Journal of Pathology*, *73*, 457–476.

Burke, H. R. (1972). Raven's Progressive Matrices: Validity, reliability and norms. *Journal of Psychology*, *82*, 253–257.

Burke, W. J., Rubin, E. H., Zorumski, C. F., & Wetzel, R. D. (1987). The safety of ECT in geriatric psychiatry. *Journal of the American Geriatrics Society*, *35*, 516–521.

Burke, W. J., Miller, J. P., Rubin, E. H., Morris, J. C., Coben, L. A., Duchek, J., Wittels, I. G., & Berg, L. (1988). Reliability of the Washington University Clinical Dementia Rating. *Archives of Neurology*, *45*, 31–32.

Burns, J. E., Elias, M. F., Hitchcock, A. G., & St. Germain, R. (1980). Corroboration of the utility of the Satz-Mogel abbreviated WAIS with hospitalized geriatric patients. *Experimental Aging Research*, *6*, 181–184.

Burns, M., Moskowitz, H., & Jaffe, J. (1986). A comparison of the effects of trazodone and amitriptyline on skills performance by geriatric subjects. *Journal of Clinical Psychiatry*, *47*, 252–254.

Buschke, H., & Fuld, P. A. (1974). Evaluating storage, retention, and retrieval in disordered memory and learning. *Neurology*, *24*, 1019–1025.

Butcher, J. N., Dahlstrom, W. G., Graham, J. R., Tellegen, A., & Kaemmer, B. (1989). *Manual for the restandardized Minnesota Multiphasic Personality Inventory: MMPI-2*. Minneapolis: University of Minnesota Press.

Butler, R. N. (1974). Successful aging and the role of the life review. *Journal of American Geriatrics Society, 22*, 529–535.

Butler, R. N., & Lewis, M. I. (Eds.). (1973). *Aging and mental health: Positive psychosocial approaches.* St. Louis: C. V. Mosby.

Butters, N., Granholm, E., Salmon, D., Grant, I., & Wolfe, J. (1987). Episodic and semantic memory: A comparison of amnestic and demented patients. *Journal of Clinical and Experimental Neuropsychology, 9*, 479–497.

Butters, N., Salmon, D. P., Cullum, C. M., Cairns, P., Troster, A. I., Jacobs, D., Moss, M., & Cermack, L. S. (1988). Differentiation of amnesic and demented patients with the Wechsler Memory Scale-Revised. *The Clinical Neuropsychologist, 2*, 121–132.

Byrne, D. C. (1977). Affect and vigilance performance in depressive illness. *Journal of Psychiatric Research, 13*, 185–191.

Byrne, E. J. (1987). Reversible dementia. *International Journal of Geriatric Psychiatry, 2*, 73–81.

Byrne, K., & Stern, S. L. (1981). Antidepressant medication in the outpatient treatment of depression: Guide for nonmedical psychotherapists. *Professional Psychology, 12*, 302–308.

Caine, E. (1981). Pseudodementia: Current concepts and future directions. *Archives of General Psychiatry, 38*, 1359–1364.

Caine, E. D. (1986). The neuropsychology of depression: The pseudodementia syndrome. In I. Grant & K. M. Adams (Eds.), *Neuropsychological assessment of neuropsychiatric disorders* (pp. 221–243). New York: Oxford University Press.

Calne, D. B., & Langston, J. W. (1983). Aetiology of Parkinson's disease. *Lancet, 2*, 1457–1459.

Calne, D. B., Crippa, D., Comi, G., Horowski, R., & Trabucchi, M. (Eds.). (1989). *Parkinsonism and aging.* New York: Raven Press.

Caltagirone, C., Carlesimo, A., Nocentini, U., & Vicari, S. (1989). Defective concept formation in Parkinsonians is independent from mental deterioration. *Journal of Neurology, Neurosurgery, and Psychiatry, 52*, 334–337.

Camp, C. J., & Stevens, A. B. (1990). Spaced-retrieval: A memory intervention for dementia of the Alzheimer's type (DAT). *Clinical Gerontologist, 10*, 58–61.

Camp, C. J., West, R. L., & Poon, L. W. (1989). Recruitment practices for psychological research in gerontology. In M. P. Lawton & A. R. Herzog (Eds.), *Special research methods for gerontology* (pp. 163–189). Amityville, NY: Baywood.

Canestrari, R. E., Jr. (1968). Age changes in acquisition. In G. A. Talland (Ed.), *Human aging and behavior* (pp. 169–188). New York: Academic Press.

Capitani, E., Sala, S. D., Lucchelli, F., Soave, P., & Spinnler, H. (1988). Perceptual attention in aging and dementia measured by Gottschaldt's Hidden Figure Test. *Journal of Gerontology: Psychological Sciences, 43*, P157–163.

Caplan, L. R., & Stein, R. W. (1986). *Stroke: A clinical approach.* Boston: Butterworths.

Cargnello, J. C., & Gurekas, R. (1987). The clinical use of a modified WAIS procedure in a geriatric population. *Journal of Clinical Psychology, 43*, 286–290.

Carlsson, A. (1986). Brain neurotransmitters in normal and pathological aging. In A. B. Scheibel & A. F. Wechsler (Eds.), *The biological substrates of Alzheimer's disease* (pp. 193–203). New York: Academic Press.

Carroll, B. J., Feinberg, M., Greden, J. F., Tarika, J., Albala, A. A., Haskett, R. F., James, N. M., Kronfol, Z., Lohr, N., Steiner, M., deVigne, J. P., & Young, E. (1981). A specific laboratory test for the diagnosis of melancholia. *Archives of General Psychiatry, 38*, 15–22.

Carughi, A., Carpenter, K. J., & Diamond, M. C. (1989). Effect of environmental enrichment during nutritional rehabilitation on body growth, blood parameters, and cerebral cortical development of rats. *Journal of Nutrition, 119*, 2005–2016.

Casey, J. E., Ferguson, G. G., Kimura, D., & Hachinski, V. C. (1989). Neuropsychological improvement versus practice effect following unilateral carotid endarterectomy in patients without stroke. *Journal of Clinical and Experimental Neuropsychology, 11*, 461–470.

Cattell, R. B. (1963). Theory of fluid and crystallized intelligence: A critical experiment. *Journal of Educational Psychology*, *54*, 1–22.
Cerella, J., Poon, L. W., & Fozard, J. L. (1982). Age and iconic read-out. *Journal of Gerontology*, *37*, 197–202.
Chandra, V., & Schoenberg, B. S. (1989). Inheritance of Alzheimer's disease: Epidemiologic evidence. *Neuroepidemiology*, *8*, 165–174.
Charness, N. (1981). Visual short-term memory and aging in chess players. *Journal of Gerontology*, *36*, 615–619.
Chase, T. N., Fedio, P., Foster, N. L., Brooks, R., Di Chiro, G., & Mansi, L. (1984). Wechsler Adult Intelligence Scale Performance. Cortical localization by fluorodeoxyglucose f18 positron emission tomography. *Archives of Neurology*, *41*, 1244–1247.
Christensen, A. L. (1975). *Luria's neuropsychological investigation*. New York: Spectrum.
Christensen, H., Hadzi-Pavlovic, D., & Jacomb, P. (1991). The psychometric differentiation of dementia from normal aging: A meta-analysis. *Psychological Assessment: A Journal of Consulting and Clinical Psychology*, *3*, 147–155.
Chui, H. C. (1989). Dementia: A review emphasizing clinicopathologic correlation and brain-behavior relationships. *Archives of Neurology*, *46*, 806–814.
Cicirelli, V. G. (1987). Locus of control and patient role adjustment of the elderly in acute-care hospitals. *Psychology and Aging*, *2*, 138–143.
Cicirelli, V. G. (1989). Feelings of attachment to siblings and well-being in later life. *Psychology and Aging*, *4*, 211–216.
Clarfield, A. M. (1988). The reversible dementias: Do they reverse? *Annals of Internal Medicine*, *109*, 476–486.
Clark, C. R., Geffen, G. M., & Geffen, L. B. (1987a). Catecholamines and attention: 1. Animal and clinical studies. *Neuroscience and Biobehavioral Reviews*, *11*, 323–352.
Clark, C. R., Geffen, G. M., & Geffen, L. B. (1987b). Catecholamines and attention: 2. Pharmacological studies in normal humans. *Neuroscience and Biobehavioral Reviews*, *11*, 353–364.
Clarkson-Smith, L., & Hartley, A. A. (1989). Relationships between physical exercise and cognitive abilities in older adults. *Psychology and Aging*, *4*, 183–189.
Clayton, P. J. (1973). The clinical morbidity of the first year of bereavement: A review. *Comprehensive Psychiatry*, *14*, 151–157.
Cohen, G. (1979). Language comprehension in old age. *Cognitive Psychology*, *11*, 412–429.
Cohen, G., & Faulkner, D. (1981). Memory for discourse in old age. *Discourse Processes*, *4*, 253–265.
Cohen, M. B., Graham, S., Lake, R. R., Metter, E. J., Fitten, J., Kulkarni, M. K., Sevrin, R., Yamada, L., Chang, C. C., Woodruff, N., & Kling, A. S. (1986). Differential diagnosis of dementia by tomographic imaging of the distribution of I-123 iodo-amphetamine. *Journal of Nuclear Medicine*, *27*, 769–774.
Cohen, N. J. (1984). Preserved learning capacity in amnesia: Evidence for multiple memory systems. In L. Squire & N. Butters (Eds.), *The neuropsychology of memory* (pp. 83–103). New York: Guilford Press.
Cohen, R. L., Sandler, S. P., & Schroeder, K. (1987). Aging and memory for words and action events: Effects of item repetition and list length. *Psychology and Aging*, *2*, 280–285.
Cohen, R. M., Weingartner, H., Smallberg, S. A., Pickar, D., & Murphy, D. L. (1982). Effort and cognition in depression. *Archives of General Psychiatry*, *39*, 593–597.
Cole, J. O., & Schatzberg, A. F. (1980). Memory difficulty and tricyclic antidepressants. In J. O. Cole (Ed.), *Psychopharmacology update* (pp. 189–195). Lexington, MA: Collamore Press.
Coleman, P. D., & Flood, D. G. (1988). Is dendritic proliferation of surviving neurons a compensatory reaction to loss of neighbors in the aging brain? In S. Finger, T. E. Le Vere, C. R. Almli, & D. G. Stein (Eds.), *Brain injury and recovery: Theoretical and controversial issues* (pp. 235–247). New York: Plenum Press.
Coleman, P. D., Higgins, G. A., & Phelps, C. H. (Eds.). (1990). *Molecular and cellular mechanisms of neuronal plasticity in normal aging and Alzheimer's disease*. Amsterdam: Elsevier.
Colligan, R. C., Osborne, D., Swenson, W. M., & Offord, M. S. (1984). Development of contemporary norms. *Mayo Clinic Proceedings*, *59*, 377–390.

Comalli, P. E. (1965). Cognitive functioning in a group of 89-90-year-old men. *Journal of Gerontology*, *20*, 14–17.

Comalli, P. E., Krus, D. M., & Wapner, S. (1965). Cognitive functions in two groups of aged: One institutionalized, the other living in the community. *Journal of Gerontology*, *20*, 9–13.

Comfort, A. (1979). *The biology of senescence*. New York, NY: Elsevier.

Cools, A. R., van den Bercken, J. H. L., Horstink, M. W. I., van Spaendonck, K. P. M., & Berger, H. J. C. (1984). Cognitive and motor shifting aptitude disorder in Parkinson's disease. *Journal of Neurology, Neurosurgery and Psychiatry*, *47*, 443–453.

Copeland, J. R. M., Kelleher, M. J., Kellett, J. M., Gourlay, A. J., Gurland, B. J., Fleiss, J. L., & Sharpe, L. (1976). A semi-structured clinical interview for the assessment of diagnosis and mental state in the elderly: The Geriatric Mental State Schedule: 1. Development and reliability. *Psychological Medicine*, *6*, 439–449.

Corkin, S., Growdon, J. H., Nissen, M. J., Huff, F. J., Freed, D. M., & Sagar, H. J. (1984). Recent advances in the neuropsychological study of Alzheimer's disease. In R. J. Wurtman, S. H. Corkin, & J. H. Growdon (Eds.), *Alzheimer's disease: Advances in basic research and therapies* (pp. 75–93). Cambridge, England: Centre for Brain Sciences and Metabolism Charitable Trust.

Cornelius, S. W., & Caspi. A. (1987). Everyday problem solving in adulthood and old age. *Psychology and Aging*, *2*, 144–153.

Costa, P. T., Jr., & Fozard, J. L. (1978). Remembering the person: Relations of individual difference variables to memory. *Experimental Aging Research*, *4*, 291–304.

Costa, P. T., Jr., Whitfield, J. R., & Stewart, D. (Eds.). (1989). *Alzheimer's disease: Abstracts of the psychological and behavioral literature*. Washington, DC: American Psychological Association.

Coughlan, A. K., & Hollows, S. E. (1984). Use of memory tests in differentiating organic disorder from depression. *British Journal of Psychiatry*, *145*, 164–167.

Craik, F. I. M. (1977). Age differences in human memory. In J. E. Birren & K. W. Schaie (Eds.), *Handbook of the psychology of aging* (pp. 384–420). New York: Van Nostrand Reinhold.

Craik, F. I. M. (1983). On the transfer of information from temporary to permanent memory. *Philosophical Transactions of the Royal Society, London, Series B*, *302*, 341–359.

Craik, F. I. M., & Byrd, M. (1982). Aging and cognitive deficits: The role of attentional processes. In F. I. M. Craik & S. Trehub (Eds.), *Aging and cognitive processes* (pp. 191–211). New York: Plenum Press.

Craik, F. I. M., & McDowd, J. M. (1987). Age differences in recall and recognition. *Journal of Experimental Psychology: Learning, Memory, and Cognition*, *13*, 474–479.

Craik, F. I. M., Byrd, M., & Swanson, J. M. (1987). Patterns of memory loss in three elderly samples. *Psychology and Aging*, *2*, 79–86.

Cronholm, R., & Ottosson, J. (1961). Memory functions in endogenous depression. *Archives of General Psychiatry*, *5*, 101–107.

Crook, T., & Larrabee, G. J. (1990). A self-rating scale for evaluating memory in everyday life. *Psychology and Aging*, *5*, 48–57.

Crook, T., Ferris, S., & McCarthy, M. (1979). The misplaced-objects task: A brief test for memory dysfunction in the aged. *Journal of the American Geriatrics Society*, *27*, 284–287.

Crook, T., Ferris, S., McCarthy, M., & Rae, D. (1980). Utility of digit recall tasks for assessing memory in the aged. *Journal of Consulting and Clinical Psychology*, *48*, 228–233.

Crook, T., Salama, M., & Gobert, J. (1986). A computerized test battery for detecting and assessing memory disorders. In A. Bes, J. Cahn, S. Hoyer, J. P. Marc-Vergenes, & H. M. Wisniewski, *Senile dementias: Early Detection* (pp. 79–85). London and Paris: John Libbey Eurotext.

Crookes, T. G., & McDonald, K. G. (1972). Benton's Visual Retention Test in the differentiation of depression and early dementia. *British Journal of Social and Clinical Psychology*, *2*, 66–69.

Crosson, B., & Warren, R. L. (1982). Use of the Luria-Nebraska Neuropsychological Battery in aphasia: A conceptual critique. *Journal of Consulting and Clinical Psychology*, *50*, 22–31.

Cummings, J. L. (1989). Dementia and depression: An evolving enigma. *Journal oofNeuropsychiatry*, *1*, 236–242.

Cummings, J. L., & Benson, D. F. (1983). *Dementia: A clinical approach*. Boston: Butterworths.

Cummings, J. L., & Benson, D. F. (1984). Subcortical dementia: Review of an emerging concept. *Archives of Neurology, 41*, 874–879.

Cummings, J. L., & Benson, D. F. (1987). The role of the nucleus basalis of Meynert in dementia: Review and reconsideration. *Alzheimer Disease and Associated Disorders, 1*, 128–145.

Cummings, J. L., & Benson, D. F. (1988). Psychological dysfunction accompanying subcortical dementias. *Annual Review of Medicine, 39*, 53–61.

Cummings, J. L., Miller, B., Hill, M. A., & Neshkes, R. (1987). Neuropsychiatric aspects of multi-infarct dementia and dementia of the Alzheimer type. *Archives of Neurology, 44*, 389–393.

Cummings, J. L., Darkins, A., Mendez, M., Hill, M. A., & Benson, D. F. (1988). Alzheimer's disease and Parkinson's disease: Comparison of speech and language alterations. *Neurology, 38*, 680–684.

Cutler, R. G., (1982). Longevity is determined by specific genes: Testing the hypothesis. In R. C. Adelman & G. S. Roth (Eds.), *Testing the theories of aging* (pp. 25–114). Boca Raton, FL: CRC Press.

Cutler, S. J., & Grams, A. E. (1988). Correlates of self-reported everyday memory problems. *Journal of Gerontology: Social Sciences, 43*, S82–90.

Danziger, W. L., & Salthouse, T. A. (1978). Age and the perception of incomplete figures. *Experimental Aging Research, 4*, 67–80.

Davidson, J. (1989). The pharmacologic treatment of psychiatric disorders in the elderly. In E. W. Busse & D. G. Blazer (Eds.), *Geriatric psychiatry* (pp. 515–542). Washington, DC: American Psychiatric Press.

Davies, A. (1968). The influence of age on Trail Making Test performance. *Journal of Clinical Psychology, 24*, 96–98.

Davies, P., & Maloney, A. J. F. (1976). Selective loss of central cholinergic neurons in Alzheimer's disease. *Lancet, 2*, 1403.

Davies, P., Katzman, R., & Terry, R. D. (1980). Reduced somatostatin-like immunoreactivity in cerebral cortex from cases of Alzheimer disease and Alzheimer senile dementia. *Nature, 288*, 279–280.

Davis, P. E., & Mumford, S. J. (1984). Cued recall and the nature of the memory disorder in dementia. *British Journal of Psychiatry, 144*, 383–386.

Dean, R. S., Gray, J. W., & Seretny, M. L. (1987). Cognitive aspects of schizophrenia and primary affective depression. *International Journal of Clinical Neuropsychology, 9*, 33–36.

DeFilippis, N. A., McCampbell, E., & Rogers, P. (1979). Development of a booklet form of the Category Test: Normative and validity data. *Journal of Clinical Neuropsychology, 1*, 339–342.

Dekaban, A. S., & Sadowsky, B. S. (1978). Changes in brain weights during the span of human life: Relation of brain weights to body heights and body weights. *Annals of Neurology, 4*, 345–356.

de Leon, M. J., George, A. E., Ferris, S. H., Christman, D. R., Fowler, J. S., Gentes, C., Brodie, J., Reisberg, B., & Wolf, A. P. (1984). Positron emission tomography and computed tomography assessments of the aging human brain. *Journal of Computer Assisted Tomography, 8*, 88–94.

de Leon, M. J., George, A. E., & Ferris, S. H. (1986). Computed tomography and positron emission tomography correlates of cognitive decline in aging and senile dementia. In L. W. Poon (Ed.), *Handbook for clinical memory assessment of older adults* (pp. 367–382). Washington, DC: American Psychological Association.

D'Elia, L. F., & Boone, K. B. (1992). *Handbook of normative data for neuropsychological assessment*. New York: Oxford University Press.

D'Elia, L., Satz, P., & Schretlen, D. (1989). Wechsler Memory Scale: A critical appraisal of the normative studies. *Journal of Clinical and Experimental Neuropsychology, 11*, 551–568.

Delis, D. C., & Kaplan, E. (1982). Assessment of aphasia with the Luria-Nebraska Neuropsychological Battery. A case critique. *Journal of Consulting and Clinical Psychology, 50*, 32–39.

Delis, D. C., & Kaplan, E. (1983). Hazards of a standardized neuropsychological test with low content validity: Comment on the Luria-Nebraska Neuropsychological Battery. *Journal of Consulting and Clinical Psychology, 51*, 396–398.

Delis, D., Direnfeld, L., Alexander, M. P., & Kaplan, E. (1982). Cognitive fluctuations associated with on-off phenomenon in Parkinson disease. *Neurology, 32*, 1049–1052.

Delis, D. C., Kramer, J. H., Kaplan, E., & Ober, B. A. (1987). *The California Verbal Learning Test, Research Edition*. New York: Psychological Corporation.

Delis, D. C., Kramer, J. H., Freeland, J., & Kaplan, E. (1988). Integrating clinical assessment with cognitive neuroscience: Construct validation of the California Verbal Learning Test. *Journal of Consulting and Clinical Psychology*, *56*, 123–130.

Demming, J. A., & Pressey, S. L. (1957). Tests "indigenous" to the adult and older years. *Journal of Counseling Psychology*, *4*, 144–148.

Denney, N. W., & Denney, D. R. (1982). The relationship between classification and questioning strategies among adults. *Journal of Gerontology*, *37*, 190–196.

Denney, N. W., & Palmer, A. M. (1981). Adult age differences on traditional and practical problem-solving measures. *Journal of Gerontology*, *36*, 323–328.

Denney, N. W., Pearce, K. A., & Palmer, A. M. (1982). A developmental study of adults' performance on traditional and practical problem-solving tasks. *Experimental Aging Research*, *8*, 115–118.

Derix, M. M. A., Hijdra, A., & Verbeeten, B. W. J., Jr. (1987). Mental changes in subcortical arteriosclerotic encephalopathy. *Clinical Neurology and Neurosurgery*, *89*, 71–78.

desRosiers, G., & Ivison, D. (1986). Paired associate learning: Normative data for differences between high and low associate word pairs. *Journal of Clinical and Experimental Neuropsychology*, *8*, 637–642.

DeVane, C. L., & Tingle, D. (1988). Psychiatric disorders. In J. C. Delafuente & R. B. Stewart (Eds.), *Therapeutics in the elderly* (pp. 185–195). Baltimore: Williams & Wilkins.

Divoll, M. K., & Greenblatt, D. J. (1987). Drug interactions and adverse drug reactions in the elderly. In C. G. Swift (Ed.), *Clinical pharmacology in the elderly* (pp. 119–148). New York: Marcel Dekker.

Doppelt, J. E., & Wallace, W. L. (1955). Standardization of the Wechsler Adult Intelligence Scale for older persons. *Journal of Abnormal and Social Psychology*, *51*, 312–330.

Dowson, J. H. (1982). Neuronal lipofuscin accumulation in ageing and Alzheimer Dementia: A pathogenic mechanism? *British Journal of Psychiatry*, *140*, 142–148.

Drachman, D. A., & Leavitt, J. (1974). Human memory and the cholinergic system. *Archives of Neurology*, *30*, 113–121.

Drachman, D. A., & Swearer, J. M. (1990). The therapy of Alzheimer's disease. In R. Porter & B. Schoenberg (Eds.), *Controlled clinical trials in neurologic disease* (pp. 361–391). Norwell, MA: Kluwer Academic.

Duara, R., Margolin, R. A., Robertson-Tchabo, E. A., London, E. D., Schwartz, M., Renfrew, J. W., Koziarz, B. J., Sundaram, M., Grady, C., Moore, A. M., Ingvar, D. H., Sokoloff, L., Weingartner, H., Kessler, R. M., Manning, R. G., Channing, M. A., Cutler, N. R., & Rapoport, S. I. (1983). Cerebral glucose utilization as measured with positron emission tomography in 21 resting healthy men between the ages of 21 and 83 years. *Brain*, *106*, 761–775.

Duara, R., Grady, C., Haxby, J., Ingvar, D., Sokoloff, L., Margolin, R. A., Manning, R. G., Cutler, N. R., & Rapoport, S. I. (1983). Human brain glucose utilization and cognitive function in relation to age. *Annals of Neurology*, *16*, 702–713.

Duffy, F. H., & McAnulty, G. (1988). Electrophysiological studies. In M. S. Albert & M. B. Moss (Eds.), *Geriatric neuropsychology* (pp. 262–289). New York: Guilford Press.

Duffy, F. H., Albert, M. S., & McAnulty, G. (1984a). Brain electrical activity in patients with presenile and senile dementia of the Alzheimer's Type. *Annals of Neurology*, *16*, 439–448.

Duffy, F. H., Albert, M. S., McAnulty, G., & Garvey, A. J. (1984b). Age-related differences in brain electrical activity of healthy subjects. *Annals of Neurology*, *16*, 430–438.

Dumbrille-Ross, A., & Tang, S. W. (1983). Noradrenergic and serotonergic receptor densities. *Psychiatry Research*, *9*, 207–215.

Dustman, R. E., Snyder, E. W., & Schlehuber, C. J. (1981). Life-span alterations in visual evoked potentials and inhibitory function. *Neurobiology of Aging*, *2*, 187–192.

Dustman, R., LaMarche, J., Cohn, N., Shearer, D. E., & Talone, J. M. (1985). Power spectral analysis and cortical coupling of EEG for young and old normal adults. *Neurobiology of Aging*, *6*, 193–198.

Duvoisin, R. C., Eldridge, R., Williams, A., Nutt, J., & Calne, D. (1981). Twin study of Parkinson disease. *Neurology*, *31*, 77–80.

Dysken, M. W., Katz, R., Stallone, F., & Kuskowski, M. (1989). Oxiracetam in the treatment of multi-infarct dementia and primary degenerative dementia. *Journal of Neuropsychiatry*, *1*, 249–252.

Earnest, P. E., Heaton, R. K., Wilkinson, W. E., & Manke, W. F. (1979). Cortical atrophy, ventricular enlargement and intellectual impairment in the aged. *Neurology*, *29*, 1138–1143.

El-Awar, M., Becker, J. T., Hammond, K. M., Nebes, R. D., & Boller, F. (1987). Learning deficit in Parkinson's disease. *Archives of Neurology*, *44*, 180–184.

Endicott, J., Spitzer, R. L., Fleiss, J. L., & Cohen, J. (1976). The Global Assessment Scale. *Archives of General Psychiatry*, *33*, 766–771.

Erber, J. T., Botwinick, J., & Storandt, M. (1981). The impact of memory on age differences in Digit Symbol performance. *Journal of Gerontology*, *36*, 586–590.

Erickson, R. C., & Scott, M. L. (1977). Clinical memory tests: A review. *Psychology Bulletin*, *84*, 1130–1149.

Erikson, E. (1959). Identify and the life cycle. *Psychological Issues*, *1*, 50–100.

Erikson, E. H., Erikson, J. M., & Kivnick, H. Q. (1986). *Vital involvement in old age*. New York: Norton.

Erkinjuntti, T. (1987). Differential diagnosis between Alzheimer's disease and vascular dementia: Evaluation of common clinical methods. *Acta Neurologica Scandinavica*, *76*, 433–442.

Ernst, J. (1987). Neuropsychological problem-solving skills in the elderly. *Psychology and Aging*, *2*, 363–365.

Escobar, J. I., Burnam, A., Karno, M., Forsythe, A., Landsverk, J., & Golding, J. M. (1986). Use of the Mini-Mental State Examination (MMSE) in a community population of mixed ethnicity. *Journal of Nervous and Mental Disease*, *174*, 607–614.

Eslinger, P. J., & Benton, A. L. (1983). Visuoperceptual performances in aging and dementia: Clinical and theoretical implications. *Journal of Clinical Neuropsychology*, *5*, 213–220.

Eslinger, P. J., & Damasio, A. R. (1986). Preserved motor learning in Alzheimer's disease: Implications for anatomy and behavior. *Journal of Neuroscience*, *6*, 3006–3009.

Eslinger, P. J., Damasio, A. R., Benton, A. L., & Van Allen, M. (1985). Neuropsychologic detection of abnormal mental decline in older persons. *Journal of the American Medical Association*, *253*, 670–674.

Eslinger, P. J., Pepin, L., & Benton, A. L. (1988). Different patterns of visual memory errors occur with aging and dementia. *Journal of Clinical and Experimental Neuropsychology*, *10*, 60–61.

Evans, D. A., Funkenstein, H. H., Albert, M. S., Scherr, P. A., Cook, N. R., Chown, M. J., Hebert, L. E., Hennekens, C. H., & Taylor, J. O. (1989). Prevalence of Alzheimer's Disease in a community population of older persons. *Journal of the American Medical Association*, *262*, 2551–2556.

Farver, P. F., & Farver, T. B. (1982). Performance of normal older adults on tests designed to measure parietal lobe functions. *American Journal of Occupational Therapy*, *36*, 444–449.

Ferris, S., Crook, T., Sathananthan, G., & Gershon, S. (1976). Reaction time as a diagnostic measure in senility. *Journal of the American Geriatrics Society*, *24*, 529–533.

Field, D., & Minkler, M. (1988). Continuity and change in social support between young-old and old-old or very-old age. *Journal of Gerontology: Psychological Sciences*, *43*, P100–106.

Filley, C. M., Kobayashi, J., & Heaton, R. K. (1987). Wechsler Intelligence Scale profiles, the cholinergic system, and Alzheimer's disease. *Journal of Clinical and Experimental Neuropsychology*, *9*, 180–186.

Finch, C. E., & Schneider, E. L. (Eds.). (1985). *Handbook of the biology of aging* (2nd ed.). New York: Van Nostrand Reinhold.

Fischer, P., Gatterer, G., Marterer, A., & Danielczyk, W. (1988). Nonspecificity of semantic impairment in dementia of Alzheimer's type. *Archives of Neurology*, *45*, 1341–1343.

Fisher, C. M. (1982). Lacunar strokes and infarcts: A review. *Neurology*, *32*, 871–876.

Flicker, C., Ferris, S. H., Crook, T., & Bartus, R. T. (1987). Implications of memory and language dysfunction in the naming deficit of senile dementia. *Brain and Language*, *31*, 187–200.

Flicker, C., Ferris, S. H., Crook, T., Reisberg, B., & Bartus, R. T. (1988). Equivalent spatial-rotation deficits in normal aging and Alzheimer's disease. *Journal of Clinical and Experimental Neuropsychology*, *10*, 387–399.

Flood, D. G., & Coleman, P. D. (1988). Neuron numbers and sizes in aging brain: Comparisons of human, monkey, and rodent data. *Neurobiology of Aging*, *9*, 453–463.

Flor-Henry, P. (1979). On certain aspects of the localization of the cerebral systems regulating and determining emotion. *Biological Psychiatry*, *14*, 677–698.

Flowers, K. A., & Robertson, C. (1985). The effect of Parkinson's disease on the ability to maintain a mental set. *Journal of Neurology, Neurosurgery, and Psychiatry*, *48*, 517–529.

Folkman, S., Lazarus, R. S., Pimley, S., & Novacek, J. (1987). Age differences in stress and coping processes. *Psychology and Aging*, *2*, 171–184.

Folstein, M. F., & McHugh, P. R. (1978). Dementia syndrome of depression. In R. Katzman, R. D. Terry, & K. L. Bick (Eds.), *Alzheimer's disease: Senile dementia and related disorders* (pp. 87–96). New York: Raven Press.

Folstein, M. F., Folstein, S. E., & McHugh, P. R. (1975). "Mini-Mental State": A practical method of grading the cognitive state of patients for the clinician. *Journal of Psychiatric Research*, *12*, 189–198.

Folstein, M. F., Anthony, J. C., Parhad, I., Duffy, B., & Gruenberg, E. M. (1985). The meaning of cognitive impairment in the elderly. *Journal of the American Geriatrics Society*, *33*, 228–235.

Ford, C. V., & Spordone, R. J. (1980). Attitudes of psychiatrists toward elderly patients. *American Journal of Psychiatry*, *137*, 571–575.

Foster, J. R. (1988). Normal aging—Biological aspects. In L. W. Lazarus (Ed.), *Essentials of geriatric psychiatry* (pp. 25–40). New York: Springer.

Fozard, J. L. (1980). The time for remembering. In L. Poon (Ed.), *Aging in the 1980s: Psychological issues* (pp. 273–291). Washington, DC: American Psychological Association.

Freed, D. M., Corkin, S., Growdon, J. H., & Nissen, M. J. (1988). Selective attention in Alzheimer's disease: CSF correlates of behavioral impairments. *Neuropsychologia*, *26*, 895–902.

Freedman, M., & Oscar-Berman, M. (1986). Comparative neuropsychology of cortical and subcortical dementia. *Canadian Journal of Neurological Sciences*, *13*, 410–414.

Friedland, R. P. (1988). Alzheimer disease: Clinical and biological heterogeneity. *Annals of Internal Medicine*, *109*, 298–311.

Friedman, A. S. (1964). Minimal effects of severe depression on cognitive functioning. *Journal of Abnormal and Social Psychology*, *69*, 237–243.

Friedman, H. S., & DiMatteo, M. R. (1989). *Health psychology*. Englewood Cliffs, NJ: Prentice-Hall.

Fries, J. F., Green, L. W., & Levine, S. (1989). Health promotion and the compression of morbidity. *The Lancet*, *1*, 481–483.

Frith, C. D., Stevens, M., Johnstone, E. C., Deakin, J. F. W., Lawler, P., & Crow, J. T. (1983). Effects of ECT and depression on various aspects of memory. *British Journal of Psychiatry*, *142*, 610–617.

Fromm, D., & Schopflocher, D. (1984). Neuropsychological test performance in depressed patients before and after drug therapy. *Biological Psychiatry*, *19*, 55–72.

Fromm-Auch, D. (1983). Neuropsychological assessment of depressed patients before and after drug therapy: Clinical profile interpretation. In P. Flor-Henry & J. Gruzelier (Eds.), *Laterality and psychopathology* (pp. 83–102). New York: Elsevier.

Fuld, P. A. (1981). *The Fuld Object-Memory Evaluation*. Chicago: Stoelting Instrument.

Fuld, P. A. (1984). Test profile of cholinergic dysfunction and of Alzheimer-type dementia. *Journal of Clinical Neuropsychology*, *6*, 380–392.

Fuld, P. A. (1986). Pathological and chemical validation of behavioral features of Alzheimer's disease. In L. W. Poon (Ed.), *Handbook for clinical memory assessment of older adults* (pp. 302–306). Washington, DC: American Psychological Association.

Fuld, P. A., Katzman, R., Davies, P., & Terry, R. O. (1982). Intrusions as a sign of Alzheimer dementia: Chemical and pathological verification. *Annals of Neurology*, *11*, 155–159.

Fuld, P. A., Muramoto, O., Blau, A., Westbrook, L., & Katzman, R. (1988). Cross-cultural and multi-ethnic dementia evaluation by mental status and memory testing. *Cortex*, *24*, 511–519.

Fuld, P. A., Masur, D. M., Blau,, A. D., Crystal, H., & Aronson, M. K. (1990). Object-Memory Evaluation for prospective detection of dementia in normal functioning elderly: Predictive and normative data. *Journal of Clinical and Experimental Neuropsychology*, *12*, 520–528.

Funkenstein, H. H. (1988). Cerebrovascular disorders. In M. S. Albert & M. B. Moss (Eds.), *Geriatric neuropsychology* (pp. 179–207). New York: Guilford Press.

Galasko, D., Klauber, M. R., Hofstetter, C. R., Salmon, D. P., Lasker, B., & Thal, L. J. (1990). The Mini-Mental State Examination in the early diagnosis of Alzheimer's Disease. *Archives of Neurology, 47*, 49–52.

Gallagher, D. (1986). Assessment of depression by interview methods and psychiatric rating scales. In L. W. Poon (Ed.), *Handbook for clinical memory assessment of older adults* (pp. 202–212). Washington, DC: American Psychological Association.

Gallagher, D., & Thompson, L. W. (1983). Depression. In P. M. Lewinsohn & Linda Teri (Eds.), *Clinical geropsychology: New directions in assessment and treatment* (pp. 7–37). New York: Pergamon Press.

Gallagher, D. E., Thompson, L. W., & Peterson, J. (1981–1982). Psychosocial factors affecting adaptation to bereavement in the elderly. *International Journal of Aging and Human Development, 14*, 79–95.

Gallagher, D., Nies, G., & Thompson, L. (1982). Reliability of the Beck Depression Inventory with older adults. *Journal of Consulting and Clinical Psychology, 50*, 152–153.

Gallagher, D., Breckenridge, J., Steinmeitz, J., & Thompson, L. (1983). The Beck Depression Inventory and Research Diagnostic Criteria: Congruence in an older population. *Journal of Clinical and Consulting Psychology, 51*, 945–946.

Gass, C. S., & Russell, E. W. (1986). Differential impact of brain damage and depression on memory test performance. *Journal of Consulting and Clinical Psychology, 54*, 261–263.

Gatz, M., & Pearson, C. G. (1988). Ageism revised and the provision of psychological services. *American Psychologist, 43*, 184–188.

Gatz, M., Popkin, S. J., Pino, C. D., & Van den Bos, G. R. (1985). Psychological interventions with older adults. In J. E. Birren & K. W. Schaie (Eds.), *Handbook of the psychology of aging* (2nd ed., pp. 755–785). New York: Van Nostrand Reinhold.

Gemmel, H. G., Sharp, P. F., Evans, N. T. S., Besson, A., Lyall, D., & Smith, F. (1984). Single photon emission tomography with 1231-isoprophylamphetamin in Alzheimer's disease and multi-infarct dementia. *Lancet, 2*, 134.

George, A. E., deLeon, M. J., Gentes, C. I., Miller, J., London, E., Budzilovich, G., Ferris, S., & Chase, N. (1986). Leukoencephalopathy in normal and pathologic aging: 1. CT of brain lucencies. *American Journal of Neuroradiology, 7*, 561–566.

German, P. S., Shapiro, S., Skinner, E. A., Von Korff, E., Klein, L. E., Turner, R. W., Teitelbaum, M. L., Burke, J., & Burns, B. (1987). Detection and management of mental health problems of older patients by primary care providers. *Journal of the American Medical Association, 257*, 489–493.

Gershon, E. S. (1983). The genetics of affective disorders. In L. Grinspoon (Ed.), *Psychiatry update* (pp. 434–457). Washington, DC: American Psychiatric Press.

Gershon, L., & Shaw, F. H. (1961). Psychiatric sequelae of chronic exposure to organophosphorous insecticides. *Lancet, 1*, 1371–1374.

Giacobini, E. (1990). The cholinergic system in Alzheimer disease. In S.-M. Aquilonius & P.-G. Gillberg (Eds.), *Cholinergic neurotransmission: Functional and clinical aspects* (pp. 321–332). Amsterdam: Elsevier.

Giaquinto, S., & Nolfe, G. (1986). The EEG in the normal elderly: A contribution to the interpretation of aging and dementia. *Electroencephalography and Clinical Neurophysiology, 63*, 540–546.

Gibb, W. R. G. (1989). Dementia and Parkinson's disease. *British Journal of Psychiatry, 154*, 596–614.

Gibson, A. J. (1981). A further analysis of memory loss in dementia and depression in the elderly. *British Journal of Clinical Psychology, 20*, 179–185.

Gilewski, J. J., & Zelinski, E. M. (1986). Questionnaire assessment of memory complaints. In L. W. Poon (Ed.), *Handbook for clinical memory assessment of older adults* (pp. 93–107). Washington, DC: American Psychological Association.

Gilleard, C. J. (1980). Wechsler Memory Scale performance of elderly psychiatric patients. *Journal of Clinical Psychology, 36*, 958–960.

Glassman, A. (1969). Indoleamines and affective disorder. *Psychosomatic Medicine, 31*, 107–114.

Glenner, G. G., & Wong, C. W. (1984). Alzheimer's disease and Down's syndrome: Sharing of a unique cerebrovascular amyloid fibril protein. *Biochemical and Biophysical Research Communication, 122*, 1131–1135.

Glosser, G., Goodglass, H., & Biber, C. (1989). Assessing visual memory disorders. *Psychological Assessment: A Journal of Consulting and Clinical Psychology, 1*, 82–91.

Godber, C., Rosenvinge, H., Wilkinson, D., & Smithies, J. (1987). Depression in old age: Prognosis after ECT. *International Journal of Geriatric Psychiatry, 2*, 19–24.

Goldberg, E. L., Comstock, G. W., & Harlow, S. D. (1988). Emotional problems in widowhood. *Journal of Gerontology: Social Sciences, 43*, S206–208.

Golden, C. J. (1978). *Stroop Color and Word Test: A manual for clinical and experimental uses*. Chicago: Stoelting.

Golden, C. J., Hammeke, T. A., & Purisch, A. D. (1980). *The Luria-Nebraska Neuropsychological Battery Manual*. Los Angeles: Western Psychological Services.

Golinkoff, M., & Sweeney, J. A. (1989). Cognitive impairments in depression. *Journal of Affective Disorders, 17*, 105–112.

Goodglass, H., & Kaplan, E. (1972). *Assessment of aphasia and related disorders*. Philadelphia: Lea & Febiger.

Goodglass, H., & Kaplan, E. (1983). *The assessment of aphasia and related orders* (2nd ed.). Philadelphia: Lea & Febiger.

Goodin, D. S., Squires, K. C., Henderson, B. H., & Starr, A. (1978). Age-related variations in evoked potentials to auditory stimuli in normal human subjects. *Electroencephalography and Clinical Neurophysiology, 44*, 447–458.

Gose, K., & Levi, G. (1985). *Dealing with memory changes as you grow older*. New York: Bantam.

Goul, W. R., & Brown, M. (1970). Effects of age and intelligence on Trail Making Test performance and validity. *Perceptual and Motor Skills, 30*, 319–326.

Gould, R. L. (1978). *Transformations: Growth and change in adult life*. New York: Simon & Schuster.

Grady, C. L., Haxby, J. V., Horwitz, B., Sundaram, M., Berg, G., Schapiro, M., Friedland, R. P., & Rapoport, S. I. (1988). Longitudinal study of the early neuropsychological and cerebral metabolic changes in dementia of the Alzheimer type. *Journal of Clinical and Experimental Neuropsychology, 10*, 576–596.

Granholm, E., & Butters, N. (1988). Associative encoding and retrieval in Alzheimer's and Huntington's disease. *Brain and Cognition, 7*, 335–347.

Grober, E. (1985). Encoding of item-specific information on Alzheimer's disease. *Journal of Clinical and Experimental Neuropsychology, 7*, 614.

Grober, E., & Buschke, H. (1987). Genuine memory deficits in dementia. *Developmental Neuropsychology, 3*, 13–36.

Grober, E., Buschke, H., Crystal, H., Bang, S., & Dresner, R. (1988). Screening for dementia by memory testing. *Neurology, 38*, 900–903.

Group for the Advancement of Psychiatry (1988). *The psychiatric treatment of Alzheimer's disease*. New York: Brunner/Mazel.

Gupta, S. R., Naheedy, M. H., Young, J. C., Ghobrial, M., Rubino, F. A., & Hindo, W. (1988). Periventricular white matter changes and dementia: Clinical, neuropsychological, radiological, and pathological correlation. *Archives of Neurology, 45*, 637–641.

Gurland, B. J. (1976). The comparative frequency of depression in various adult age groups. *Journal of Gerontology, 31*, 283–292.

Gurland, B. J., & Cross, P. S. (1982). Epidemiology of psychopathology in old age. *Psychiatric Clinics of North America, 5*, 11–26.

Gurland, B. J., & Wilder, D. E. (1984). The CARE interview revisited: Development of an efficient, systematic clinical assessment. *Journal of Gerontology, 2*, 129–137.

Guttentag, R. E., & Hunt, R. R. (1988). Adult age differences in memory for imagined and performed actions. *Journal of Gerontology: Psychological Science, 43*, P107–108.

Guttman, R. (1981). Performance on the Raven Progressive Matrices as a function of age, education, and sex. *Educational Gerontology*, *7*, 49–55.

Haaland, K. Y., Linn, R. T., Hunt, W. C., & Goodwin, J. S. (1983). A normative study of Russell's variant of the Wechsler Memory Scale in a healthy elderly population. *Journal of Consulting and Clinical Psychology*, *51*, 878–881.

Haaland, K. Y., Vranes, L. F., Goodwin, J. S., & Garry, P. J. (1987). Wisconsin Card Sort Test performance in a healthy elderly population. *Journal of Gerontology*, *42*, 345–346.

Haan, H., & Day, D. (1974). A longitudinal study of change and sameness in personality development: Adolescence to later adulthood. *International Journal of Aging and Human Development*, *5*, 11–39.

Hachinski, V. C., Lassen, N. A., & Marshall, J. (1974). Multi-infarct dementia: A cause of mental deterioration in the elderly. *The Lancet*, *2*, 207–209.

Hachinski, V. C., Iliff, L. D., Zilhka, E., Du Boulay, G. H., McAllister, V. L., Marshall, J., Russell, R. W., & Symon, L. (1975). Cerebral blood flow in dementia. *Archives of Neurology*, *32*, 632–637.

Hakim, A. M., & Mathieson, G. (1979). Dementia in Parkinson disease: A neuropathological study. *Neurology*, *29*, 1209–1214.

Halaris, A. (1986–1987). Antidepressant drug therapy in the elderly: Enhancing safety and compliance. *International Journal of Psychiatry in Medicine*, *16*, 1–19.

Halstead, W. C. (1947). *Brain and intelligence: A quantitative study of the frontal lobes*. Chicago: University of Chicago.

Halstead, W. C., & Wepman, J. M. (1959). The Halstead-Wepman aphasia screening test. *Journal of Speech and Hearing Disorders*, *14*, 9–15.

Hamilton, M. (1967). Development of a rating scale for primary depressive illness. *British Journal of Social and Clinical Psychology*, *6*, 278–296.

Hammeke, T. A., Golden, C. J., & Purisch, A. D. (1978). A standardized, short, and comprehensive neuropsychological test battery based on the Luria Neuropsychological Evaluation. *International Journal of Neuroscience*, *8*, 135–141.

Handel, M., Albert, M., Kaplan, E., Moss, M., & Hurwitz, I. (1985, February). *Lateralization of cognitive processes in depression*. Paper presented at a meeting of the International Neuropsychological Society, San Diego.

Hannay, H. J., & Levin, H. S. (1985). Selective Reminding Test: An examination of the equivalence of four forms. *Journal of Clinical and Experimental Neuropsychology*, *7*, 251–263.

Hannay, H. J., Levin, H. S., & Grossman, R. G. (1979). Impaired recognition memory after head injury. *Cortex*, *15*, 269–283.

Harbaugh, R. E., Roberts, D. W., Coombs, D. W., Saunders, R. L., & Reeder, T. M. (1984). Preliminary report: Intracranial cholinergic drug infusion in patients with Alzheimer's disease. *Neurosurgery*, *15*, 514–518.

Harman, D. (1968). Free radical theory of aging: Effect of free radical reaction inhibitors on the mortality rate of male LAF-1 mice. *Journal of Gerontology*, *23*, 476–482.

Harris, L. (1975). *The myth and reality of aging in America*. Washington, DC: National Council on Aging.

Harrison, M. J. G., Thomas, D. J., Du Boulay, G. H., & Marshall, J. (1979). Multi-infarct dementia. *Journal of Neurological Science*, *40*, 97–103.

Hart, R. P., Kwentus, J. A., Hamer, R. M., & Taylor, J. R. (1987a). Selective reminding procedure in depression and dementia. *Psychology and Aging*, *2*, 111–115.

Hart, R. P., Kwentus, J. A., Taylor, J. R., & Harkins, S. W. (1987b). Rate of forgetting in dementia and depression. *Journal of Consulting and Clinical Psychology*, *55*, 101–105.

Hart, R. P., Kwentus, J. A., Wade, J. B., & Hamer, R. M. (1987c). Digit Symbol performance in mild dementia and depression. *Journal of Consulting and Clinical Psychology*, *55*, 236–238.

Hart, S. (1988). Language and dementia: A review. *Psychological Medicine*, *18*, 99–112.

Hasher, L., & Zacks, R. T. (1979). Automatic and effortful processes in memory. *Journal of Experimental Psychology: General*, *120*, 301–309.

Hasher, L., & Zacks, R. T. (1984). Automaticity processing of fundamental information: The case of frequency of occurrence. *American Psychologist, 39*, 1372–1388.

Hassinger, M., & La Rue, A. (1986, August). *Independence of mood and cognition in geriatric depression*. Paper presented at a meeting of the American Psychological Association, Washington, DC.

Hassinger, M., Smith, G., & La Rue, A. (1989). Assessing depression in older adults. In T. Hunt & C. J. Lindley (Eds.), *Testing older adults* (pp. 92–121). Austin, TX: Pro-Ed.

Hathaway, S. R., & McKinley, J. C. (1943). *The Minnesota Multiphasic Personality Inventory Manual*. Minneapolis: University of Minnesota Press.

Haug, M. (1979). Doctor-patient relationships and the older patient. *Journal of Gerontology, 34*, 853–860.

Hayslip, B., Kennelly, K., & Maloy, R. (1989, November). *Fatigue, depression, and cognitive performance among aged persons*. Paper presented at a meeting of the Gerontological Society of America Meeting, Minneapolis.

Heaton, R. K. (1981). *A manual for the Wisconsin Card Sorting Test*. Odessa, FL: Psychological Assessment Resources.

Heaton, R. K., & Crowley, T. J. (1981). Effects of psychiatric disorders and their somatic treatments on neuropsychological test results. In W. B. Filskov & T. J. Boll (Eds.), *Handbook of clinical neuropsychology* (pp. 481–525). New York: Wiley-Interscience.

Heaton, R. K., & Pendleton, M. G. (1981). Use of neuropsychological tests to predict adult patients' everyday functioning. *Journal of Consulting and Clinical Psychology, 49*, 807–821.

Heaton, R. K., Baade, L. E., & Johnson, K. L. (1978). Neuropsychological test results associated with psychiatric disorders in adults. *Psychological Bulletin, 85*, 141–162.

Heaton, R. K., Grant, I., & Matthews, C. G. (1986). Differences in neuropsychological test performance associated with age, education, and sex. In I. Grant & K. M. Adams (Eds.), *Neuropsychological assessment of neuropsychiatric disorders* (pp. 100–120). New York: Oxford University Press.

Heaton, R. K., Grant, I., & Matthews, C. G. (1991). *Comprehensive norms for an expanded Halstead-Reitan Battery*. Odessa, FL: Psychological Assessment Resources.

Helkala, E.-L., Laulumaa, V., Soininen, H., & Riekkinen, P. J. (1988). Recall and recognition memory in patients with Alzheimer's and Parkinson's diseases. *Annals of Neurology, 24*, 214–217.

Hely, M. A., Morris, J. G. J., Rail, D., Reid, W. G. J., O'Sullivan, D. J., Williamson, P. M., Genge, S., & Broe, G. A. (1989). The Sydney Multicentre Study of Parkinson's disease: A report on the first 3 years. *Journal of Neurology, Neurosurgery, and Psychiatry, 52*, 324–328.

Hemsi, L. K., Whitehead, A., & Post, F. (1968). Cognitive functioning and cerebral arousal in elderly depressives and dements. *Journal of Psychosomatic Research, 12*, 145–156.

Henderson, V. W., Mack, W., & Williams, B. W. (1989). Spatial disorientation in Alzheimer's disease. *Archives of Neurology, 46*, 391–394.

Henry, G. M., Weingartner, H., & Murphy, D. L. (1973). Influence of affective states and psychoactive drugs on verbal learning and memory. *American Journal of Psychiatry, 130*, 966–971.

Hertzog, C., & Schaie, K. W. (1986). Stability and change in adult intelligence: 1. Analysis of longitudinal covariance structures. *Psychology and Aging, 1*, 159–171.

Hertzog, C., & Schaie, K. W. (1988). Stability and change in adult intelligence: 2. Simultaneous analysis of longitudinal means and covariance structures. *Psychology and Aging, 3*, 122–130.

Heston, L. L. (1988). Morbid risk in first-degree relatives of persons with Alzheimer's disease. *Archives of General Psychiatry, 45*, 97–98.

Heston, L. L., Mastri, A. R., Anderson, V. E., & White, J. (1981). Dementia of the Alzheimer type. *Archives of General Psychiatry, 38*, 1085–1090.

Heyman, A., Wilkinson, W. E., Stafford, J. A., Helms, M. J., Sigmon, A. H., & Weinberg, T. (1984). Alzheimer's disease: A study of epidemiological aspects. *Annals of Neurology, 15*, 335–341.

Hier, D. B., Hagenlocker, K., & Shindler, A. G. (1985). Language disintegration in dementia: Effects of etiology and severity. *Brain and Language, 25*, 117–133.

Hietanen, M., & Teravainen, H. (1986). Cognitive performance in early Parkinson's disease. *Acta Neurologica Scandinavica, 73*, 151–159.

Hietanen, M., & Teravainen, H. (1988). The effect of age of disease onset on neuropsychological performance in Parkinson's disease. *Journal of Neurology, Neurosurgery, and Psychiatry*, *51*, 244–249.

Hochanadel, G., & Kaplan, E. (1984). Neuropsychology of normal aging. In M. L. Albert (Ed.), *Clinical neurology of aging* (pp. 231–244). New York: Oxford University Press.

Hoehn, M. M., & Yahr, M. D. (1967). Parkinsonism: Onset, progression, and mortality. *Neurology*, *17*, 427–442.

Hoffman, G. M. A., Gonze, J. C., & Mendlewicz, J. (1985). Speech pause time as a method for the evaluation of psychomotor retardation in depressive illness. *British Journal of Psychiatry*, *146*, 535–538.

Hooper, N. E. (1958). *The Hooper Visual Organization Test*. Los Angeles: Western Psychological Services.

Horn, J. L. (1970). Organization of data on life-span development of human abilities. In L. R. Goulet & P. B. Baltes (Eds.), *Life-span developmental psychology: Research and theory* (pp. 423–466). New York: Academic Press.

Horn, J. L. (1982). The aging of human abilities. In B. B. Wolman (Ed.), *Handbook of developmental psychology* (pp. 847–870). New York: Prentice-Hall.

Horn, J. L. (1985). Remodeling old models of intelligence. In B. B. Wolman (Ed.), *Handbook of intelligence* (pp. 267–300). New York: Wiley.

Houlihan, J. P., Abrahams, J. P., La Rue, A. A., Jarvik, L. F. (1985). Qualitative differences in vocabulary performance of Alzheimer versus depressed patients. *Developmental Neuropsychology*, *1*, 139–144.

Howard, D. V., & Howard, H. H. (1989). Age differences in learning serial patterns: Direct versus indirect measures. *Psychology and Aging*, *4*, 357–364.

Howes, J. L., & Katz, A. N. (1988). Assessing remote memory with an improved public events questionnaire. *Psychology and Aging*, *3*, 142–150.

Huber, S. J., Shuttleworth, E. C., Paulson, G. W., Bellchambers, M. J. G., & Clapp, L. E. (1986). Cortical vs. subcortical dementia. *Archives of Neurology*, *43*, 392–394.

Huber, S. J., Freidenberg, D. O., Shuttleworth, E. C., Paulson, G. W., & Christy, J. A. (1989). Neuropsychological impairments associated with severity of Parkinson's disease. *Journal of Neuropsychiatry*, *1*, 155–158.

Huff, F. J., Corkin, S., & Growdon, J. H. (1986). Semantic impairment and anomia in Alzheimer's disease. *Brain and Language*, *28*, 235–249.

Huff, F. J., Becker, J. T., Belle, S. H., Nebes, R. D., Holland, A. L., & Boller, F. (1987). Cognitive deficits and clinical diagnosis of Alzheimer's disease. *Neurology*, *37*, 1119–1124.

Hughes, C. P., Berg, L., Danziger, W. L., Coben, L. A., & Martin, R. L. (1982). A new clinical scale for the staging of dementia. *British Journal of Psychiatry*, *140*, 566–572.

Hulicka, I. M. (1966). Age differences in Wechsler Memory Scale scores. *Journal of Genetic Psychology*, *109*, 135–145.

Hulicka, I. M., & Grossman, J. L. (1967). Age group comparisons for the use of mediators in paired-associate learning. *Journal of Gerontology*, *22*, 46–51.

Hunt, E. (1983). Attention and intelligence. *Journal of Educational Psychology*, *75*, 471–490.

Hyer, L., & Blazer, D. G. (1982). Depressive symptoms: Impact and problems in long-term care facilities. *International Journal of Behavioral Geriatrics*, *1*, 33–44.

Hyman, B. T., Van Hoesen, G. W., Damasio, A. R., & Barnes, C. L. (1984). Alzheimer's disease: Cell-specific pathology isolates the hippocampal formation. *Science*, *225*, 1168–1170.

Hyman, B. T., Van Hoesen, G. W., & Damasio, A. R. (1990). Memory-related neural systems in Alzheimer's disease: An anatomic study. *Neurology*, *40*, 1721–1730.

Ingersoll-Dayton, B., & Antonucci, T. C. (1988). Reciprocal and nonreciprocal social support: Contrasting sides of intimate relationships. *Journal of Gerontology: Social Sciences*, *43*, S65–73.

Inglis, J. (1959). Learning, retention, and conceptual usage in elderly patients with memory disorder. *Journal of Abnormal and Social Psychology*, *159*, 210–215.

Ivnik, R. J., Malec, J. F., Tangalos, E. G., Petersen, R. C., Kokmen, E., & Kurland, L. T. (1990). The Auditory-Verbal Learning Test (AVLT): Norms for ages 55 years and older. *Psychological Assessment: A Journal of Consulting and Clinical Psychology*, *2*, 304–312.

Ivnik, R. J., Malec, J. F., Smith, G. E., Tangalos, E. G., Petersen, R. C., & Kurland, L. T. (1992). Mayo's older Americans normative studies: WAIS-R norms for ages 56 to 97. *The Clinical Neuropsychologist, 6* (Suppl), 1–30.

Jackson, J. E., & Ramsdell, J. W. (1988). Use of the Mini-Mental State Examination (MMSE) to screen for dementia in elderly outpatients. *Journal of the American Geriatric Society, 36*, 662.

Jacobs, J. W., Bernhard, M. R., Delgado, A., & Strain, J. J. (1977). Screening for organic mental syndromes in the medically ill. *Annals of Internal Medicine, 86*, 40–46.

Janowsky, D. S. (1980). The cholinergic nervous system in depression. In J. Mendels & J. D. Amsterdam (Eds.), *The psychobiology of affective disorders* (pp. 83–89). New York: Karger.

Jansen, W., Bruckner, G. W., & Jansen, P. (1985). The treatment of senile dementia associated with cerebrovascular insufficiency: A comparative study of Buflomedil and dihydrogenated ergot alkaloids. *Journal of Internal Medicine Research, 13*, 48–53.

Jarvik, L. F. (1988). Aging of the brain: How can we prevent it? *The Gerontologist, 28*, 739–747.

Jarvik, L. F., & Bank, L. (1983). Aging twins: Longitudinal psychometric data. In K. W. Schaie (Ed.), *Longitudinal studies of adult psychological development* (pp. 40–63). New York: Guilford Press.

Jarvik, L. F., & Blum, J. E. (1971). Cognitive declines as predictors of mortality in twin pairs: A twenty-year longitudinal study of aging. In E. Palmore & F. C. Jeffers (Eds.), *Prediction of life span* (pp. 199–211). Lexington, MA: D. C. Heath.

Jarvik, L. F., & Small, G. W. (1988). *Parentcare*. New York: Crown Publishers.

Jarvik, L. F., & Winograd, C. H. (Eds.). (1988). *Treatments for the Alzheimer patient: The long haul*. New York: Springer.

Jarvik, L. F., Ruth, V., & Matsuyama, S. S. (1980). Organic brain syndrome and aging: A six-year follow-up of surviving twins. *Archives of General Psychiatry, 37*, 280–286.

Jarvik, L. F., Mintz, J., Steuer, J., & Gerner, R. (1982). Treating geriatric depression: A 26-week interim analysis. *Journal of the American Geriatrics Society, 30*, 713–717.

Jernigan, T. L., Zatz, L. M., Feinberg, I., & Fein, G. (1980). Measurement of cerebral atrophy in the aged by computed tomography. In L. W. Poon (Ed.), *Aging in the 1980s: Psychological issues* (pp. 86–94). Washington, DC: American Psychological Association.

Joachim, C. L., & Selkoe, D. J. (1989). Minireview: Amyloid protein in Alzheimer's Disease. *Journal of Gerontology: Biological Sciences, 44*, B77–82.

Joachim, C. L., Morris, J. H., & Selkoe, D. J. (1988). Clinically diagnosed Alzheimer's disease: Autopsy results in 150 cases. *Annals of Neurology, 24*, 50–56.

Joachim, C. L., Mori, H., & Selkoe, D. J. (1989). Amyloid beta-protein deposition in tissues other than brain in Alzheimer's disease. *Nature, 341*, 226–230.

John, E. R., Prichep, L. S., Fridman, J., & Easton, P. (1988). Neurometrics: Computer-assisted differential diagnosis of brain dysfunctions. *Science, 239*, 117–232.

Johnson, M. H., & Magaro, P. A. (1987). Effects of mood and severity of memory processes in depression and mania. *Psychological Bulletin, 101*, 28–40.

Johnson, T. E. (1988). Minireview: Genetic specification of life span: Processes, problems, and potentials. *Journal of Gerontology: Biological Sciences, 43*, B87–92.

Jordan, S. W. (1971). Central nervous system. *Human Pathology, 2*, 561.

Jorm, A. F. (1985). Subtypes of Alzheimer's dementia. A conceptual analysis and critical review. *Psychological Medicine, 15*, 543–553.

Jorm, A. F., Korten, A. E., & Henderson, A. S. (1987). The prevalence of dementia: A quantitative integration of the literature. *Acta Psychiatrica Scandinavica, 76*, 465–479.

Kahn, R. L., Goldfarb, A. I., Pollock, M., & Peck, A. (1960). Brief objective measures for the determination of mental status in the aged. *American Journal of Psychiatry, 117*, 326–328.

Kahn, R. L., Zarit, S. H., Hilbert, N. M., & Niederehe, M. A. (1975). Memory complaint and impairment in the aged: The effect of depression and altered brain function. *Archives of General Psychiatry, 32*, 1569–1573.

Kane, R. A., & Kane, R. L., (1981). *Assessing the elderly: A practical guide to measurement*. Lexington, MA: Lexington Books.

Kane, R. L., Parsons, O. A., Goldstein, G., & Moses, J. A., Jr. (1987). Diagnostic accuracy of the Halstead-Reitan and Luria-Nebraska Neuropsychological Batteries: Performance of clinical raters. *Journal of Consulting and Clinical Psychology*, *55*, 783–784.

Kaplan, E. F., Goodglass, H., & Weintraub, S. (1978). *The Boston Naming Test*. Boston: E. Kaplan & H. Goodglass.

Kaplan, E., Goodglass, H., & Weintraub, S. (1983). *The Boston Naming Test* (rev. ed.). Philadelphia: Lea & Febiger.

Karp, D. A. (1988). A decade of reminders: Changing age consciousness between fifty and sixty years old. *The Gerontologist*, *28*, 727–738.

Kaszniak, A. W. (1986). The neuropsychology of dementia. In I. Grant & K. Adams (Eds.), *Neuropsychological assessment of neuropsychiatric disorders* (pp. 172–220). New York: Oxford University Press.

Kaszniak, A. W., Garron, D. C., Fox, J. H., Bergen, D., & Huckman, M. (1979). Cerebral atrophy: EEG slowing, age, education, and cognitive functioning in suspected dementia. *Neurology*, *29*, 1273–1279.

Kaszniak, A. W., Poon, L. W., & Riege, W. (1986). Assessing memory deficits: An information-processing approach. In L. W. Poon (Ed.), *Handbook for clinical memory assessment of older adults* (pp. 168–188). Washington, DC: American Psychological Association.

Katz, D. I., Alexander, M. P., & Mandell, A. M. (1987). Dementia following strokes in the mesencephalon and diencephalon. *Archives of Neurology*, *44*, 1127–1133.

Katz, I. R., Greenberg, W. H., Barr, G. A., Garbarino, C., Buckley, P., & Smith, D. (1985). Screening for cognitive toxicity of anticholinergic drugs. *Journal of Clinical Psychiatry*, *46*, 323–326.

Katz, R., & Horowitz, G. R. (1982). Electroencephalogram in the septuagenarian: Studies in a normal geriatric population. *Journal of the American Geriatrics Society*, *3*, 273–275.

Katzman, R. (1986). Alzheimer's disease. *New England Journal of Medicine*, *314*, 964–973.

Katzman, R., Brown, T., Fuld, P., Peck, A., Schechter, R., & Schimmel, H. (1983). Validation of a short orientation-memory-concentration test of cognitive impairment. *American Journal of Psychiatry*, *140*, 734–739.

Katzman, R., Terry, R., DeTeresa, R., Brown, T., Davies, P., Fuld, P., Renbing, X., & Peck, A. (1988). Clinical, pathological, and neurochemical changes in dementia: A subgroup with preserved mental status and numerous neocortical plaques. *Annals of Neurology*, *23*, 138–144.

Katzman, R., & Rowe, J. W. (Eds.) (1992). *Principles of geriatric neurology*. Philadelphia: F. A. Davis.

Kausler, D. H. (1982). *Experimental psychology and human aging*. New York: Wiley.

Kay, D. W. K. (1989). Genetics, Alzheimer's disease and senile dementia. *British Journal of Psychiatry*, *154*, 311–320.

Kemper, S. (1986). Imitation of complex syntactic constructions by elderly adults. *Applied Psycholinguistics*, *7*, 277–288.

Kemper, T. (1984). Neuroanatomical and neuropathological changes in normal aging and in dementia. In M. L. Albert (Ed.), *Clinical neurology of aging* (pp. 9–52). New York: Oxford University Press.

Kendig, H. L., Coles, R., Pittelkow, Y., & Wilson, S. (1988). Confidants and family structure in old age. *Journal of Gerontology: Social Sciences*, *43*, S31–40.

Kennedy, K. J. (1981). Age effects on Trail Making Test performance. *Perceptual and Motor Skills*, *52*, 671–675.

Kertesz, A. (1985) Aphasia. In P. J. Vinken, G. W. Bruyn, & H. L. Klawans (Eds.), *Handbook of clinical neurology: Clinical neuropsychology* (pp. 287–331). New York: Elsevier.

Kessler, I. I., & Diamond, E. L. (1971). Epidemiologic studies on Parkinson's disease: 1. Smoking and Parkinson's disease: A survey and explanatory hypothesis. *American Journal of Epidemiology*, *94*, 16–25.

Khachaturian, Z. S. (1985). Diagnosis of Alzheimer's disease. *Archives of Neurology*, *41*, 491–496.

Kiernan, R. J., Mueller, J., Langston, J. W., & Van Dyke, C. (1987). The Neurobehavioral Cognitive Status Examination: A brief but quantitative approach to cognitive assessment. *Annals of Internal Medicine*, *107*, 481–485.

Kiloh, L. G. (1961). Pseudo-dementia. *Acta Psychiatrica Scandinavica*, *37*, 336–351.

Kincannon, J. C. (1968). Prediction of the standard MMPI scale scores from 71 items: The Mini-Mult. *Journal of Consulting and Clinical Psychology*, *32*, 319–325.

King, D., Caine, E., Salzman, L., & Conwell, Y. (1988). *Neuropsychological and event-related potential measures of information processing: A comparative study of late-life depression, Alzheimer's disease and normal aging*. Paper presented at a meeting of the International Neuropsychological Society, New Orleans.

Kirshner, H. S., Webb, W. G., & Kelly, M. P. (1984a). The naming disorder of dementia. *Neuropsychologia*, *22*, 23–30.

Kirshner, H. S., Webb, W. G., Kelly, M. P., & Wells, C. E. (1984b). Language disturbance: An initial symptom of cortical degeneration and dementia. *Archives of Neurology*, *41*, 491–496.

Kitagawa, Y., Meyer, J. S., Tachibana, H., Mortel, K. F., & Rogers, R. L. (1984). CT-CBF correlations of cognitive deficits in multi-infarct dementia. *Stroke*, *15*, 1000–1009.

Kite, M. E., & Johnson, B. T. (1988). Attitudes toward older and younger adults: A meta-analysis. *Psychology and Aging*, *3*, 233–244.

Kleemeier, R. W. (1961, September). *Intellectual changes in the senium, or death and the I. Q*. Paper presented at a meeting of the Division on Maturity and Old Age, American Psychological Association, New York.

Klesges, R. C., & Troster, A. I. (1987). A review of premorbid indices of intellectual and neuropsychological functioning: What have we learned in the past five years? *International Journal of Clinical Neuropsychology*, *9*, 1–11.

Klisz, D. (1978). Neuropsychology and medical disorders. In M. Storandt, I. C. Seigler, & M. F. Elias (Eds.), *The clinical psychology of aging* (pp. 71–95). New York: Plenum Press.

Klonoff, H., & Kennedy, M. (1965). Memory and perceptual functioning in octogenarians and nonagenarians in the community. *Journal of Gerontology*, *20*, 328–333.

Klonoff, H., & Kennedy, M. (1966). A comparative study of cognitive functioning in old age. *Journal of Gerontology*, *21*, 239–243.

Knight, B. G. (1986). *Psychotherapy with the older adult*. Beverly Hills, CA: Sage.

Knight, B. (1988). Factors influencing therapist-rated change in older adults. *Journal of Gerontology: Psychological Sciences*, *43*, P111–112.

Knopman, D. S.., & Ryberg, S. (1989). A verbal memory test with high predictive accuracy for dementia of the Alzheimer type. *Archives of Neurology*, *46*, 141–145.

Kolb, B., & Whishaw, I. (1984). *Fundamentals of human neuropsychology*, (2nd ed.). San Francisco: Freeman.

Koller, W. C. (1984). Disturbance of recent memory function in Parkinsonian patients on anticholinergic therapy. *Cortex*, *20*, 307–311.

Koller, W. C. (1987). Classification of Parkinsonism. In W. C. Koller (Ed.), *Handbook of Parkinson's Disease* (pp. 51–80). New York: Marcel Dekker.

Kopelman, M. D. (1986). Clinical tests of memory. *British Journal of Psychiatry*, *148*, 517–525.

Koponen, H., Hurri, L., Stenback, U.,. Mattila, E., Soininen, H., & Riekkinen, P. J. (1989a). Computed tomography findings in delirium. *Journal of Nervous and Mental Disease*, *177*, 226–231.

Koponen, H., Partanen, J., Paakkonen, A., Mattila, E., & Riekkinen, P. J. (1989b). EEG spectral analysis in delirium. *Journal of Neurology, Neurosurgery, and Psychiatry*, *52*, 980–985.

Kovar, M. B. (1986). Aging in the eighties, age 65 years and over living alone, contacts with family, friends and neighbors. *Advancedata*, *116*, Washington, DC: National Center for Health Statistics.

Kral, V. A. (1983). The relationship between senile dementia (Alzheimer type) and depression. *Canadian Journal of Psychiatry*, *28*, 304–306.

Kral, V. A., & Emery, O. B. (1989). Long-term follow--up of depressive pseudodementia of the aged. *Canadian Journal of Psychiatry*, *34*, 445–446.

Kramer, B. A. (1987). Electroconvulsive therapy use in geriatric depression. *Journal of Nervous and Mental Disease*, *175*, 233–235.

Kramer, J. H., Delis, D. C., Blusewicz, M. J., Brandt, J., Ober, B. A., & Strauss, M. (1988). Verbal memory errors in Alzheimer's and Huntington's dementias. *Developmental Neuropsychology*, *4*, 1–15.

Kramer-Ginzberg, E., Mohs, R. C., Aryan, M., Lobel, D., Silverman, J. M., Davidson, M., & Davis, K. L. (1988). Predictors of course for Alzheimer patients in a longitudinal study: A preliminary report. *Psychopharmacology Bulletin*, *24*, 458–462.

Krause, N. (1986). Stress and sex differences in depressive symptoms among older adults. *Journal of Gerontology*, *41*, 727–731.

Krause, N. (1987). Life stress, social support, and self-esteem in an elderly population. *Psychology and Aging*, *2*, 349–356.

Krause, N. (1988). Stressful life events and physician utilization. *Journal of Gerontology: Social Sciences*, *43*, S53–61.

Kubanis, P., & Zornetzer, S. F. (1981). Age-related behavioral and neurobiological changes: A review with an emphasis on memory. *Behavioral and Neural Biology*, *31*, 115–172.

Kuhl, D. E., Metter, E. J., Riege, W. H., & Phelps, M. E. (1982). Effects of human aging on patterns of local cerebral glucose utilization determined by the F-18 Fluoro-deoxyglucose method. *Journal of Cerebral Blood Flow and Metabolism*, *2*, 163–171.

Kuhl, D. E., Metter, E. J., Riege, W. H., Hawkins, J. C., Mazziotta, J. C., Phelps, M. E., & Kling, A. S. (1983). Local cerebral glucose utilization in elderly patients with depression, multi-infarct dementia, and Alzheimer's disease. *Journal of Cerebral Blood Flow and Metabolism*, *3*, s494–s495.

Kuhl, D. E., Metter, E. J., Riege, W. H., & Hawkins, R. A. (1984). The effect of normal aging on patterns of local cerebral glucose utilization. *Annals of Neurology*, *15*, S133–137.

Kuhl, D. E., Metter, E. J., & Riege, W. H. (1985). Patterns of cerebral glucose utilization in depression, multiple infarct dementia, and Alzheimer's disease. In L. Sokoloff (Ed.), *Brain imaging and brain functions* (pp. 211–226). New York: Raven Press.

Kuhl, D. E., Small, G. W., Riege, W. H., Fujikawa, D. G., Metter, E. J., Benson, D.F., Ashford, J. W., Mazziotta, J. C., Maltese, A., & Dorsey, D. A. (1987). Cerebral metabolic patterns before the diagnosis of probable Alzheimer's disease. *Journal of Cerebral Blood Flow and Metabolism*, *7* (Suppl. 1), S–406.

Kuypers, J. A., & Bengtson, V. L. (1973). Social breakdown and competence: A model of normal aging. *Human Development*, *16*, 181–201.

Kynette, D., & Kemper, S. (1986). Aging and the loss of grammatical forms: A cross-sectional study of language performance. *Language and Communication*, *6*, 65–72.

Labouvie-Vief, G. (1985). Intelligence and cognition. In J. E. Birren & K. W. Schaie (Eds.), *Handbook of the psychology of aging* (2nd ed., pp. 500–530) New York: Van Nostrand Reinhold.

Labouvie-Vief, G., & Gonda, J. N. (1976). Cognitive strategy training and intellectual performance in the elderly. *Journal of Gerontology*, *31*, 327–332.

Ladurner, G., Iliff, L. D., & Lechner, H. (1982). Clinical factors associated with dementia in ischaemic stroke. *Journal of Neurology, Neurosurgery, and Psychiatry*, *45*, 97–101.

Lang, A. E., (1987). Genetics. In W. C. Koller (Ed.), *Handbook of Parkinson's disease* (pp. 81–98). New York: Marcel Dekker.

Langer, E. J., & Rodin, J. (1976). The effects of choice and enhanced personal responsibility for the aged. *Journal of Personality and Social Psychology*, *34*, 191–198.

Langston, J. W. (1989). Current theories on the cause of Parkinson's disease. *Journal of Neurology, Neurosurgery, and Psychiatry*. (Special Supplement), 13–17.

Langston, J. W., & Forno, L. S. (1978). The hypothalamus in Parkinson's disease. *Annals of Neurology*, *3*, 129–133.

Langston, J. W., Ballard, P., Tetrud, J. W., & Irwin, I. (1983). Chronic Parkinsonism in humans due to a product of meperidine-analog synthesis. *Science*, *219*, 979–980.

Lapp, D. C. (1987). *Don't forget!* New York: McGraw-Hill.

Larrabee, G. J., & Crook, T. H. (1989). Dimensions of everyday memory in age-associated memory impairment. *Psychological Assessment: A Journal of Consulting and Clinical Psychology*, *1*, 92–97.

Larson, E. B., Reifler, B. V., Sumi, S. M., Canfield, C. G., & Chinn, N. M. (1985). Diagnostic evaluation of 200 elderly outpatients with suspected dementia. *Journal of Gerontology*, *40*, 536–543.

La Rue, A. (1989). Patterns of performance on the Fuld Object Memory Evaluation in elderly inpatients. *Journal of Clinical and Experimental Neuropsychology*, *11*, 409–422.

La Rue, A. (1992). Adult development and aging. In A. Puente & R. McCaffrey (Eds.), *Handbook of neuropsychological assessment: A biopsychosocial perspective* (pp. 81–119). New York: Plenum Press.

La Rue, A., & D'Elia, L. (1985). Anxiety and problem solving in middle-aged and elderly adults. *Experimental Aging Research*, *11*, 215–220.

La Rue, A., & McCreary, C. (1991). Emerging issues in the health care of the elderly. In J. Sweet, R. Rozensky, & S. Tovian (Eds.), *Handbook of clinical psychology in medical settings* (pp. 227–248). New York: Plenum Press.

La Rue, A., & Waldbaum, A. (1980, February). *Aging vs. illness as predictors of Piagetian problem solving in older adults*. Paper presented at a meeting of the 10th Annual Interdisciplinary International Conference on Piagetian Theory and the Helping Professions, Los Angeles.

La Rue, A., Dessonville, E., & Jarvik, L. F. (1985). Aging and mental disorders. In J. E. Birren & K. W. Schaie (Eds.), *Handbook of the psychology of aging* (2nd ed., pp. 664–702). New York: Van Nostrand Reinhold.

La Rue, A., D'Elia, L. F., Clark, E. O., Spar, J. E., & Jarvik, L. F. (1986a). Clinical tests of memory in dementia, depression, and healthy aging. *Psychology and Aging*, *1*, 69–77.

La Rue, A., Spar, J., & Hill, C. (1986b). Cognitive impairment in late-life depression: Clinical correlates and treatment implications. *Journal of Affective Disorders*, *11*, 179–184.

La Rue, A., Watson, J., Plotkin, D., Larson, E., & Kukull, W. (1988, November). *Caregiver's reports of dementia symptoms: Perspectives on reliability*. Paper presented at a meeting of the Gerontological Society Meeting, San Francisco.

La Rue, A., Goodman, S., & Spar, J. E. (1992a). Risk factors for memory impairment in geriatric depression. *Neuropsychiatry, Neuropsychology, and Behavioral Neurology*, 5 (in press).

La Rue, A., Yang, J., & Osato, S. (1992b). Neuropsychological assessment. In J. E. Birren, R. B. Sloan, & G. Cohen (Eds.), *Handbook of mental health and aging* (2nd ed.), (pp. 643–670). New York: Academic Press.

Lawton, M. P. (1986). Contextual perspectives: Psychosocial influences. In L. W. Poon (Ed.), *Handbook for clinical memory assessment of older adults* (pp. 32–42). Washington, DC: American Psychological Association.

Lawton, M. P., & Brody, E. M. (1969). Assessment of older people: Self-maintaining and instrumental activities of daily living. *The Gerontologist*, *9*, 179–186.

Lawton, M. P., Whelihan, W. M., & Belsky, J. M. (1980). Personality tests and their uses with older adults. In J. E. Birren & R. B. Sloane (Eds.), *Handbook of mental health and aging* (pp. 537–553). Englewood Cliffs, NJ: Prentice-Hall.

Layton, B. C. (1975). Perceptual noise and aging. *Psychological Bulletin*, *82*, 875–883.

Lazarus, R. S., & DeLongis, A. (1983). Psychological stress and coping in aging. *American Psychologist*, *38*, 245–254.

Le Breck, D. B., & Baron, A. (1987). Age and practice effects in continuous recognition memory. *Journal of Gerontology*, *42*, 89–91.

Lees, A. J. (1987). Monoamine oxidase inhibitors. In W. C. Koller (Ed.), *Handbook of Parkinson's Disease* (pp. 403–420). New York: Marcel Dekker.

Lees, A. J., & Smith, E. (1983). Cognitive deficits in the early stages of Parkinson's disease. *Brain*, *106*, 257–270.

Lesser, R. P., Fahn, S., Snider, S. R., Cote, L. J., Isgreen, W. P., & Barrett, R. E. (1979). Analysis of the clinical problems in Parkinsonism and the complications of long-term levodopa therapy. *Neurology*, *29*, 1253–1260.

Leuchter, A., Spar, J. E., Walter, D. O., & Weiner, H. (1987). Electroencephalographic spectra and coherence in the diagnosis of Alzheimer's type and multi-infarct dementia. *Archives of General Psychiatry*, *44*, 993–998.

Levine, D. N., & Grek, A. (1984). The anatomic basis of delusions after right cerebral infarction. *Neurology*, *34*, 577–582.

Levinson, D. (1986). A conception of adult development. *American Psychologist*, *41*, 3–13.

Levinson, D., Darrow, C., Klein, E., Levinson, M., & McKee, B. (1978). *The seasons of a man's life*. New York: Knopf.

LeWitt, P. A. (1987). Therapy with dopaminergic drugs in Parkinson disease. In W. C. Koller (Ed.), *Handbook of Parkinson's disease* (pp. 381–402). New York: Marcel Dekker.

Lezak, M. D. (1983). *Neuropsychological assessment* (2nd ed.). New York: Oxford University Press.

Lezak, M. D. (1984). An individualized approach to neuropsychological assessment. In P. E. Logue & J. M. Schear, *Clinical neuropsychology: A multidisciplinary approach* (pp. 29–49). Springfield, IL: Charles C Thomas.

Lieberman, H. R., & Abou-Nader, T. M. (1986). Possible dietary strategies to reduce cognitive deficits in old age. In D. F. Swaab, E. Fliers, M. Miroran, W. A. Van Gool & F. Van Haaren (Eds.), *Aging of the brain and Alzheimer's disease* (pp. 461–471). Amsterdam: Elsevier.

Lindvall, O. (1989). Transplantation into the human brain: Present status and future possibilities. *Journal of Neurology, Neurosurgery, and Psychiatry* (Special Supplement), 39–54.

Lipowski, Z. J. (1980). *Delirium: Acute brain failure in man*. Springfield, IL: Charles C Thomas.

Lipowski, Z. J. (1983). The need to integrate liaison psychiatry and geropsychiatry. *American Journal of Psychiatry*, *140*, 1003–1005.

Lipowski, Z. J. (1987). Delirium (acute confusional states). *Journal of the American Medical Association*, *258*, 1789–1792.

Liston, E. H. (1982). Delirium in the aged. In L. F. Jarvik & G. W. Small (Eds.), *The psychiatric clinics of North America* (Vol. 5, pp. 49–66). Philadelphia: W. B. Saunders.

Liston, E. (1989). Delirium. In B. Karasu (Ed.), *Treatments of Psychiatric Disorders* (Vol. 2, p. 806). Washington, DC: American Psychiatric Association.

Liston, E. H., & La Rue, A. (1983a). Clinical differentiation of primary degenerative and multi-infarct dementia: A critical review of the evidence. Part I: Clinical studies. *Biological Psychiatry*, *18*, 1451–1465.

Liston, E. H., & La Rue, A. (1983b). Clinical differentiation of primary degenerative and multi-infarct dementia: A critical review of the evidence: Part 2. Pathological studies. *Biological Psychiatry*, *18*, 1467–1484.

Lloyd, G. G., & Lishman, W. A. (1975). Effect of depression on the speed of recall of pleasant and unpleasant experiences. *Psychological Medicine*, *5*, 173–180.

Loeb, C. (1980). Clinical diagnosis of multi-infarct dementia. In L. Amaducci, A. N. Davidson, & P. Antuono (Eds.), *Aging of the brain and dementia* (pp. 251–260). New York: Raven Press.

Loeb, C. (1988a). Clinical criteria for diagnosis and classification of vascular and multi-infarct dementia. In J. S. Meyer, J. Marshall, H. Lechner, & J. F. Toole (Eds.), *Vascular and multi-infarct dementia* (pp. 13–22). Mount Kisco, NY: Futura Publishing.

Loeb, C. (1988b). Intellectual function, transient ischemic attacks and vascular and multi-infarct dementia. In J. S. Meyer, J. Marshall, H. Lechner, & J. F. Toole (Eds.), *Vascular and multi-infarct dementia* (pp. 23–34). Mount Kisco, NY: Futura Publishing.

Loeb, C., & Gandolfo, C. (1983). Diagnostic evaluation of degenerative and vascular dementia. *Stroke*, *14*, 399–401.

Loewenstein, D. A., Amigo, E., Duara, R., Guterman, A., Hurwitz, D., Berkowitz, N., Wilkie, F., Weinberg, G., Black, B., Gittelman, B., & Eisdorfer, C. (1989a). A new scale for the assessment of functional status in Alzheimer's Disease and related disorders. *Journal of Gerontology: Psychological Sciences*, *44*, 114–121.

Loewenstein, D. A., Barker, W. W., Chang, J.-Y., Apicella, A., Yoshii, F., Kothari, P., Levin, B., & Duara, R. (1989b). Predominant left hemisphere metabolic dysfunction in dementia. *Archives of Neurology*, *46*, 146–152.

Loewenstein, D. A., Wilkie, F., Eisdorfer, C., Guterman, A., & Berkowitz, N. (1989c). An analysis of intrusive error types in Alzheimer's disease and related disorders. *Developmental Neuropsychology*, *5*, 115–126.

Loewenstein, D. A., D'Elia, L., Guterman, A., Eisdorfer, C., Wilkie, F., La Rue, A., Mintzer, J., & Duara, R. (1991). The occurrence of different intrusive errors in patients with Alzheimer disease, multiple cerebral infarctions and major depression. *Brain and Cognition*, *16*, 104–117.

Logsdon, R. G., Teri, L., Williams, D. E., Vitiello, M. V., & Prinz, P. N. (1989). The WAIS-R profile: A diagnostic tool for Alzheimer's disease? *Journal of Clinical and Experimental Neuropsychology*, *11*, 892–898.

Loranger, A. W., & Misiak, H. (1960). The performance of aged females on five nonlanguage tests of intellectual functions. *Journal of Clinical Psychology*, *16*, 189–191.

Loring, D. W., & Papanicolaou, A. C. (1987). Memory assessment in neuropsychology: Theoretical considerations and practical utility. *Journal of Clinical and Experimental Neuropsychology*, *9*, 340–358.

Loring, D. W., Levin, H. S., Papanicolaou, A. C., Larrabee, G. J., & Eisenberg, H. M. (1984). Auditory evoked potentials in senescent forgetfulness. *International Journal of Neuroscience*, *24*, 131–141.

Lowenthal, M. F., & Haven, C. (1968). Interaction and adaptation: Intimacy as a critical variable. *American Sociological Review*, *33*, 20–30.

Lubin, B., Larsen, R. M., & Matarazzo, J. D. (1984). Patterns of psychological test usage in the United States: 1935–1982. *American Psychologist*, *39*, 451–454.

Luria, A. (1974). *The working brain*. London: Penguin.

Luria, A. (1980). *Higher cortical functions in man* (2nd ed.). New York: Basic Books.

Luria, A. R., & Majovski, L. V. (1977). Basic approaches used in American and Soviet clinical neuropsychology. *American Psychologist*, *32*, 959–968.

Maas, J. W. (1975). Biogenic amines and depression: Biochemical and pharmacological separation of two subtypes of depression. *Archives of General Psychiatrist*, *32*, 1357–1361.

Mace, N., & Rabins, P. (1981). *The 36 hour day*. Baltimore: Johns Hopkins University Press.

Mace, N. L. (1989). *Dementia care: Patient, family and community*. Baltimore: Johns Hopkins University Press.

Macht, M. L., & Buschke, H. (1983). Age differences in cognitive effort in recall. *Journal of Gerontology*, *38*, 695–700.

Mack, J. L., & Carlson, N. J. (1978). Conceptual deficits and aging: The Category Test. *Perceptual and Motor Skills*, *46*, 123–128.

Madden, J. J., Luhan, J. A., Kaplan, L. A., & Manfredi, H. M. (1952). Nondementing psychoses in older persons. *Journal of the American Medical Association*, *150*, 1567–1572.

Makinodan, T. (1974). Cellular basis of immunosenescence. *Molecular and cellular mechanisms of aging* (Vol. 27, pp. 153–166). Paris: INSERM.

Manton, K. G., Siegler, I. C., & Woodbury, M. A. (1986). Patterns of intellectual development in later life. *Journal of Gerontology*, *41*, 486–499.

Marcopulos, B. A. (1989). Pseudodementia, dementia, and depression: Test differentiation. In T. Hunt & C. J. Lindley (Eds.), *Testing older adults* (pp. 70–91). Austin, TX: Pro-ed.

Marcopulos, B. A., & Graves, R. (1987, February). *Effect of antidepressants on cognitive test performance in the elderly*. Paper presented at a meeting of the 15th Annual International Neuropsychological Society Meeting, Washington, DC.

Margolis, R. B., & Scialfa, C. T. (1984). Age differences in Wechsler Memory Scale performance. *Journal of Clinical Psychology*, *40*, 1442–1449.

Marshall, J. (1988). Vascular and multi-infarct dementia. Do they exist? In J. S. Meyer, J. Marshall, H. Lechner, & J. F. Toole (Eds.), *Vascular and multi-infarct dementia* (pp. 1–4). New York: Futura Publishing.

Martin, A., & Fedio, P. (1983). Word production and comprehension in Alzheimer's disease: The breakdown of semantic knowledge. *Brain and Language*, *19*, 124–141.

Martin, A., Browers, P., Cox, C., Teleska, P., Fedio, P., Foster, N. L., & Chase, T. H. (1986). Towards a behavioral typology of Alzheimer's patients. *Journal of Clinical and Experimental Neuropsychology*, *8*, 594–610.

Martin, W. R. W., & Palmer, M. R. (1989). The nigrostriatal system in aging and Parkinsonism: In vivo studies with positron emission tomography. In D. B. Calne, D. Crippa, G. Comi, R. Horowski, & M. Trabucci (Eds.), *Parkinsonism and aging* (pp. 165–172). New York: Raven Press.

Marttila, R. J. (1987). Epidemiology. In W. C. Koller (Ed.), *Handbook of Parkinson's disease* (pp. 35–50). New York: Marcel Dekker.

Marvel, G. A., Golden, C. J., Hammeke, T., Purisch, A., & Osmon, D. (1979). Relationship of age and education to performance on a standardized version of Luria's neuropsychological tests in different patient populations. *International Journal of Neuroscience*, *9*, 63–70.

Mason, C. F., & Ganzler, H. (1964). Adult norms for the Shipley Institute of Living Scale and Hooper Visual Organization Test based on age and education. *Journal of Gerontology*, *19*, 419–424.

Masur, D. M., Fuld, P. A., Blau, A., Levin, H. S., & Aronson, M. K. (1989). Distinguishing normal and demented elderly with the Selective Reminding Test. *Journal of Clinical and Experimental Neuropsychology*, *11*, 615–630.

Masur, D. M., Fuld, P. A., Blau, A. D., Crystal, H., & Aronson, M. K. (1990). Predicting development of dementia in the elderly with the Selective Reminding Test. *Journal of Clinical and Experimental Neuropsychology*, *12*, 529–538.

Matarazzo, J. D. (1972). *Wechsler's measurement and appraisal of adult intelligence* (5th ed.). Baltimore: Williams & Wilkins.

Matarazzo, J. D., & Herman, D. O. (1984). Base rate data for the WAIS-R: Test-retest stability and VIQ-PIQ differences. *Journal of Clinical Neuropsychology*, *6*, 351–366.

Matarazzo, J. D., & Prifitera, A. (1989). Subtest scatter and premorbid intelligence: Lessons from the WAIS-R standardization sample. *Psychological Assessment: A Journal of Consulting and Clinical Psychology*, *1*, 186–191.

Matarazzo, J. D., Daniel, M. H., Prifitera, A., & Herman, D. O. (1988). Inter-subtest scatter in the WAIS-R standardization sample. *Journal of Clinical Psychology*, *44*, 940–950.

Matsuyama, H., & Nakamura, S. (1978). Senile changes in the brain in the Japanese: Incidence of Alzheimer's neurofibrillary change and senile plaque. In R. Katzman, R. D. Terry, & K. L. Bick (Eds.), *Alzheimer's disease: Senile dementia and related disorders* (pp. 287–297). New York: Raven Press.

Matsuyama, S. S., & Jarvik, L. F. (1989). Hypothesis: Microtubules, a key to Alzheimer disease. *Proceedings of the National Academy of Sciences*, *86*, 8152–8156.

Mattis, S. (1976). Mental status examination for organic mental syndrome in the elderly patient. In L. Bellak & T. B. Karasu (Eds.), *Geriatric psychiatry* (pp. 79–121). New York: Grune & Stratton.

Mayeux, R. (1987). Mental state. In W. D. Keller (Ed.), *Handbook of Parkinson's disease* (pp. 127–144). New York: Marcel Dekker.

Mayeux, R., Stern, Y., Rosenstein, R., Marder, K., Hauser, A., Cote, L., & Fahn, S. (1988). An estimate of the prevalence of dementia in idiopathic Parkinson's disease. *Archives of Neurology*, *45*, 260–262.

Mazziotta, J. C., Maltese, A., & Dorsey, D. A. (1987). Cerebral metabolic patterns before the diagnosis of probable Alzheimer's disease. *Journal of Cerebral Blood Flow Metabolism*, *7* (Suppl. 1), S-406.

McAllister, T. W. (1983). Overview: Pseudodementia. *American Journal of Psychiatry*, *140*, 528–533.

McAllister, T. W., & Price, T. R. P. (1982). Severe depressive pseudodementia with and without dementia. *American Journal of Psychiatry*, *139*, 626–629.

McCarthy, M., Ferris, S. H., Clark, E., & Crook, T. (1981). Acquisition and retention of categorized material in normal aging and senile dementia. *Experimental Aging Research*, *7*, 127–135.

McCarty, S. M., Siegler, I. C., & Logue, P. E. (1982). Cross-sectional and longitudinal patterns of three Wechsler Memory Scale subtests. *Journal of Gerontology*, *37*, 169–175.

McCrae, R. R., & Costa, P. T., Jr. (1984). *Emerging lives, enduring dispositions: Personality in adulthood.* Boston: Little, Brown.

McCue, M., Shelly, C., & Goldstein, G. (1985). A proposed short form of the Luria-Nebraska Neuropsychological Battery oriented toward assessment of the elderly. *International Journal of Clinical Neuropsychology*, *7*, 96–101.

McCue, M., Goldstein, G., & Shelly, C. (1989). The application of a short from of the Luria-Nebraska Neuropsychological Battery to discrimination between dementia and depression in the elderly. *International Journal of Clinical Neuropsychology*, *11*, 21–29.

McDermott, P. A., Glutting, J. J., Jones, J. N., & Noonan, J. V. (1989). Typology and prevailing composition of core profiles in the WAIS-R standardization sample. *Psychological Assessment: A Journal of Consulting and Clinical Psychology, 1*, 118–125.

McFie, J. (1975). *Assessment of organic intellectual impairment*. London: Academic Press.

McGeer, E. G., & McGeer, P. L. (1975). Age changes in the human for some enzymes associated with metabolism of catecholamines, GABA, and acetylcholine. In J. M. Ordy & K. R. Brizzee (Eds.), *Neurobiology of aging* (pp. 287–305). New York: Plenum Press.

McGeer, E. G., & McGeer, P. L. (1976). Neurotransmitter metabolism and the aging brain. In R. D. Terry & S. Gershon (Eds.), *Neurobiology of aging* (pp. 389–404). New York: Raven Press.

McGeer, P.L., Itagaki, S., Akiyama, H., & McGeer, E. G. (1988). Rate of cell death in parkinsonism indicates active neuropathological process. *Annals of Neurology, 24*, 574–576.

McInnes, W. D., Gillen, R. W., Golden, C. J., Graber, B., Cole, J. K., Uhl, H. S. M., & Greenhouse, A. H. (1983). Aging and performance on the Luria-Nebraska Neuropsychological Battery. *International Journal of Neuroscience, 19*, 179–190.

McKay, S., & Ramsey, R. (1983). Correlation of the Wechsler Memory Scale and the Luria-Nebraska Memory Scale. *Clinical Neuropsychology, 5*, 168–170.

McKay, S. E., Golden, C. J., Moses, J. A., Jr., Fishburne, F., & Wisniewski, A. (1981). Correlation of the Luria-Nebraska Neuropsychological Battery with the WAIS. *Journal of Consulting Clinical Psychology, 49*, 940–946.

McKenna, P., & Warrington, E. K. (1986). The analytical approach to neuropsychological assessment. In I. Grant & K. M. Adams (Eds.), *Neuropsychological assessment of neuropsychiatric disorders* (pp. 31–47). New York: Oxford University Press.

McKhann, G., Drachman, D., Folstein, M., Katzman, R., Price, D., & Stadlan, E. M. (1984). Clinical diagnosis of Alzheimer's disease: Report of the NINCDS-ADRDA Work Group. *Neurology, 34*, 939–944.

McLean, J. E., Reynolds, C. R., & Kaufman, A. S. (1990). WAIS-R subtest scatter using the Profile Variability Index. *Psychological Assessment: A Journal of Consulting and Clinical Psychology, 2*, 289–292.

McNeal, E. T., & Cimbolic, P. (1986). Antidepressants and biochemical theories of depression. *Psychological Bulletin, 99*, 361–374.

McSweeny, A. J., Grant, I., Heaton, R. K., Prigatano, G. P., Adams, K. M. (1985). Relationship of neuropsychological status to everyday functioning in healthy and chronically ill persons. *Journal of Clinical and Experimental Neuropsychology, 7*, 281–291.

Mendels, J., Stinnett, J. L., Burns, D., & Frazer, A. (1975). Amine precursors and depression. *Archives of General Psychiatry, 32*, 22–30.

Merriam, A. E., Aronson, M. K., Gaston, P., Wey, S.-L., & Katz, I. (1988). The psychiatric symptoms of Alzheimer's disease. *Journal of the American Geriatric Society, 36*, 7–12.

Mesulam, M.-M. (1979). Acute behavioral derangements without hemiplegia in cerebrovascular accidents. *Primary Care, 6*, 813–821.

Metter, E. J. (1988). Positron tomography and cerebral blood flow studies. In M. S. Albert & M. B. Moss (Eds.), *Geriatric neuropsychology* (pp. 228–261). New York: Guilford Press.

Meyer, J. S., & Shaw, T. G. (1984). Cerebral blood flow in aging. In M. L. Albert (Ed.), *Clinical neurology of aging* (pp. 178–196). New York: Oxford University Press.

Meyer, J. S., Judd, B. W., Tawaklna, T., Rogers, R. L., & Mortel, K. F. (1986). Improved cognition after control of risk factors for multi-infarct dementia. *Journal of the American Medical Association, 256*, 2203–2209.

Meyer, J. S., McClintic, K. L., Rogers, R. L., Sims, P., & Mortel, K. F. (1988a). Aetiological considerations and risk factors for multi-infarct dementia. *Journal of Neurology, Neurosurgery, and Psychiatry, 51*, 1489–1497.

Meyer, J. S., McClintic, K., Sims, P., Rogers, R. L., & Mortel, K. F. (1988b). Etiology, prevention, and treatment of vascular and multi-infarct dementia. In J. S. Meyer, J. Marshall, H. Lechner, & J. F. Toole (Eds.), *Vascular and multi-infarct dementia* (pp. 129–147). Mount Kisco, NY: Futura Publishing.

Meyer, J. S., Rogers, R. L., McClintic, K., Mortel, K. F., & Lotfi, J. (1989). Randomized clinical trial of daily aspirin therapy in multi-infarct dementia. *Journal of the American Geriatrics Society*, *37*, 549–555.

Milberg, W. P., Hebben, N., & Kaplan, E. (1986). The Boston process approach to neuropsychological assessment. In I. Grant & K. M. Adams (Eds.), *Neuropsychological assessment of neuropsychiatric disorders* (pp. 65–86). New York: Oxford University Press.

Miller, A. K. H., Alston, R. L., & Corsellis, J. A. N. (1980). Variations with age in the volumes of grey and white matter in the cerebral hemispheres of man: Measurements with an image analyzer. *Neuropathology and Applied Neurobiology*, *6*, 119–132.

Miller, E. (1974). Psychomotor performance in presenile dementia. *Psychological Medicine*, *4*, 65–68.

Miller, E. (1975). Impaired recall and the memory disturbance in presenile dementia. *British Journal of Social and Clinical Psychology*, *14*, 73–79.

Miller, E. (1980). Cognitive assessment of the older adult. In J. E. Birren & R. B. Sloane (Eds.), *Handbook of mental health and aging* (pp. 520–536). Englewood Cliffs, NJ: Prentice-Hall.

Miller, E., & Lewis, P. (1977). Recognition memory in elderly patients with depression and dementia: A signal detection analysis. *Journal of Abnormal Psychology*, *86*, 84–86.

Miller, W. R. (1975). Psychological deficit in depression. *Psychological Bulletin*, *82*, 238–260.

Minkler, M. (1989). Gold in gray: Reflections on business' discovery of the elderly market. *The Gerontologist*, *29*, 17–23.

Mirsen, T., & Hachinski, V. (1988). Epidemiology and classification of vascular and multi-infarct dementia. In J. S. Meyer, J. Marshall, H. Lechner, & J. F. Toole (Eds.). *Vascular and multi-infarct dementia* (pp. 61–76). Mount Kisco, NY: Futura Publishing.

Mishkin, M., Malamut, M., & Bachevalier, J. (1984). Memories and habits: Two neural systems. In G. Lynch, J. L. McGaugh, & N. M. Weinberger (Eds.), *Neurobiology of learning and memory* (pp. 65–77). New York: Guilford Press.

Mitrushina, M., & Satz, P. (in press). Test-retest reliability of WAIS-R Satz-Mogel short form in a normal elderly sample. *International Journal of Clinical Neuropsychology*.

Mitrushina, M., Satz, P., Chervinsky, A., & D'Elia, L. (1991). Performance of four age groups of normal elderly on Rey Auditory-Verbal Learning Test. *Journal of Clinical Psychology*, *47*, 351–357.

Mittenberg, W., Seidenberg, M., O'Leary, D. S., & DiGiulio, D. V. (1989). Changes in cerebral functioning associated with normal aging. *Journal of Clinical and Experimental Neuropsychology*, *11*, 918–932.

Moehle, K. A, & Long, C. J. (1989). Models of aging and neuropsychological test performance decline with aging. *Journal of Gerontology: Psychological Sciences*, *44*, 176–177.

Mohs, R. C., Breitner, J. C. S., Silverman, J. M., & Davis, K. L. (1987). Alzheimer's Disease: Morbid risk among first-degree relatives approximates 50% by 90 years of age. *Archives of General Psychiatry*, *44*, 405–408.

Montgomery, K. M. (1982). *A normative study of neuropsychological test performance of a normal elderly sample*. Unpublished master's thesis, University of Victoria, British Columbia.

Moran, L. J., & Mefferd, R. B., Jr., (1959). Repetitive psychometric measures. *Psychological Reports*, *5*, 269–275.

Morgan, D. (1988). Age differences in social network participation. *Journal of Gerontology: Social Sciences*, *43*, S129–137.

Morrell, R. W., Park, D. C., & Poon, L. W. (1989). Quality of instructions on prescription drug labels: Effects on memory and comprehension in young and old adults. *The Gerontologist*, *29*, 345–354.

Morris, J. C., McKeel, D. W., Jr., Fulling, K., Torack, R. M., & Berg, L. (1988). Validation of clinical diagnostic criteria for Alzheimer's disease. *Annals of Neurology*, *24*, 17–22.

Morris, R. G., & Baddeley, A. D. (1988). Primary and working memory functioning in Alzheimer-type dementia. *Journal of Clinical and Experimental Neuropsychology*, *10*, 279–296.

Mortimer, J. A., Schuman, L. M., & French, L. R. (1981). Epidemiology of dementing illness. In J. A. Mortimer & L. M. Schuman (Eds.), *The epidemiology of dementia* (pp. 3–23). New York: Oxford University Press.

Mortimer, J. A., Pirozzolo, F. J., Hansch, E. C., & Webster, D. D. (1982). Relationship of motor symptoms to intellectual deficits in Parkinson disease. *Neurology*, *32*, 133–137.

Mortimer, J. A., French, L. R., Hutton, J. T., & Schuman, L. M. (1985). Head injury as a risk factor for Alzheimer's disease. *Neurology*, *35*, 264–267.

Mortimer, J. A., Jun, S.-P., Kuskowski, M. A., & Webster, D. D. (1987). Subtypes of Parkinson's disease defined by intellectual impairment. *Journal of Neural Transmission*, *24*, 101–104.

Moscovitch, M. (1982). A neuropsychological approach to perception and memory in normal and pathological aging. In F. I. M. Craik & S. Trehub (Eds.), *Aging and cognitive processes* (pp. 55–98). New York: Plenum Press.

Moss, M. B., & Albert, M. S. (1988). Alzheimer's disease and other dementing disorders. In M. S. Albert & Mark B. Moss (Eds.), *Geriatric Neuropsychology* (pp. 145–178). New York: Guilford Press.

Moss, M. B., Albert, M. S., Butters, N., & Payne, M. (1986). Differential patterns of memory loss among patients with Alzheimer's disease, Huntington's disease and alcoholic Korsakoff's syndrome. *Archives of Neurology*, *43*, 239–246.

Mullis, R., Holcomb, P., Diner, B., & Dykman, R. A. (1985). The effects of aging on the P3 component of the visual event-related potential. *Electroencephalography and Clinical Neurophysiology*, *62*, 141–149.

Murphy, D. L., & Weingartner, H. (1973). Catecholamines and memory: Enhanced verbal learning during L-dopa administration. *Psychopharmacology Bulletin*, *27*, 319–326.

Murphy, E. (1983). The prognosis of depression in old age. *British Journal of Psychiatry*, *142*, 111–119.

Murray, H. A. (1943). *The Thematic Apperception Test*. Cambridge: Harvard University Press.

Murrell, S. A., & Himmelfarb, S. (1989). Effects of attachment bereavement and pre-event conditions on subsequent depressive symptoms in older adults. *Psychology and Aging*, *4*, 166–172.

Nadeau, S. E., Malloy, P. F., & Andrew, M. E. (1988). A crossover trial of bromocriptine in the treatment of vascular dementia. *Annals of Neurology*, *24*, 270–272.

Nahmias, C., Garnett, E. S., Firnau, G., & Lang, A. (1985). Striatal dopamine distribution in parkinsonian patients during life. *Journal of Neurological Sciences*, *69*, 223–230.

National Center for Health Statistics (1986). *Health, United States, 1986*. (DHHS Publication No. PHS 87-1232). Washington, DC: Department of Health and Human Services.

National Center for Health Statistics (1987a). Current estimates from the National Health Interview Survey, United States, 1986. *Vital and Health Statistics*, Series 10, No. 164.

National Center for Health Statistics. (1987b). Family use of health care, United States, 1980. *National Medical Care Utilization and Expenditure Survey*. (DHHS Publication No. 87-20210). Washington, DC: Department of Health and Human Services.

National Center for Health Statistics (1987c). Utilization of short-stay hospitals, United States, 1985, annual summary. *Vital and Health Statistics*, Series 13, No. 91.

National Institutes of Health (1987). Differential diagnosis of dementing diseases. *Consensus Development Conference Statement*, *6*, 1–27.

National Institute on Aging Task Force. (1980). Senility reconsidered. *Journal of the American Medical Association*, *244*, 259–263.

Naugle, R. I., Cullum, C. M., Bigler, E. D., & Massman, P. J. (1985). Neuropsychological and computerized axial tomography volume characteristics of empirically derived dementia subgroups. *Journal of Nervous and Mental Disease*, *173*, 596–604.

Nebes, R. D, & Andrews-Kulis, M. S. (1976). The effect of age on the speed of sentence formation and incidental learning. *Experimental Aging Research*, *2*, 315–331.

Nee, L. E., Eldridge, R., Sunderland, T., Thomas, C. G., Katz, D., Thompson, K. E., Weingartner, H., Weiss, H., Julian, C., & Cohen, R. (1987). Dementia of the Alzheimer type: Clinical and family study of 22 twin pairs. *Neurology*, *37*, 359–363.

Nelson, H. E. (1982). *Nelson Adult Reading Test manual*. London: National Hospital for Nervous Diseases.

Nelson, H. E., & McKenna, P. (1975). The use of current reading ability in the assessment of dementia. *British Journal of Social and Clinical Psychology*, *14*, 259–267.

Nelson, L. D., Satz, P., Mitrushina, M., Van Gorp, W., Cicchetti, D., Lewis, R., & Van Lancker, D. (1989). Development and validation of the Neuropsychology Behavior and Affect Profile. *Psychological Assessment: A Journal of Consulting and Clinical Psychology*, *1*, 266–272.

Nesselroade, J. R., & Labouvie, E. W. (1985). Experimental design in research on aging. In J. E. Birren & K. W. Schaie (Eds.), *Handbook of the psychology of aging* (2nd ed., pp. 35–60). New York: Van Nostrand Reinhold.

Neugarten, B. (1977). Personality and aging. In J. E. Birren & K. W. Schaie (Eds.), *Handbook of the psychology of aging* (pp. 626–249). New York: Van Nostrand Reinhold.

Neugarten, B. L. (1970). Adaptation and the life cycle. *Journal of Geriatric Psychiatry*, *4*, 71–85.

Neville, H. J., & Folstein, M. F. (1979). Performance on three cognitive tasks by patients with dementia, depression or Korsakov's syndrome. *Gerontology*, *25*, 285–290.

Newman, R. P., Weingartner, H., & Smallberg, S. A. (1984). Effortful and automatic memory effects of dopamine. *Neurology*, *34*, 805–807.

Newmann, J. P. (1989). Aging and depression. *Psychology and Aging*, *4*, 150–165.

Nicholas, M., Obler, L. K., Albert, M. L, & Goodglass, H. (1985). Lexical retrieval in healthy aging. *Cortex*, *21*, 595–606.

Niederehe, G. (1986). Depression and memory impairment in the aged. In L. W. Poon (Ed.), *Handbook for clinical memory assessment of older adults* (pp. 226–237). Washington, DC: American Psychological Association.

Niederehe, G., & Yoder, C. (1989). Metamemory perceptions in depressions of young and older adults. *Journal of Nervous and Mental Disease*, *177*, 4–14.

Nolen-Hoeksema, S. (1987). Sex differences in unipolar depression: Evidence and theory. *Psychological Bulletin*, *101*, 259–282.

Norris, J. T., Gallagher, D., Wilson, A., & Winograd, C. H. (1987). Assessment of depression in geriatric medical outpatients: The validity of two screening measures. *Journal of the American Geriatrics Society*, *35*, 989–995.

Nott, P. N., & Fleminger, J. J. (1975). Presenile dementia: The difficulties of early diagnosis. *Acta Psychiatrica Scandinavica*, *51*, 210–217.

Ober, B. A., Koss, E., Friedland, R. P., & Delis, D. C. (1985). Processes of verbal memory failure in Alzheimer type dementia. *Brain and Cognition*, *4*, 90–103.

Ober, B. A., Dronkers, N. F., Koss, E., Delis, D. C., & Friedland, R. P. (1986). Retrieval from semantic memory in Alzheimer-type dementia. *Journal of Clinical and Experimental Neuropsychology*, *8*, 75–92.

Obeso, J. A., & Martinez-Lage, J. M. (1987). Anticholinergics and amantadine. In W. C. Koller (Ed.), *Handbook of Parkinson's disease* (pp. 309–316). New York: Marcel Dekker.

Obler, L. K. (1980). Narrative discourse style in the elderly. In L. K. Obler & M. L. Albert (Eds.), *Language and communication in the elderly* (pp. 75–90). Lexington, MA: D. C. Heath.

Obler, L. K., & Albert, M. L. (1981). Language and aging: A neurobehavioral analysis. In D. S. Beasley & G. A. Davis (Eds.), *Aging: Communication processes and disorders* (pp. 107–121). New York: Grune & Stratton.

Obler, L. K., & Albert, M. L. (1985). Language skills across adulthood. In J. E. Birren & K. W. Schaie (Eds.), *Handbook of the psychology of aging* (2nd ed., pp. 463–473). New York: Van Nostrand Reinhold.

Obler, L. K., Fein, D., Nicholas, M., & Albert, M. L. (1981a). *Syntactic comprehension in aging*. Paper presented at a meeting of the Academy of Aphasia, Pittsburgh.

Obler, L., Albert, M. L., & Goodglass, H. (1981b). *The word finding difficulties of aging and dementia*. Paper presented at a meeting of the Annual Meeting of Gerontological Society of America, Toronto.

O'Brien, M. D. (1988). Vascular dementia is underdiagnosed. *Archives of Neurology*, *45*, 797–798.

Obrist, W. D. (1963). The electroencephalogram of healthy aged males. In J. E. Birren, R. N. Butler, S. W. Greenhouse, L. Sokoloff, & M. Yarrow (Eds.), *Human aging: A biological and behavioral study* (pp. 79–93). Washington, DC: U.S. Government Printing Office.

Obrist, W. D. (1975). Cerebral physiology of the aged. Relation to psychological function. In N. R. Burch & H. L. Altschuler (Eds.), *Behavior and brain electrical activity* (pp. 421–430). New York: Plenum Press.

Offenbach, S. I. A. (1974). A developmental study of hypothesis testing and cue selection strategies. *Developmental Psychology*, *10*, 484–490.

Olszewski, J. (1962). Subcortical arteriosclerotic encephalopathy. *World Neurology*, *3*, 359–374.

Orgel, L. E. (1963). The maintenance of the accuracy of protein synthesis and its relevance to aging. *Proceedings of the National Academy of Sciences*, *49*, 517–521.

Osato, S., La Rue, A., & Yang, J. (1989, November). *Screening for cognitive deficits in older psychiatric patients*. Paper presented at a meeting of the Annual meeting of the Gerontological Society of America, Minneapolis.

Osborne, D. P., Brown, E. R., & Randt, C. T. (1982). Qualitative changes in memory function: Aging and dementia. In S. Corkin, K. L. Davis, J. H. Growdin, E. Usdin, & R. J. Wurtman (Eds.), *Alzheimer's disease: A report of progress in research* (pp. 165–169). New York: Raven Press.

Osterrieth, P. A. (1944). Le test de copie d'une figure complexe. *Archives de Psychologie*, *30*, 206–356.

Ouslander, J. G. (1981). Drug therapy in the elderly. *Annals of Internal Medicine*, *95*, 711–722.

Overall, J. E., & Gomez-Mont, F. (1974). The MMPI-168 for psychiatric screening. *Educational and Psychological Measurement*, *34*, 315–319.

Overall, J. E., & Gorham, D. R. (1962). The Brief Psychiatric Rating Scale. *Psychological Reports*, *10*, 799–812.

Padgett, R. J., & Ratner, H. H. (1987). Older and younger adults' memory for structured and unstructured events. *Experimental Aging Research*, *13*, 133–139.

Parker, K. (1983). Factor analysis of the WAIS-R at nine age levels between 16 and 74 years. *Journal of Consulting and Clinical Psychology*, *51*, 302–308.

Parmelee, P. A., Katz, I. R., & Lawton, M. P. (1989). Depression among institutionalized aged: Assessment and prevalence estimation. *Journal of Gerontology: Medical Sciences*, *44*, M22–29.

Passeri, M., & Cucinotta, D. (1989). Ateroid in the clinical treatment of multi-infarct dementia; Modern problems of pharmacopsychiatry. *Modern Problems of Pharmacopsychiatry*, *23*, 85–94.

Perez, F. I., Gay, J. R. A., Taylor, R. L., & Rivera, V. M. (1975a). Patterns of memory performance in the neurologically impaired aged. *Canadian Journal of Neurological Sciences*, *2*, 347–355.

Perez, F. I., Rivera, V. M., Meyer, J. S., Gay, J. R. A., Taylor, R. L., & Mathew, N. T. (1975b). Analysis of intellectual and cognitive performance in patients with multi-infarct dementia, vertebrobasilar insufficiency with dementia, and Alzheimer's disease. *Journal of Neurological and Neurosurgical Psychiatry*, *38*, 533–540.

Perez, F. I., Mathew, N. T., Stump, D. A., & Meyer, J. S. (1977). Regional cerebral blood flow statistical patterns and psychological performance in multi-infarct dementia and Alzheimer's disease. *Canadian Journal of Neurological Sciences*, *4*, 53–62.

Perl, D. P., & Brody, A. R. (1980). Alzheimer's disease: X-ray spectrometric evidence of aluminum accumulation in neurofibrillary tangle-bearing neurons. *Science*, *208*, 297–299.

Perlmutter, M. (1988). Cognitive potential throughout life. In J. E. Birren & V. L. Bengtson (Eds.), *Emergent theories of aging* (pp. 247–268). New York: Springer.

Perlmutter, M., & Mitchell, D. B. (1982). The appearance and disappearance of age differences in adult memory. In F. I. M. Craik & S. Trehub (Eds.), *Aging and cognitive processes* (pp. 127–143). New York: Plenum Press.

Perry, E. K., Tomlinson, B. E., Blessed, G., Bergmann, K., Gibson, P. H., & Perry, R. H. (1978). Correlation of cholinergic abnormalities with senile plaques and mental test scores in senile dementia. *British Medical Journal*, *2*, 1457–1459.

Perry, E. K., Curtis, M., Dick, D. J., Candy, J. M., Atack, J. R., Bloxham, C. A., Blessed, G., Fairbairn, A., Tomlinson, B. E., & Perry, E. T. (1985). Cholinergic correlates of cognitive impairment in Parkinson's disease: Comparisons with Alzheimer's disease. *Journal of Neurology, Neurosurgery and Psychiatry*, *48*, 413–421.

Perry, R. H., Tomlinson, B. E., Candy, J. M., Blessed, G., Foster, J. F., Bloxham, C. A., & Perry, E. R. (1983). Cortical cholinergic deficit in mentally impaired Parkinsonian patients. *Lancet*, *2*, 789–790.

Pfeiffer, E. A. (1975). A short portable mental status questionnaire for the assessment of organic brain deficit in elderly patients. *Journal of the American Geriatric Society*, *23*, 433–441.

Pharmaceutical Manufacturers Association. (1989, January). *New medicines in development for older Americans*. Available from Author, 1100 15th Street, NW, Washington, DC 20005.

Phelps, M. E., & Mazziotta, J. C. (1985). Positron emission tomography: Human brain function and biochemistry. *Science*, *228*, 799–809.

Phifer, J. F., & Murrell, S. A. (1986). Etiologic factors in the onset of depressive symptoms in older adults. *Journal of Abnormal Psychology*, *95*, 282–291.

Piedmont, R. L., Sokolove, R. L., & Fleming, M. Z. (1989). An examination of some diagnostic strategies involving the Wechsler Intelligence Scales. *Psychological Assessment: A Journal of Consulting and Clinical Psychology*, *1*, 181–185.

Piersma, H. L. (1986). Wechsler Memory Scale performance in geropsychiatric patients. *Journal of Clinical Psychology*, *42*, 323–327.

Pillon, B., Dubois, B., Lhermitte, F., & Agid, Y. (1986). Heterogeneity of cognitive impairment in progressive supranuclear palsy, Parkinson's disease, and Alzheimer's disease. *Neurology*, *36*, 1179–1185.

Pillon, B., Dubois, B., Cusimano, G., Bonnet, A.-M., Lhermitte, F. L., & Agid, Y. (1989). Does cognitive impairment in Parkinson's disease result from non-dopaminergic lesions? *Journal of Neurology, Neurosurgery, and Psychiatry*, *52*, 201–206.

Pirozzolo, F. J., & Hansch, E. C. (1981). Oculomotor reaction time in dementia reflects degree of cerebral dysfunction. *Science*, *214*, 349–351.

Pirozzolo, F. J., Hansch, E. C., Mortimer, J. A., Webster, D. D., & Kuskowski, A. (1982). Dementia in Parkinson disease: A neuropsychological analysis. *Brain and Cognition*, *1*, 71–83.

Pirozzolo, F. J., Swihart, A. A., Rey, G., Jankovic, J., & Mortimer, J. A. (1988). Cognitive impairments associated with Parkinson's disease and other movement disorders. In J. Jankovic & E. Tolosa (Eds.), *Parkinson's disease and movement disorders* (pp. 425–440). Baltimore: Urban & Schwarzenberg.

Plemons, J. K., Willis, S. L., & Baltes, P. B. (1978). Modifiability of fluid intelligence in aging: A short-term longitudinal training approach. *Journal of Gerontology*, *33*, 224–231.

Plude, D. J., Milberg, W. P., & Cerella, J. (1986). Age differences in depicting and perceiving tridimensionality in simple line drawings. *Experimental Aging Research*, *12*, 221–225.

Poon, L. W. (Ed.), (1986). *Handbook for clinical memory assessment of older adults*. Washington, DC: American Psychological Association.

Poon, L. W., & Fozard, J. L. (1980). Age and word frequency effects in continuous recognition memory. *Journal of Gerontology*, *35*, 77–86.

Poon, L. W., Krauss, I. K., & Bowles, N. J. (1984). On subject selection in cognitive research. *Experimental Aging Research*, *10*, 43–50.

Poon, L. W., Rubin, D. C., & Wilson, B. C. (Eds.). (1989). *Everyday cognition in adulthood and late life*. New York: Cambridge University Press.

Popkin, S. J., Gallagher, D., Thompson, L. W., & Moore, M. (1982). Memory complaint and performance in normal and depressed older adults. *Experimental Aging Research*, *8*, 141–145.

Post, F. (1966). Somatic and psychic factors in the treatment of elderly psychiatric patients. *Journal of Psychosomatic Research*, *10*, 13–19.

Powell, A. L., Cummings, J. L., Hill, M. A., & Benson, F. (1988). Speech and language alterations in multi-infarct dementia. *Neurology*, *38*, 717–719.

Price, L. H., Fein, G., & Feinberg, I. (1980). Neuropsychological assessment of cognitive functioning in the elderly. In L. W. Poon (Ed.), *Aging in the 1980s: Psychological issues* (pp. 78–85). Washington, DC: American Psychological Association.

Purisch, A. D., & Sbordone, R. J. (1986). The Luria-Nebraska Neuropsychological Battery. In G. Goldstein & R. E. Tarter (Eds.), *Advances in clinical neuropsychology* (pp. 291–316). New York: Plenum Press.

Quereshi, M. Y., & Erstad, D. (1990). A comparison of the WAIS and the WAIS-R for ages 61–91 years. *Psychological Assessment: A Journal of Consulting and Clinical Psychology*, *2*, 293–297.

Query, W. T., & Megran, J. (1983). Age-related norms for AVLT in a male patient population. *Journal of Clinical Psychology*, *39*, 136–138.

Quinn, N. P. (1987). Levodopa. In W. C. Koller (Ed.), *Handbook of Parkinson's disease* (pp. 317–338). New York: Marcel Dekker.

Rabbitt, P. M. A. (1979). Some experiments and a model for changes in attentional selectivity with old age. In F. Hoffmeister & C. Muller (Eds.), *Brain function in old age* (pp. 82–94). Berlin: Springer-Verlag.

Rabinowitz, J. C., Craik, F. I. M., & Ackerman, B. P. (1982). A processing resource account of age differences in recall. *Canadian Journal of Psychology*, *36*, 325–344.

Rabins, P. V. (1983). Reversible dementia and the misdiagnosis of dementia: A review. *Hospital and Community Psychiatry*, *34*, 830–835.

Rabins, P. V., & Folstein, M. F. (1982). Delirium and dementia: Diagnostic criteria and fatality rates. *British Journal of Psychiatry*, *140*, 149–153.

Rabins, P. V., Merchant, A., & Nestadt, G. (1984). Criteria for diagnosing reversible dementia caused by depression: Validation by 2-year follow-up. *British Journal of Psychiatry*, *144*, 488–492.

Rajput, A. H., Offord, K. P., Beard, C. M., & Kurland, L. T. (1984). Epidemiology of parkinsonism: Incidence, classification, and mortality. *Annals of Neurology*, *16*, 278–282.

Randt, C. T., Brown, E. R, & Osborne, D. P. (1980). A memory test for longitudinal measurement of mild to moderate deficits. *Clinical Neuropsychology*, *2*, 184–194.

Rao, S. M., Mittenberg, W., Bernardin, L., Haughton, V., & Leo, G. J. (1989). Neuropsychological test findings in subjects with leukoaraiosis. *Archives of Neurology*, *46*, 40–44.

Rapp, S. R., & Davis, K. M. (1989). Geriatric depression: Physicians' knowledge, perceptions, and diagnostic practices. *The Gerontologist*, *29*, 242–257.

Rapp, S. R., Parisi, S. A., & Walsh, D. A. (1988a). Psychological dysfunction and physical health among elderly medical inpatients. *Journal of Consulting and Clinical Psychology*, *56*, 851–855.

Rapp, S. R., Parisi, S. A., Walsh, D. A., & Wallace, C. E. (1988b). Detecting depression in elderly medical inpatients. *Journal of Consulting and Clinical Psychology*, *56*, 509–513.

Raskin, A. (1986). Partialing out the effects of depression and age on cognitive functions: Experimental data and methodologic issues. In L. W. Poon (Ed.), *Handbook for clinical memory assessment of older adults* (pp. 244–256). Washington, DC: American Psychological Association.

Raskin, A., Friedman, A. S., & DiMascio, A. (1982). Cognitive and performance deficits in depression. *Psychopharmacology Bulletin*, *18*, 196–202.

Raskin, A., & Crook, T. (1988). Relative's assessment of global symptomatology (RAGS). *Psychopharmacology Bulletin*, *24*, 759–763.

Raven, J. C. (1960). *Guide to the Standard Progressive Matrices*. London: H. K. Lewis.

Raven, J. C. (1965). *Guide to using the Coloured Progressive Matrices*. New York: Psychological Corporation.

Read, D. E. (1988). Age-related changes in performance on a visual-closure task. *Journal of Clinical and Experimental Neuropsychology*, *10*, 451–466.

Reding, M., Haycox, J., & Blass, J. (1985). Depression in patients referred to a dementia clinic. A three-year prospective study. *Archives of Neurology*, *42*, 894–896.

Reed, H. B. C., & Reitan, R. M. (1963). Changes in psychological test performances associated with the normal aging process. *Journal of Gerontology*, *18*, 271–274.

Reed, B. R., Jagust, W. J., & Seab, J. P. (1988, February). *Differences in rates of confabulatory intrusions in Alzheimer's disease and multiinfarct dementia*. Paper presented at a meeting of the International Neuropsychological Society, New Orleans.

Reed, B. R., Jagust, W. J., & Seab, J. P. (1989). Mental status as a predictor of daily function in progressive dementia. *The Gerontologist*, *29*, 804–807.

Regier, D. A., Myers, J. K., Kramer, M., Robins, L. N., Blazer, D. G., Hough, R. L., Eaton, W. W., & Locke, B. Z. (1984). The NIMH epidemiological catchment area program. *Archives of General Psychiatry*, *41*, 934–941.

Regier, D. A., Boyd, J. H., Burke, J. D., Jr., Rae, D. S., Myers, J. K., Kramer, M., Robins, L. N., George, L. K., Karno, M., & Locke, B. Z. (1988). One-month prevalence of mental disorders in the United States. *Archives of General Psychiatry*, *45*, 977–986.

Reich, J. W., Zautra, A. J., & Guarnaccia, C. A. (1989). Effects of disability and bereavement on the mental health and recovery of older adults. *Psychology and Aging*, *4*, 57–65.

Reichel, W. (1989). *Clinical aspects of aging* (3rd ed.). Baltimore, MD: Williams & Wilkins.

Reifler, B. V., Larson, E., & Hanley, R. (1982). Coexistence of cognitive impairment and depression in geriatric outpatients. *American Journal of Psychiatry, 139*, 623–629.

Reifler, B. V., Larson, E., Teri, L., & Poulsen, M. (1986). Dementia of the Alzheimer's type and depression. *Journal of the American Geriatric Society, 34*, 855–859.

Reisberg, B. (1985). Alzheimer's disease update. *Psychiatric Annals, 15*, 319–322.

Reisberg, B., Ferris, S. H., de Leon, M. J., & Crook, T. (1982a). The global deterioration scale for assessment of primary degenerative dementia. *American Journal of Psychiatry, 139*, 1136–1139.

Reisberg, B., Ferris, S. H., Georgotas, A., de Leon, M. J., & Schneck, M. K. (1982b). Relationship between cognition and mood in geriatric depression. *Psychopharmacology Bulletin, 18*, 191–193.

Reisberg, B., Borenstein, J., Salob, S. P., Ferris, S. H., Franssen, E, & Georgotas, A. (1987). Behavioral symptoms in Alzheimer's disease: Phenomenology and treatment. *Journal of Clinical Psychiatry, 48* (Suppl.), 9–15.

Reitan, R. M. (1955). The distribution according to age of a psychologic measure dependent upon organic brain functions. *Journal of Gerontology, 10*, 338–340.

Reitan, R. M. (1958). Validity of the Trail Making Test as an indicator of organic brain damage. *Perceptual and Motor Skills, 19*, 199–206.

Reitan, R. M. (1986). Theoretical and methodological bases of the Halstead-Reitan Neuropsychological Test Battery. In I. Grant & K. M. Adams (Eds.), *Neuropsychological assessment of neuropsychiatric disorders* (pp. 3–30). New York: Oxford University Press.

Reitan, R. M., & Davison, L. A. (Eds.). (1974). *Clinical neuropsychology: Current status and applications*. New York: Winston/Wiley.

Reitan, R. M., & Wolfson, D. (1985). *The Halstead-Reitan Neuropsychological Test Battery*. Tempe, AZ: Neuropsychology Press.

Reus, V. I., Silberman, E., Post, R. M., & Weingartner, H. (1979). D-amphetamine: Effects on memory in a depressed population. *Biological Psychiatry, 14*, 345–356.

Revenson, T. A. (1989). Compassionate stereotyping of elderly patients by physicians: Revising the social contact hypothesis. *Psychology and Aging, 4*, 230–234.

Rey, A. (1941). L'examen psychologique dans les cas d'encephalopathie traumatique. *Archives de Psychologie, 28*, 286–340.

Rey, A. (1964). *L'examen clinque en psychologie*. Paris: Presses Universitaires de France.

Rey, A. (1968). *Epreuves mnesiques et d'apprentissage*. Paris: Delachaux & Niestle.

Reynolds, C. F., III, Perel, M. M., Kupfer, D. J., Zimmer, B., Stack, J. A., & Hoch, C. C. (1987). Open-trial response to antidepressant treatment in elderly patients with mixed depression and cognitive impairment. *Psychiatry Research, 21*, 111–122.

Reynolds, C. F., Hoch, C. C., Kupfer, D. J., Buysse, D. J., Houck, P. R., Stack, J. A., & Campbell, D. W. (1988). Bedside differentiation of depressive pseudodementia from dementia. *American Journal of Psychiatry, 145*, 1099–1103.

Rezek, D. L., Morris, J. C., Fulling, K. H., & Gado, M. H. (1987). Periventricular white matter lucencies in senile dementia of the Alzheimer type and in normal aging. *Neurology, 37*, 1365–1368.

Ricaurte, G. A., Langston, J. W., Irwin, I., DeLanney, L. E., & Forno, L. S. (1985). The neurotoxic effect of MPTP on the dopaminergic cells of the substantia nigra in mice is age-related. *Society of Neurosciences Abstracts, 11*, 631.

Richards, P. M., & Ruff, R. M. (1989). Motivational effects on neuropsychological functioning: Comparison of depressed versus nondepressed individuals. *Journal of Consulting and Clinical Psychology, 57*, 396–402.

Riege, W. H., & Metter, E. J. (1988). Cognitive and brain imaging measures of Alzheimer's disease. *Neurobiology of Aging, 9*, 69–86.

Riege, W. H., Harker, J. O., & Metter, E. J. (1986). Clinical validators: Brain lesions and brain imaging. In L. W. Poon (Ed.), *Handbook for clinical memory assessment of older adults* (pp. 314–336). Washington, DC: American Psychological Association.

Riegel, K. F., & Riegel, R. M. (1972). Development, drop, and death. *Developmental Psychology*, *6*, 309–316.

Riklan, M., Reynolds, C. M., & Stellar, S. (1989). Correlates of memory in Parkinson's disease. *Journal of Nervous and Mental Disease*, *177*, 237–240.

Roark, A. C. (1989, May 4). Most older persons say they're happy with lives. *Los Angeles Times*, pp. 1, 24–25.

Robertson-Tchabo, E. A., Hausman, C. P., & Arenberg, D. (1976). A classical mnemonic for old learners: A trip that works. *Educational Gerontology*, *1*, 215–226.

Robiner, W. N. (1987). An experimental inquiry into transference roles and age. *Psychology and Aging*, *2*, 306–311.

Robins, L. N., Helzer, J. E., Croughan, J., & Ratcliff, K. S. (1981). National Institute of Mental Health Diagnostic Interview Schedule: Its history, characteristics, and validity. *Archives of General Psychiatry*, *38*, 381–389.

Robinson, D. S., Nies, A., Davies, H. M., Bunney, W. E., Davis, J. M., Colburn, R. W., Bourne, H. R., Shaw, D. M., & Coppen, A. J. (1972). Ageing, monoamines and monoamine-oxidase levels. *Lancet*, *1*, 290–291.

Robinson, R. G. (1986). Post-stroke mood disorders. *Hospital Practice*, *21*, 83–89.

Roca, R. P. (1987). Bedside cognitive examination. *Psychosomatics*, *28*, 71–76.

Rocca, W. A., Amaducci, L. A., & Schoenberg, B. S. (1986). Epidemiology of clinically diagnosed Alzheimer's disease. *Annals of Neurology*, *19*, 415–424.

Rogers, J., & Bloom, F. E. (1985). Neurotransmitter metabolism and function in the aging central nervous system. In C. E. Finch & E. L. Schneider (Eds.), *Handbook of the biology of aging* (2nd ed., pp. 645–691). New York: Van Nostrand Reinhold.

Rogers, R. L., Meyer, J. S., Mortel, K. F., Mahurin, R. K., & Judd, B. W. (1986). Decreased cerebral blood flow precedes multi-infarct dementia, but follows senile dementia of Alzheimer type. *Neurology*, *36*, 1–6.

Romano, J., & Engel, G. L. (1944). Delirium. I. Electroencephalographic data. *Archives of Neurological Psychiatry*, *51*, 376–377.

Ron, M. A., Toone, B. K., Garralda, M. E., & Lishman, W. A. (1979). Diagnostic accuracy in presenile dementia. *British Journal of Psychiatry*, *134*, 161–168.

Rorschach, H. (1942). *Psychodiagnostics*. New York: Grune & Stratton.

Rosen, W. G. (1980). Verbal fluency in aging and dementia. *Journal of Clinical Neuropsychology*, *2*, 135–146.

Rosen, W. G. (1983). Neuropsychological investigation of memory, visuoconstructional, visuoperceptual, and language abilities in senile dementia of the Alzheimer type. In R. Mayeux & W. G. Rosen (Eds.), *The dementias* (pp. 65–73). New York: Raven Press.

Rosen, W. G., Terry, R. D., Fuld, P. A., Katzman, R., & Peck, A. (1980). Pathological verification of ischemic score in differentiation of dementias. *Annals of Neurology*, *7*, 486–488.

Rosen, W. G., Mohs, R. C., & Davis, K. L. (1984). A new rating scale for Alzheimer's disease. *American Journal of Psychiatry*, *141*, 1356–1364.

Roses, A. D., Pericak-Vance, M. A., Dawson, D. V., Haynes, C. S., Kaplan, E. B., Gaskell, P. C., Jr., Heyman, A., Clark, C. M., & Earl, N. L. (1988). Standard likelihood linkage analysis in late-onset Alzheimer's disease. *Alzheimer Disease and Associated Disorders*, *2*, 275.

Rossor, M. N., Emson, P. C., Mountjoy, C. Q., Roth, M., & Iversen, L. L. (1980). Reduced amounts of immunoreactive somatostatin in the temporal cortex in senile dementia of Alzheimer type. *Neuroscience Letters*, *20*, 373–377.

Roth, M. (1955). The natural history of mental disorder in old age. *Journal of Mental Science*, *101*, 281–301.

Roth, M., & Kay, D. W. K. (1956). Affective disorder arising in the senium: 2. Physical disability as an aetiological factor. *Journal of Mental Science*, *102*, 141–150.

Rothschild, D. (1942). Neuropathologic changes in arteriosclerotic psychoses and their psychiatric significance. *Archives of Neurological Psychiatry*, *48*, 417–436.

Rovner, B. W., Kafonek, S., Filipp, L., Lucas, M. J., & Folstein, M. F. (1986). Prevalence of mental illness in a community nursing home. *American Journal of Psychiatry*, *143*, 1446–1449.

Roybal, E. R. (1988). Mental health and aging: The need for an expanded Federal response. *American Psychologist*, *43*, 189–194.

Roy-Byrne, P. P., Weingartner, H., Bierer, L. M., Thompson, K., & Post, R. M. (1986). Effortful and automatic cognitive processes in depression. *Archives of General Psychiatry*, *43*, 265–267.

Rubin, E. H., Morris, J. C., Storandt, M., & Berg, L. (1987). Behavioral changes in patients with mild senile dementia of the Alzheimer's type. *Psychiatry Research*, *21*, 55–62.

Rubin, E. H., Morris, J. C., Grant, E. A., & Vendegna, T. (1989). Very mild senile dementia of the Alzheimer type: 1. Clinical assessment. *Archives of Neurology*, *46*, 379–382.

Ruff, R. M., Evans, R. W., & Light, R. H. (1986). Automatic detection vs. controlled search: A paper-and-pencil approach. *Perceptual and Motor Skills*, *62*, 407–416.

Ruff, R. M., Light, R. H., & Quayhagen, M. (1988). Selective reminding tests: A normative study of verbal learning in adults. *Journal of Clinical and Experimental Neuropsychology*, *11*, 539–550.

Ruhm, C. J. (1989). Why older Americans stop working. *The Gerontologist*, *29*, 294–299.

Rush, A. J., Weissenburger, Vinson, D. B., & Giles, D. E. (1983). Neuropsychological dysfunctions in unipolar nonpsychotic major depressions. *Journal of Affective Disorders*, *5*, 281–287.

Russell, E. W. (1984). Theory and development of pattern analysis methods related to the Halstead-Reitan Battery. In P. E. Logue & J. M. Schear (Eds.), *Clinical neuropsychology: A multidisciplinary approach* (pp. 50–98). Springfield, IL: Charles C Thomas.

Russell, E. W. (1988). Renorming Russell's version of the Wechsler Memory Scale. *Journal of Clinical and Experimental Neuropsychology*, *10*, 235–249.

Russell, E. W., Neuringer, C., & Goldstein, G. (1970). *Assessment of brain damage: A neuropsychological key approach*. New York: Wiley-Interscience.

Russell, R. W. (1988). Brain "transplants," neurotrophic factors and behavior. *Alzheimer Disease and Associated Disorders*, *2*, 77–95.

Ryan, J. J., Georgemiller, R. J., & McKinney, B. E. (1984). Application of the four-subtest WAIS-R short form with an older clinical sample. *Journal of Clinical Psychology*, *40*, 1033–1036.

Ryan, J. J., Paolo, A. M., & Brungardt, T. M. (1990). Standardization of the Wechsler Adult Intelligence Scale-Revised for persons 75 years and older. *Psychological Assessment: A Journal of Consulting and Clinical Psychology*, *2*, 404–411.

Ryff, C. D. (1989). In the eye of the beholder: Views of psychological well-being among middle-aged and older adults. *Psychology and Aging*, *4*, 195–210.

Sacks, O. (1990). *Awakenings*. New York: HarperPerennial.

Sadeh, M., Braham, J., & Modan, M. (1982). Effects of anticholinergic drugs on memory in Parkinson's disease. *Archives of Neurology*, *39*, 666–667.

Sagar, H. J., Cohen, N. J., Sullivan, E. V., Corkin, S., & Growdon, J. H. (1988). Remote memory function in Alzheimer's disease and Parkinson's disease. *Brain*, *111*, 185–206.

Salmon, D. P., Granholm, E., McCullough, D., Butters, N., & Grant, I. (1989). Recognition memory span in mildly and moderately demented patients with Alzheimer's disease. *Journal of Clinical and Experimental Neuropsychology*, *11*, 429–443.

Salthouse, T. A. (1985). Speed of behavior and its implications for cognition. In J. E. Birren & K. W. Schaie (Eds.), *Handbook of the psychology of aging* (2nd ed., pp. 400–426). New York: Van Nostrand Reinhold.

Sanders, J. A. C., Sterns, H. L., Smith, M., & Sanders, R. E. (1975). Enhancement of conjunctive concept attainment in older adults. *Developmental Psychology*, *11*, 824–829.

Sands, L. P., & Meredith, W. (1989). Effects of sensory and motor functioning on adult intellectual performance. *Journal of Gerontology*, *44*, P56–58.

Sands, L. P., Terry, H., & Meredith, W. (1989). Change and stability in adult intellectual functioning assessed by Wechsler item responses. *Psychology and Aging*, *4*, 79–87.

Satz, P., & Mogel, S. (1962). An abbreviation of the WAIS for clinical use. *Journal of Clinical Psychology*, *18*, 77–79.

Satz, P., Van Gorp, W. G., Soper, H. V., & Mitrushina, M. (1987). A WAIS-R marker for dementia for the

Alzheimer type? An empirical and statistical induction test. *Journal of Clinical and Experimental Neuropsychology*, *9*, 767–774.

Savard, R. J., Rey, A. C., & Post, R. M. (1980). Halstead-Reitan Category Test in bipolar and unipolar affective disorders. *Journal of Nervous and Mental Disease*, *168*, 297–303.

Saxton, J., McGonigle-Gibson, K. L., Swihart, A. A., Miller, V. J., & Boller, F. (1990). Assessment of the severely impaired patient: Description and validation of a new neuropsychological test battery. *Psychological Assessment: A Journal of Consulting and Clinical Psychology*, *2*, 298–303.

Sbordone, R. J., & Caldwell, A. (1979). ODB-168. *Clinical Neuropsychology*, *1*, 38–41.

Schacter, D. L. (1987). Memory, amnesia, and frontal lobe dysfunction. *Psychobiology*, *15*, 21–36.

Schaie, K. W. (1983). The Seattle Longitudinal Study: A 21-year exploration of exploration of psychometric intelligence in adulthood. In K. W. Schaie (Ed.), *Longitudinal studies of adult psychological development* (pp. 64–135). New York: Guilford Press.

Schaie, K. W., & Hertzog, C. (1985). Measurement in the psychology of adulthood and aging. In J. E. Birren, & K. W. Schaie (Eds.), *Handbook of the psychology of aging* (2nd ed., pp. 61–92). New York: Van Nostrand Reinhold.

Schaie, K. W., & Labouvie-Vief, G. (1974). Generational versus ontogenetic components of change in adult cognitive behavior: A fourteen-year cross-sequential study. *Developmental Psychology*, *10*, 305–320.

Schaie, K. W., & Schaie, J. P. (1977). Clinical assessment and aging. In J. E. Birren & K. W. Schaie (Eds.), *Handbook of the psychology of aging* (pp. 692–723). New York: Van Nostrand Reinhold.

Schear, J. M. (1984). Neuropsychological assessment of the elderly in clinical practice. In P. E. Logue & J. M. Schear (Eds.), *Clinical neuropsychology: A multidisciplinary approach* (pp. 199–236). Springfield, IL: Charles C Thomas.

Scheibel, A. B. (1992). Structural changes in the aging brain. In J. E. Birren, R. B. Sloane, & G. Cohen (Eds.), *Handbook of mental health and aging* (2nd ed., pp. 147–173). New York: Academic Press.

Scheibel, A. B., & Wechsler, A. F. (Eds.). (1986). *The biological substrates of Alzheimer's disease*. New York: Academic Press.

Scheibel, M. E., Lindsay, R. D., Tomiyasu, U., & Scheibel, A. B. (1975). Progressive dendritic changes in aging human cortex. *Experimental Neurology*, *47*, 392–403.

Scheibel, M. E., Lindsay, R. D., Tomiyasu, U., & Scheibel, A. B. (1976). Progressive dendritic changes in the human limbic system. *Experimental Neurology*, *53*, 420–430.

Schellenberg, G. D., Bird, T. D., Wijsman, E. M., Moore, D. K., Boehnke, M., Bryant, E. M., Lampe, T. H., Nochlin, D., Sumi, S. M., Deeb, S. S., Beyreuther, K., & Martin, G. M. (1988). Absence of linkage of chromosome 21q21 markers of familial Alzheimer's disease. *Science*, *241*, 1507–1508.

Schildkraut, J. J. (1965). The catecholamine hypothesis of affective disorders: A review of supporting evidence. *American Journal of Psychiatry*, *122*, 509–522.

Schneider, E. L. (1987). Theories of aging: A perspective. In H. R. Warner, R. N. Butler, R. L. Sprott, & R. L. Schneider (Eds.), *Modern biological theories of aging* (pp. 1–4). New York: Raven Press.

Schneider, E. L., & Rowe, J. W. (Eds.). (1989). *Handbook of the biology of aging* (3rd ed.). New York: Academic Press.

Schoenberg, B. S. (1988). Epidemiology of vascular and multi-infarct dementia. In J. S. Meyer, J. Marshall, H. Lechner, & J. F. Toole (Eds.), *Vascular and multi-infarct dementia* (pp. 47–60). Mount Kosco, NY: Futura Publishing.

Schwamm, L. H., Van Dyke, C., Kiernan, R. J., Merrin, E. L., & Mueller, J. (1987). The Neurobehavioral Cognitive Status Examination: Comparison with the Cognitive Capacity Screening Examination and the Mini-Mental State Examination in a neurosurgical population. *Annals of Internal Medicine*, *107*, 486–491.

Scogin, F., & Bienias, J. L. (1988). A three-year follow-up of older adult participants in a memory-skills training program. *Psychology and Aging*, *3*, 334–337.

Scogin, F., Storandt, M., & Lott, L. (1985). Memory-skills training, memory complaints, and depression in older adults. *Journal of Gerontology*, *40*, 562–568.

Scogin, F., Beutler, L., Corbishley, A., & Hamblin, D. (1987, November). *Reliability and validity of the Short*

Form Beck Depression Inventory with older adults. Paper presented at a meeting of the Annual Convention of the Gerontological Society of America, Washington, DC.

Segal, J. L., Thompson, J. F., & Floyd, R. A. (1979). Drug utilization and prescribing patterns in a skilled nursing facility: The need for a rational approach to therapeutics. *Journal of the American Geriatrics Society*, *27*, 1171–1122.

Shapiro, S., Skinner, E. A., Kessler, L. G., Von Korff, M., German, P. S., Tischler, G. L., Leaf, P. J., Benham, L., Cottler, L., & Regier, D. A. (1984). Utilization of health and mental health services. *Archives of General Psychiatry*, *41*, 971–978.

Sharps, M. J., & Gollin, E. S. (1988). Aging and free recall for objects located in space. *Journal of Gerontology: Psychological Sciences*, *43*, 8–11.

Sherrill, R. E. (1985). Comparison of three short forms of the Category Test. *Journal of Clinical and Experimental Neuropsychology*, *7*, 231–238.

Shimamura, A. P., Salmon, D. P., Squire, L. R., & Butters, H. (1987). Memory dysfunction and word priming in dementia and amnesia. *Behavioral Neuroscience*, *101*, 347–351.

Shindler, A. G., Caplan, L. R., & Hier, D. B. (1984). Intrusions and perseverations. *Brain and Language*, *23*, 148–158.

Shock, N. W. (1977). Biological theories of aging. In J. E. Birren, & K. W. Schaie (Eds.), *Handbook of the psychology of aging* (pp. 103–115). New York: Van Nostrand Reinhold.

Shoulson, I. (1989). Experimental therapeutics directed at the pathogenesis of Parkinson's disease. In D. B. Calne (Ed.), *Drugs for treatment of Parkinson's disease* (pp. 289–305). New York: Springer-Verlag.

Shuerger, J. M., & Witt, A. C. (1989). The temporal stability of individually tested intelligence. *Journal of Clinical Psychology*, *45*, 294–302.

Siegfried, K. R., Jansen, W., & Pahnke, K. (1984). Cognitive dysfunction in depression: Difference between depressed and nondepressed elderly patients and differential cognitive effects of Nomifensine. *Drug Development Research*, *4*, 533–553.

Siegler, I. C., (1975). The terminal drop hypothesis: Fact or artifact? *Experimental Aging Research*, *1*, 169–185.

Silberman, E. K., Weingartner, H., & Post, R. M. (1983a). Thinking disorder in depression. *Archives of General Psychiatry*, *40*, 775–780.

Silberman, E. K., Weingartner, H., Stillman, R., Chen, H. I., & Post, R. M. (1983b). Altered lateralization of cognitive processes in depressed women. *American Journal of Psychiatry*, *140*, 1340–1344.

Silfverskiold, P., & Risberg, J. (1989). Regional cerebral blood flow in depression and mania. *Archives of General Psychiatry*, *46*, 253–259.

Silverstein, A. B. (1982). Two- and four-subtest short forms of the Wechsler Adult Intelligence Scale-Revised. *Journal of Clinical Psychology*, *41*, 676–680.

Simons, R. (1983–1984). Specificity and substitution in the social networks of the elderly. *International Journal of Aging and Human Development*, *18*, 121–139.

Simonson, W. (1984). *Medications and the elderly: A guide for promoting proper use*. Rockville, MD: Aspen.

Slater, E., & Roth, M. (1969). *Clinical psychiatry* (3rd ed.). Baltimore: Williams & Wilkins.

Sluss, T. K., Gruenberg, E. M., Rabins, P., & Kramer, M. (1982). Distribution of focal signs in a group of demented men. *Neuropsychobiology*, *8*, 109–112.

Small, G. W., & Fawzy, F. I. (1988). Psychiatric consultation for the medically ill elderly in the general hospital: Need for a collaborative model of care. *Psychosomatics*, *29*, 94–103.

Smyer, M. A., Zarit, S. H., & Qualls, S. H. (1990). Psychological intervention with the aging individual. In J. E. Birren & K. W. Schaie (Eds.), *Handbook of the psychology of aging* (3rd ed., pp. 376–403). New York: Academic Press.

Snow, W. G., Tierney, M. C., Zorzitto, M. L., Fisher, R. H., & Reid, D. W. (1989). WAIS-R Test-retest reliability in a normal elderly sample. *Journal of Clinical and Experimental Neuropsychology*, *11*, 423–428.

Spar, J. E., & La Rue, A. (1983). Major depression in the elderly: DSM-III criteria and the dexamethasone suppression test as predictors of treatment response. *American Journal of Psychiatry*, *140*, 844–847.

Spar, J. E., & La Rue, A. (1990). *Concise guide to geriatric psychiatry*. Washington, DC: American Psychiatric Press.

Spielberger, C. D., Gorusch, R. L., & Lushene, R. E. (1970). *State Trait Anxiety Inventory manual*. Palo Alto, CA: Consulting Psychologists Press.

Spiers, P. (1981). Have they come to praise Luria or to bury him? The Luria-Nebraska Battery controversy. *Journal of Consulting and Clinical Psychology*, *49*, 331–341.

Spitzer, R. L., & Endicott, J. (1977). *Schedule for Affective Disorders and Schizophrenia—Life-time version (SADS-L)*. New York: New York State Psychiatric Institute.

Spitzer, R. L., & Williams, J. B. W. (1986). *Structured clinical interview for DSM-III-R*. New York: Biometric Research Department, New York State Psychiatric Institute.

Spitzer, R. L., Endicott, J., & Robbins, E. (1978). Research Diagnostic Criteria: Rationale and reliability. *Archives of General Psychiatry*, *35*, 773–782.

Spreen, O., & Benton, A. L. (1965). Comparative studies of some psychological tests for cerebral damage. *Journal of Nervous and Mental Disease*, *140*, 323–333.

Squire, L. R. (1974). Remote memory as affected by aging. *Neuropsychologia*, *12*, 429–435.

Squire, L. R. (1986). Mechanisms of memory. *Science*, *232*, 1612–1619.

Stafford, J. L., Albert, M. S., Naeser, M. A., Sandor, T., & Garvey, A. J. (1988). Age-related differences in computed tomographic scan measurements. *Archives of Neurology*, *45*, 409–415.

Stankov, L. (1988). Aging, attention, and intelligence. *Psychology and Aging*, *3*, 59–74.

Starkstein, S. E., & Robinson, R. G. (1989). Affective disorders and cerebral vascular disease. *British Journal of Psychiatry*, *154*, 170–182.

Starkstein, S. E., Bolduc, P. L., Preziosi, T. J., & Robinson, R. G. (1989a). Cognitive impairments in different stages of Parkinson's disease. *Journal of Neuropsychiatry*, *1*, 243–248.

Starkstein, S. E., Esteguy, M., Berthier, M. L., Garcia, H., & Leiguarda, R. (1989b). Evoked potentials, reaction time and cognitive performance in on and off phases of Parkinson's disease. *Journal of Neurology, Neurosurgery, and Psychiatry*, *52*, 338–340.

Stengel, E. (1943). A study on the symptomatology and differential diagnosis of Alzheimer's disease and Pick's disease. *Journal of Mental Science*, *89*, 1–20.

Sternberg, D. E., & Jarvik, M. E. (1976). Memory functions in depression. *Archives of General Psychiatry*, *33*, 219–224.

Steuer, J., La Rue, A., Blum, J. E., & Jarvik, L. F. (1980). "Critical loss" in the eighth and ninth decades. *Journal of Gerontology*, *36*, 211–213.

Stewart, R. B. (1988). Adverse drug reactions. In J. C. Delafuente & R. B. Stewart (Eds.), *Therapeutics in the elderly* (pp. 121–131). Baltimore: Williams & Wilkins.

St. George-Hyslop, P. H., Tanzi, R. E., Polinsky, R. J., Haines, J. L., Nee, L., Watkins, P. C., Myers, R. H., Feldman, R. G., Pollen, D., Drachman, D., Growdon, J., Bruni, A., Foncin, J. F., Salmon, D., Frommelt, P., Amaducci, L., Sorbi, S., Piacentini, S., Steward, G. D., Hobbs, W. J., Conneally, P. M., & Gusella, J. F. (1987). The genetic defect causing familial Alzheimer's disease maps on chromosome 21. *Science*, *235*, 885–890.

Stones, M. J., & Kozma, A. (1988). Physical activity, age, and cognitive/motor performance. In M. J. Stones & A. Kozma (Eds.), *Cognitive development in adulthood: Progress in cognitive development research* (pp. 273–322). New York: Springer-Verlag.

Storandt, M. (1977). Age, ability level, and method of administering and scoring the WAIS. *Journal of Gerontology*, *32*, 175–178.

Storandt, M., & Futterman, A. (1982). Stimulus size and performance on two subtests of the Wechsler Adult Intelligence Scale by younger and older adults. *Journal of Gerontology*, *37*, 602–603.

Storandt, M., & Hill, R. D. (1989). Very mild senile dementia of the Alzheimer type: 2. Psychometric test performance. *Archives of Neurology*, *46*, 383–386.

Storandt, M., Botwinick, J., Danziger, W. L., Berg, L., & Hughes, C. P. (1984). Psychometric differentiation of mild senile dementia of the Alzheimer type. *Archives of Neurology*, *41*, 497–499.

Storandt, M., Botwinick, J., & Danziger, W. L. (1986). Longitudinal changes: Patients with mild SDAT and matched healthy controls. In L. W. Poon (Ed.)., *Handbook for clinical memory assessment of older adults* (pp. 277–284). Washington, DC: American Psychological Association.

Stoudemire, A., Hill, C. D., Kaplan, W., Hill, D., Morris, R., Cohen-Cole, S., & Houpt, J. L. (1988). Clinical issues in the assessment of dementia and depression in the elderly. *Psychiatric Medicine*, *6*, 40–49.

Strehler, B. L. (1964). On the histochemistry and ultrastructure of age pigment. In B. L. Strehler (Ed.), *Advances in gerontological research* (Vol. 1, pp. 343–383) New York: Academic Press.

Stromgren, L. S. (1977). The influence of depression on memory. *Acta Psychiatrica Scandanavica*, *56*, 109–128.

Strub, R. L., & Black, F. W. (1977). *The mental status examination in neurology*. Philadelphia: F. A. Davis.

Strub, R. L., & Black, F. W. (1988). *Neurobehavioral disorders: A clinical approach*. Philadelphia: F. A. Davis.

Stuss, D. T., & Benson, D. F. (1984). Neuropsychological studies of the frontal lobes. *Psychological Bulletin*, *95*, 3–28.

Summers, W. K., Majovski, L. V., Marsh, G. M., Tachiki, K., & Kling, A. (1986). Oral tetrahydroamino-acridine in long-term treatment of senile dementia, Alzheimer type. *New England Journal of Medicine*, *315*, 1241–1245.

Sunderland, T., Tariot, P., Murphy, D. L., Weingartner, H., Meuller, E. A., & Cohen, R. M. (1985). Scopolamine challenges in Alzheimer's disease. *Psychopharmacology*, *87*, 247–249.

Sunderland, T., Alterman, I. S., Yount, D., Hill, J. L., Tariot, P. N., Newhouse, P. A., Mueller, E. A., Mellow, A. M., & Cohen, R. M. (1988). A new scale for the assessment of depressed mood in demented patients. *American Journal of Psychiatry*, *145*, 955–959.

Sweet, J. J., Moberg, P. J., & Tovian, S. M. (1990). Evaluation of Wechsler Adult Intelligence Scale–Revised premorbid IQ formulas in clinical populations. *Psychological Assessment: A Journal of Consulting and Clinical Psychology*, *2*, 41–44.

Sweet, J. J., Rozensky, R. H., & Tovian, S. M. (Eds.) (1991). *Handbook of clinical psychology in medical settings*. New York: Plenum Press.

Swihart, A. A., Panisset, M., Becker, J. T., Beyer, J. R., & Boller, F. (1989). Semantics, syntactics, and the Token Test in Alzheimer's disease. *Developmental Neuropsychology*, *5*, 69–78.

Tanaka, Y., Tanaka, O., Mizuno, Y., & Yoshida, M. (1989). A radiologic study of dynamic processes in lacunar dementia. *Stroke*, *20*, 1488–1493.

Tariot, P. N., Cohen, R. M., Welkowitz, J. A., Sunderland, T., Newhouse, P. A., Murphy, D. L., & Weingartner, H. (1988). Multiple-dose arecoline infusions in Alzheimer's disease. *Archives of General Psychiatry*, *45*, 901–905.

Taub, H. A. (1979). Comprehension and memory of prose materials by young and old adults. *Experimental Aging Research*, *5*, 3–13.

Taylor, A. E., Saint-Cyr, J. A., & Lang, A. E. (1986). Frontal lobe dysfunction in Parkinson's Disease. *Brain*, *109*, 845–883.

Taylor, A. E., Saint-Cyr, J. A., & Lang, A. E. (1987). Parkinson's disease: Cognitive changes in relation to treatment response. *Brain*, *110*, 35–51.

Taylor, M. A., & Abrams, R. (1987). Cognitive impairment patterns in schizophrenia and affective disorder. *Journal of Neurology, Neurosurgery, and Psychiatry*, *50*, 895–899.

Taylor, M. A., Greenspan, B., & Abrams, R. (1979). Lateralized neuropsychological dysfunction in affective disorder and schizophrenia. *American Journal of Psychiatry*, *136*, 1031–1034.

Teng, E. L., & Chui, H. C. (1987). The modified Mini-Mental State (3MS) Examination. *Journal of Clinical Psychiatry*, *48*, 314–318.

Teng, E. L., Chui, H. C., Schneider, L. S., & Metzger, L. E. (1987). Alzheimer's dementia: Performance on the Mini-Mental State Examination. *Journal of Consulting and Clinical Psychology*, *55*, 96–100.

Terri, L., & Gallagher-Thompson, D. (1991). Cognitive-behavioral interventions for treatment of depression in Alzheimer's patients. *The Gerontologist*, *31*, 413–416.

Terry, R. D. (1976). Dementia: A brief and selective review. *Archives of Neurology*, *33*, 1–4.

Terry, R. D. (Ed.). (1988). *Aging and the brain*. New York: Raven Press.

Terry, R. D., & Hansen, L. A. (1988). Some morphometric aspects of Alzheimer disease and of normal aging. In R. D. Terry (Ed.), *Aging and the brain* (pp. 109–114). New York: Raven Press.

Terry, R. D., Peck, A., DeTeresa, R., Schechter, R., & Horoupian, D. S. (1981). Some morphometric aspects of the brain in senile dementia of the Alzheimer type. *Annals of Neurology, 10*, 184–192.

Terry, R. D., Hansen, L. A., DeTeresa, R., Davies, P., Tobias, H., & Katzman, R. (1987). Senile dementia of the Alzheimer type without neocortical neurofibrillary tangles. *Journal of Neuropathological Experiments in Neurology, 46*, 262–286.

Tetrud, J. W., & Langston, W. J. (1989). The effect of Deprenyl (Selegiline) on the natural history of Parkinson's disease. *Science, 245*, 519–245.

Thompson, A. P. (1987). Methodological issues in the clinical evaluation of two- and four-subtest short forms of the WAIS-R. *Journal of Clinical Psychology, 43*, 142–145.

Thompson, L. W., Gallagher, D., & Breckenridge, J. S. (1987). Comparative effectiveness of psychotherapies for depressed elders. *Journal of Consulting and Clinical Psychology, 55*, 385–390.

Thurstone, L. L., & Thurstone, T. G. (1949). *SRA Primary Mental Abilities*. Chicago: Science Research Associates.

Tierney, M. C., Snow, W. G., Reid, D. W., Zorzitto, M. L., & Fisher, R. H. (1987). Psychometric differentiation of dementia: Replication and extension of the findings of Storandt and coworkers. *Archives of Neurology, 44*, 720–722.

Tierney, M. C., Fisher, R. H., Lewis, A. J., Zorzitto, M. L., Snow, W. G., Reid, D. W., & Nieuwstraten, P. (1988). The NINCDS-ADRDA work group criteria for the clinical diagnosis of probable Alzheimer's disease: A clinicopathologic study of 57 cases. *Neurology, 38*, 359–364.

Timiras, P. S. (1988). *Physiological basis of geriatrics*. New York: Macmillan.

Tomlinson, B. E., & Kitchener, D. (1972). Granulovacuolar degeneration of hippocampal pyramidal cells. *Journal of Pathology, 106*, 165–185.

Tomlinson, B. E., Blessed, G., & Roth, M. (1968). Observations on the brains of nondemented old people. *Journal of Neurological Science, 7*, 331–356.

Tomlinson, B. E., Blessed, G., & Roth, M. (1970). Observations on the brains of demented old people. *Journal of Neurological Science, 11*, 205–242.

Tomonago, M. (1979). On the morphological changes in locus coeruleus in the senile human brain. *Japanese Journal of Geriatrics, 16*, 545–550.

Tomonago, M. (1981). Cerebral amyloid angiopathy in the elderly. *Journal of the American Geriatrics Society, 29*, 151–157.

Toner, J., Gurland, B., & Teresi, J. (1988). Comparison of self-administered and rater-administered methods of assessing levels of severity of depression in elderly patients. *Journal of Gerontology: Psychological Sciences, 43*, P136–140.

Torres, F. (1988). Contributions of electrophysiological methods for establishing diagnosis and prognosis in stroke and vascular and multi-infarct dementia. In J. S. Meyer, J. Marshall, H. Lechner, & J. F. Toole (Eds.), *Vascular and multi-infarct dementia* (pp. 157–166). Mount Kisco, NY: Futura Publishing.

Trahan, D. E., & Larrabee, G. J. (1988). *Continuous Visual Memory Test: Professional manual*. Odessa, FL: Psychological Assessment Resources.

Trahan, D. E., Larrabee, G. J., & Levin, H. S. (1986). Age-related differences in recognition memory for pictures. *Experimental Aging Research, 12*, 147–150.

Treat, N. J., Poon, L. W., & Fozard, J. L. (1981). Age, imagery, and practice in paired-associate learning. *Experimental Aging Research, 7*, 337–342.

Trimble, M. R. (1987). Anticonvulsant drugs and cognitive function: A review of the literature. *Epilepsia, 28* (Suppl. 3), S37–S45.

Trzepacz, P. T., Baker, R. W., & Greenhouse, J. (1988). A symptom rating scale for delirium. *Psychiatry Research, 23*, 89–97.

Trzepacz, P. T., Sclabassi, R. J., & Van Thiel, D. H. (1989). Delirium: A subcortical phenomenon? *Journal of Neuropsychiatry, 1*, 283–290.

Turner, R. J., & Noh, S. (1988). Physical disability and depression: A longitudinal analysis. *Journal of Health and Social Behavior*, *29*, 23–37.

Tuszynski, M. H., Petito, C. K., & Levy, D. E. (1989). Risk factors and clinical manifestations of pathologically verified lacunar infarctions. *Stroke*, *20*, 990–999.

Ulatowska, H. K., Hayaski, M. M., Cannito, M. P., & Fleming, S. G. (1986). Disruption of reference. *Brain and Language*, *28*, 24–41.

U.S. Bureau of the Census. (1987). Estimates of the population of the United States, by age, sex and race: 1980–1986. *Current Population Reports* (Series P-25, No. 1000). Washington, DC: Author.

U.S. Congress, Office of Technology Assessment (1987). *Losing a million minds: Confronting the tragedy of Alzheimer's disease and other dementias* (OTA-BA-323). Washington, DC: U.S. Government Printing Office.

U.S. Senate Special Committee on Aging. (1987–1988). *Aging America: Trends and projections*. Washington, DC: Department of Health and Human Services.

Valliant, G. E. (1977). *Adaptation to life*. Boston: Little, Brown.

VandenBos, G. R., & Stapp, J. (1983). Service providers in psychology: Results of the 1982 APA Human Resources Survey. *American Psychologist*, *38*, 1330–1352.

Van Gorp, W. G., Satz, P., & Mitrushina, M. (1990). Neuropsychological processes associated with normal aging. *Developmental Neuropsychology*, *6*, 279–290.

Vicente, P., Kennelly, D., Golden, C. J., Kane, R., Sweet, J., Moses, J. A., Cardellino, J. P., Templeton, R., & Graber, B. (1980). The relationship of the Halstead-Reitan Neuropsychological Battery to the Luria-Nebraska Neuropsychological Battery: Preliminary report. *Clinical Neuropsychology*, *2*, 140–141.

Vincent, K. R. (1979). The modified WAIS: An alternative to short forms. *Journal of Clinical Psychology*, *35*, 624–625.

Vincent, K. R., & Cox, J. A. (1974). A reevaluation of Raven's Standard Progressive Matrices. *Journal of Psychology*, *88*, 299–303.

Vitaliano, P. P., Breen, A. R., Albert, M. S., Russo, J., & Prinz, P. N. (1984). Memory, attention, and functional status in community-residing Alzheimer type dementia patients and optimally healthy aged individuals. *Journal of Gerontology*, *39*, 58–64.

Volkmar, F. R., & Greenough, W. T. (1972). Rearing complexity affects branching of dendrites in the visual cortex of the rat. *Science*, *176*, 1445–1447.

von Ammon-Cavanaugh, S., & Wettstein, R. M. (1983). The relationship between severity of depression, cognitive dysfunction, and age in medical inpatients. *American Journal of Psychiatry*, *140*, 495–496.

Walford, R. L. (1969). *The immunologic theory of aging*. Copenhagen: Munksgaard.

Walford, R. L. (1983). *Maximum life span*. New York: Norton.

Walsh, D. A., Till, R. E., & Williams, M. V. (1978). Age differences in peripheral perception processing: A monoptic backward masking investigation. *Journal of Experimental Psychology: Human Perception and Performance*, *4*, 232–243.

Wang, H. S., & Busse, E. W. (1969). EEG of healthy old persons—A longitudinal study: 1. Dominant background activity and occipital rhythm. *Journal of Gerontology*, *24*, 419–426.

Ward, C. D., Duvoisin, R. C., Ince, S. E., Nutt, J. D., Eldridge, R., & Calne, D. B. (1983). Parkinson's disease in 65 pairs of twins and in a set of quadruplets. *Neurology*, *33*, 815–824.

Ward, C. D., Duvoisin, R. C., Ince, S. E., Nutt, J. D., Eldridge, R., & Calne, D. B. (1984). Parkinson's disease in twins. *Advances in Neurology*, *40*, 341–344.

Warner, H. R., Butler, R. N., Sprott, R. L., & Schneider, E. L. (Eds.). (1987). *Modern biological theories of aging*. New York: Raven Press.

Warrington, E. K., & Sanders, H. I. (1971). The fate of old memories. *Quarterly Journal of Experimental Psychology*, *23*, 432–442.

Watts, F. N., & Sharrock, R. (1985). Description and measurement of concentration problems in depressed patients. *Psychological Medicine*, *15*, 317–326.

Watts, F. N., Morris, L., & MacLeod, A. K. (1987). Recognition memory in depression. *Journal of Abnormal Psychology*, *96*, 273–275.

Wechsler, D. (1944). *The measurement of adult intelligence*. Baltimore: Williams & Wilkins.

Wechsler, D. (1945). A standardized memory scale for clinical use. *Journal of Psychology, 19*, 87–95.

Wechsler, D. (1955). *Wechsler Adult Intelligence Scale*. New York: Psychological Corporation.

Wechsler, D. (1958). *The measurement and appraisal of adult intelligence* (4th ed.). Baltimore: Williams & Wilkins.

Wechsler, D. (1981). *Wechsler Adult Intelligence Scale—Revised*. New York: Psychological Corporation.

Wechsler, D. (1987). *Wechsler Memory Scale—Revised*. New York: Psychological Corporation.

Weicker, W. (1987, October). *Diagnosis of delirium in older adults*. Paper presented at a meeting of the Canadian Gerontological Society, Calgary, Alberta.

Weiner, W. J., & Goetz, C. (Eds.). (1989). *Neurology for the non-neurologist* (2nd ed.). Philadelphia: J. B. Lippincott.

Weingartner, H. (1984). Psychobiological determinants of memory failures. In L. R. Squire & N. Butters (Eds.), *Neuropsychology of memory* (pp. 203–212). New York: Guilford Press.

Weingartner, H., & Silberman, E. (1982). Models of cognitive impairment: Cognitive changes in depression. *Psychopharmacology Bulletin, 18*, 27–42.

Weingartner, H., Cohen, R. M., Murphy, D. L., Martello, J., & Gerdt, C. (1981a). Cognitive processes in depression. *Archives of General Psychiatry, 38*, 42–47.

Weingartner, H., Kaye, W., Smallberg, S. A., Ebert, M. H., Gillin, J. C., & Sitaram, N. (1981b). Memory failures in progressive idiopathic dementia. *Journal of Abnormal Psychology, 90*, 187–196.

Weingartner, H., Burns, S., Diebel, R., Le Witt, P. A. (1984). Cognitive impairments in Parkinson's disease: Distinguishing between effort-demanding and automatic cognitive processes. *Psychiatry Research, 11*, 223–235.

Weinstein, H. C., Hijdra, A., van Royen, E. A., & Derix, M. M. A. (1989). Determination of cerebral blood flow by SPECT: A valuable tool in the investigation of dementia? *Clinical Neurology and Neurosurgery, 91*, 13–19.

Weishaus, S., & Field, D. (1988). Half century of marriage: Continuity or change. *Journal of Marriage and the Family, 50*, 763–774.

Weisman, M. M., & Klerman, G. L. (1977). Sex differences and the epidemiology of depression. *Archives of General Psychiatry, 34*, 98–111.

Weisman, M. M., Kidd, K. K., & Prusoff, B. A. (1982). Variability in rates of affective disorders in relatives of depressed and normal probands. *Archives of General Psychiatry, 39*, 1397–1403.

Welford, A. T. (1958). *Aging and human skill*. London: Oxford University Press.

Wells, C. E. (1979). Pseudodementia. *American Journal of Psychiatry, 136*, 895–900.

Wells, C. E. (1983). Differential diagnosis of Alzheimer's dementia: Affective disorder. In B. Reisberg (Ed.), *Alzheimer's disease: The standard reference* (pp. 193–198). New York: Free Press.

Wells, C. E., & Buchanan, D. C. (1977). The clinical use of psychological testing in evaluation for dementia. In C. E. Wells (Ed.), *Dementia* (2nd ed., pp. 189–204). Philadelphia: F. A. Davis.

Wenk, G. L. (1988). Amnesia and Alzheimer's disease: Which neurotransmitter system is responsible? *Neurobiology of Aging, 9*, 640–641.

West, R. (1985). *Memory fitness over 40*. Gainesville, FL: Triad.

West, R. L. (1986). Everyday memory and aging. *Developmental Neuropsychology, 2*, 323–344.

White, N., & Cunningham, W. R. (1988). Is terminal drop pervasive or specific? *Journal of Gerontology: Psychological Sciences, 43*, P141–144.

Whitehead, A. (1973). Verbal learning and memory in elderly depressives. *British Journal of Psychiatry, 123*, 203–208.

Whitehead, A. (1974). Factors in the learning deficit of elderly depressives. *British Journal of Social and Clinical Psychology, 13*, 201–208.

Whitehouse, P. J. (1986). The concept of subcortical and cortical dementia: Another look. *Annals of Neurology, 19*, 1–6.

Whitehouse, P. J. (1987). Neurotransmitter receptor alterations in Alzheimer disease: A review. *Alzheimer Disease and Associated Disorders, 1*, 9–18.

Whitehouse, P. J., & Au, K. S. (1986). Cholinergic receptors in aging and Alzheimer's Disease. *Progress in Neuropsychopharmacology and Biological Psychiatry, 10*, 665–676.

Whitehouse, P. J., Price, D. L., Struble, R. G., Clark, A. W., Coyle, J. T., & DeLong, M. R. (1982). Alzheimer's disease and senile dementia: Loss of neurons in the basal forebrain. *Science, 215*, 1237–1239.

Whitehouse, P. J., Hedreen, J. C., White, C. L., & Price, D. L. (1983). Basal forebrain neurons in the dementia of Parkinson's disease. *Annals of Neurology, 13*, 243–248.

Wiederhold, W. C. (1988). *Neurology for non-neurologists* (2nd ed.). New York: Grune & Stratton.

Wiens, A. N., McMinn, M. R., & Crossen, J. R. (1988). Rey Auditory-Verbal Learning Test: Development of norms for healthy young adults. *The Clinical Neuropsychologist, 2*, 67–87.

Williams, A., Denney, N. W., & Schadler, M. (1983). Elderly adults' perception of their own cognitive development during the adult years. *International Journal of Aging and Human Development, 16*, 147–158.

Williams, J. B. W. (1988). A structured interview guide for the Hamilton Depression Rating Scale. *Archives of General Psychiatry, 45*, 742–747.

Williams, J. M. G., & Scott, J. (1988). Autobiographical memory in depression. *Psychological Medicine, 18*, 689–695.

Williams, M. (1956). Spatial disorientation in senile dementia. *Journal of Mental Science, 102*, 291–299.

Willis, L., Yeo, R. A., Thomas, P., & Garry, P. J. (1988). Differential declines in cognitive function with aging: The possible role of health status. *Developmental Neuropsychology, 4*, 23–28.

Willis, S. L., & Schaie, K. W. (1986). Training the elderly on the ability factors of spatial orientation and inductive reasoning. *Psychology and Aging, 1*, 239–247.

Wilson, B. A., Cockburn, J., & Baddeley, A. D. (1985). *The Rivermead Behavioural Memory Test*. Titchfield, England: Thames Valley Test Company.

Wilson, B., Cockburn, J., Baddeley, A., & Hiorns, R. (1989). The development and validation of a test battery for detecting and monitoring everyday memory problems. *Journal of Clinical and Experimental Neuropsychology, 11*, 855–870.

Wilson, J. R., DeFries, J. C., McClearn, G. E., Vandenberg, S. G., Johnson, R. C., & Rashad, M. N. (1975). Cognitive abilities: Use of family data as a control to assess sex and age differences in two ethnic groups. *International Journal of Aging and Human Development, 6*, 261–176.

Wilson, R. S., Rosenbaum, G., Brown, G., Rourke, D., Whitman, D., & Gisell, J. (1978). An index of premorbid intelligence. *Journal of Consulting and Clinical Psychology, 46*, 1554–1555.

Wilson, R. S., Bacon, L. D., Fox, J. H., & Kaszniak, A. W. (1983). Primary memory and secondary memory in dementia of the Alzheimer type. *Journal of Clinical Neuropsychology, 5*, 337–344.

Wolfe, J., Granholm, E., Butters, N., Saunders, E., & Janowsky, D. (1987). Verbal memory deficits associated with major affective disorders: A comparison of unipolar and bipolar patients. *Journal of Affective Disorders, 13*, 83–92.

Wolk, R. L., & Wolk, R. B. (1971). *The Gerontological Apperception Test*. New York: Behavioral Publications.

Wolters, E. Ch. & Calne, D. B. (1989). Is Parkinson's disease related to aging? In D. B. Calne, D. Crippa, G. Comi, R. Horowski, & M. Trabucchi (Eds.), *Parkinsonism and aging* (pp. 125–132). New York: Raven Press.

Woodward, N. J., & Wallston, B. S. (1987). Age and health care beliefs: Self-efficacy as a mediator of low desire for control. *Psychology and Aging, 2*, 3–8.

Wurtman, R. J., Corkin, S., Ritter-Walker, E., & Growdon, J. H. (Eds.). (1990). *Alzheimer's disease*. New York: Raven Press.

Yesavage, J. A. (1986). The use of self-rating depression scales in the elderly. In L. W. Poon (Ed.), *Handbook for clinical memory assessment of older adults* (pp. 213–217). Washington, DC: American Psychological Association.

Yesavage, J., Brink, T., Rose, T., Lum, O., Huang, O., Adey, V., & Leirer, V. (1983a). Development and validation of a geriatric depression screening scale: A preliminary report. *Journal of Psychiatric Research, 17*, 37–49.

Yesavage, J. A., Rose, T. L., & Bower, G. H. (1983b). Interactive imagery and affective judgments improve face-name learning in the elderly. *Journal of Gerontology, 38*, 197–203.

Young, R. C., Manley, M. W., & Alexopoulos, G. S. (1985). "I don't know" responses in elderly depressives and in dementia. *Journal of the American Geriatrics Society, 33*, 253–257.

Zarantonello, M. M. (1988). Comparability of the WAIS and the WAIS-R: A consideration of level of neuropsychological impairment. *Journal of Consulting and Clinical Psychology, 56*, 295–297.

Zarit, S. H., Miller, N. E., & Kahn, R. L. (1978). Brain function, intellectual impairment and education in the aged. *Journal of the American Geriatric Society, 26*, 58–67.

Zarit, S. H., Cole, K. D., & Guider, R. L. (1981). Memory training strategies and subjective complains of memory in the aged. *The Gerontologist, 21*, 158–164.

Zarit, S. H., Orr, N. K., & Zarit, J. M. (1985). *The hidden victims of Alzheimer's disease: Families under stress*. New York: New York University Press.

Zelinski, E. M., Gilewski, M. J., & Anthony-Bergstone, C. R. (1990). Memory functioning questionnaire: Concurrent validity with memory performance and self-reported memory failures. *Psychology and Aging, 5*, 388–399.

Zornetzer, S. (1985). Catecholamine system involvement in age-related memory dysfunction. *Annals of the New York Academy of Sciences, 444*, 242–254.

Zubenko, G. S., Moossy,J., Martinez, A. J., Rao, G. R., Kopp, U., & Hanin, I., (1989). A brain regional analysis of morphologic and cholinergic abnormalities in Alzheimer's disease. *Archives ofNeurology, 46*, 634–639.

Index

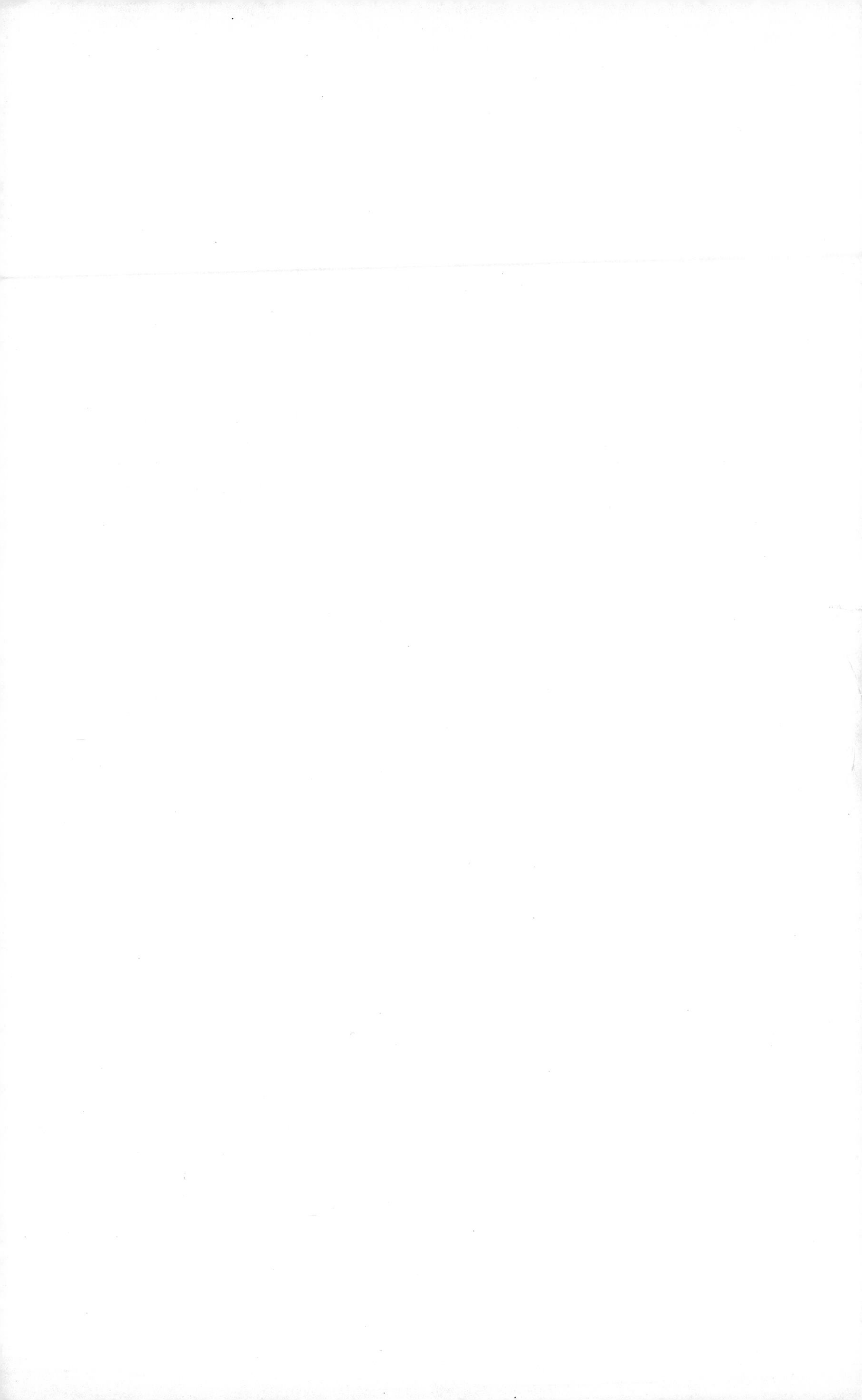